Clinics in Developmental Medicine

DOWN SYNDROME: CURRENT PERSPECTIVES

Clinics in Developmental Medicine

Down Syndrome Current Perspectives

Edited by

RICHARD W NEWTON
Royal Manchester Children's Hospital
Manchester
UK

SHIELA PURI
University of Leeds
UK

LIZ MARDER
Nottingham Children's Hospital
Nottingham University Hospitals NHS Trust
Nottingham
UK

2015
Mac Keith Press

© 2015 Mac Keith Press
6 Market Road, London, N7 9PW

Editor: Hilary M. Hart
Managing Director: Ann-Marie Halligan
Commissioning and Production Editor: Udoka Ohuonu
Project Management: Lumina Datamatics

First published in this edition in 2015

British Library Cataloguing-in-Publication data
A catalogue record for this book is available from the British Library

Cover: Main image, Michael Newton - 'Thumbs up to life'. Top circle, Billie-Jo Bailey at school, © Richard Bailey. Middle circle, Prisca Byera, courtesy of Mariana Melo Lima (www.marianamelolima.com). Bottom circle, Feet typical of Down syndrome. Photograph by Katy Francis of her own feet. Used with permission.

ISBN: 978-1-909962-47-7

Typeset by Lumina Datamatics, Chennai, India

Printed by Berforts, Information Press, Eynsham, Oxford, UK

Mac Keith Press is supported by Scope

DEDICATION

We would like to dedicate this book to:
Our families . . .
Davina, Aiysha, Rajiv, Pooja and Sunil
Surinder, Joe and Hannah
Judith, Sarah, Mike, Jenny, Chris and Will . . .
for their love and giving us the opportunity and encouragement
to complete this work;
to parents everywhere as they help their children with Down syndrome
reach their potential;
to people working in medicine, education and social care who offer those
families support in the light of current knowledge; and
to the Down's Syndrome Association and like organizations everywhere
for their continuing important work.

CONTENTS

AUTHORS' APPOINTMENTS

Sarah Almond
Locum Consultant Paediatric Surgeon,
Royal Manchester Children's Hospital, UK

Tiina Annus
Research Assistant, Cambridge Intellectual
and Developmental Disabilites Research Group,
Department of Psychiatry,
University of Cambridge, UK

Peter Arkwright
Consultant Paediatric Immunologist,
Department of Immunology,
Royal Manchester Children's Hospital, UK

Gillian Bird
Training Services Manager, Down's Syndrome
Association, Teddington, UK

Lesley Black
Down's Syndrome Association,
Teddington, UK

Arjan Bouman
Clinical Geneticist in Training, Department of
Clinical Genetics, Academic Medical Center,
University of Amsterdam, The Netherlands

Pat Charleton
Chairman DSMIG (UK and Ireland); Associate
Specialist Paediatrician, Department of
Community Child Health, Royal Aberdeen
Children's Hospital, Aberdeen, UK

Natali Chung
Consultant Cardiologist, Adult Congenital
Heart Disease, Guy's and St Thomas' Hospital
NHS, Foundation Trust, London, UK

Sheila M. Clark
Consultant Dermatologist, Leeds Teaching and
Mid Yorkshire Teaching Hospitals NHS Trust,
Member of the British Association of
Dermatologists and the British Society for
Paediatric Dermatology, UK

Jennifer Dennis
Retired Paediatrician, and Specialist
Advisor to Down Syndrome Medical Interest
Group (UK and Ireland),
Oxford, UK

Malcolm Donaldson
Honorary Senior Research Fellow
Glasgow University, UK

Hazel Evans	Consultant Respiratory Paediatrician, Southampton General Hospital, Tremona Road, Southampton, UK
Janet Gardner-Medwin	ARC Clinical Senior in Paediatric Rheumatology Royal Hospital for Sick Children Glasgow, UK
Peter Gillett	Consultant Paediatric Gastroenterologist, Royal Hospital for Sick Children, Edinburgh, UK
Christine Hardie	Associate Specialist in Community Paediatrics, Ashurst Child and Family Health Centre, Southampton, UK
Raoul Hennekam	Professor of Pediatrics and Translational Genetics, Department of Pediatrics, Academic Medical Center, University of Amsterdam, The Netherlands
Sheila Heslam	Services Director, Down's Syndrome Association, Teddington, UK
Hilary Hoey	Emeritus Professor of Paediatrics University of Dublin, Trinity College, and Consultant Paediatric Endocrinologist, National Children's Hospital, Dublin; Dean of the Faculty of Paediatrics and Vice President of the Royal College of Physicians of Ireland, Dublin, Ireland
Anthony Holland	Health Foundation Chair in Learning Disabilities, Cambridge Intellectual and Developmental Disabilities Research Group, Department of Psychiatry, University of Cambridge, UK
Patricia D Jackson	Paediatrician, Honorary Senior Fellow, University of Edinburgh, UK
Beki James	Consultant Paediatric Haematologist, Leeds Children's Hospital, Leeds General Infirmary, UK
Kath Leyland	Consultant Community Paediatrician, Royal Hospital for Sick Children, Yorkhill, Glasgow, UK
Liz Marder	Consultant Paediatrician and Pathway Lead Clinician for Children and Young People, Nottingham Children's Hospital, Nottingham University Hospitals NHS Trust, UK
Lou Marsden	Down's Syndrome Association, Teddington, UK

Claire McCall Associate Specialist in Paediatrics,
Nottingham Children's Hospital,
Nottingham University Hospitals NHS Trust, UK

Liz McDermott Consultant Immunologist,
Nottingham University Hospitals NHS Trust, UK

Marian McGowan Consultant Paediatrician,
Child Development Centre,
St George's Hospital London, London, UK

Emma McNeill Clinical Fellow in Otolaryngology,
Freeman Hospital,
Newcastle-upon-Tyne, UK

Stuart Mills Information Officer, Down's Syndrome
Association, Teddington, UK

Joan Morris Director of the National Down Syndrome
Cytogenetic Register, Centre for Environmental
and Preventive Medicine, Wolfson Institute of
Preventive Medicine; the London School of
Medicine and Dentistry, Queen Mary University
of London, UK

Richard Newton Honorary Consultant Paediatric Neurologist,
Royal Manchester Children's Hospital, UK

June Nunn Professor of Special Care Dentistry and Dean
of the School of Dental Science, Trinity
College, Dublin, Ireland

Emma Pascall Department of Congenital Heart Disease,
Bristol Royal Hospital for Children, Bristol, UK

Katy Pike Clinical Lecturer,
University of Southampton and NIHR
Southampton Research Unit, University
Hospital Southampton NHS Foundation Trust, UK

Rajiv Puri Consultant Urological Surgeon, Yorkshire Clinic,
Bradford, UK

Shiela Puri Consultant Paediatrician in Community Child
Health, Children and Family Services, NHS
Leeds Community Healthcare, St James's
University Hospital, Child Development Centre,
Leeds, UK

Vanda Ridley Information Services Manager, Down's
Syndrome Association, Teddington, UK

Laura Savage	Dermatology Specialist Registrar, Leeds Centre for Dermatology, Chapel Allerton Hospital, Chapeltown Road, Leeds, UK
Patrick Sheehan	Consultant & Honorary Senior Lecturer in Paediatric Otolaryngology, St Georges Hospital and Medical School, London, UK
Sally Shott	Professor, Department of Otolaryngology Head and Neck Surgery, Children's Hospital Medical Center, University of Cincinnati, Cincinnati, Ohio, USA
Fiona Straw	Consultant Paediatrician, Nottingham Children's Hospital, Nottingham University Hospitals NHS Trust, UK
Sally Tennant	Consultant Paediatric Orthopaedic Surgeon, Royal National Orthopaedic Hospital and St Mary's Hospital Paddington, London, UK
Maureen Todd	Senior Research Nurse, Glasgow Clinical Research Facility, Western Infirmary, Glasgow; University of Glasgow, UK
Robert Tulloh	Consultant in Paediatric Cardiology, Bristol Royal Hospital for Children, Upper Maudlin Street, Bristol, UK
Jeremy Turk	Professor of Developmental Psychiatry, Institute of Psychiatry, King's College, University of London, and Consultant Child & Adolescent Psychiatrist, South London & Maudsley NHS Foundation Trust, London UK
Liam Reese Wilson	Research Assistant, Cambridge Intellectual and Developmental Disabilites Research Group, Department of Psychiatry, University of Cambridge, UK
Maggie Woodhouse	Senior Lecturer and Optometrist, School of Optometry & Vision Sciences Cardiff University, Maindy Road, Cardiff, UK

FOREWORD

The prospects for individuals born with Down syndrome today are better than ever and many should expect to live long, healthy lives filled with the experiences and challenges most of us take for granted. Of course, this has not always been the case. Many individuals born with Down syndrome within living memory were denied treatment for remediable conditions simply on the basis of their genetic condition. I recall the teenager with severe pulmonary hypertension as a result of an untreated cardiac lesion and the cardiologist's letter justifying the decision not to treat as 'being in his best interest' in some way. Thankfully, such situations are no longer acceptable in contemporary medicine, but the spectre of previous discrimination and medical patriarchy hangs over and shames our profession.

Therefore, as both a paediatrician caring for children with Down syndrome and as the parent of a young person with Down syndrome, I am delighted to welcome this excellent book, which provides a comprehensive guide to the delivery of healthcare for children and young people with Down syndrome, within the context of promoting health and well-being.

The book covers the fascinating genetic aspects of the syndrome (Why do some children have cardiac defects while others do not, yet all have Down syndrome?) followed by consideration of the perinatal aspects of diagnosis, counselling and management. We are reminded how to impart a diagnosis and pitfalls to avoid. Memories of the ward round with the consultant reciting a list of possible complications to the newborn infant's stunned parents return to make me cringe even now.

The book includes a system-by-system guide, using case examples to illustrate important topics, with key learning points highlighted for easy reference.

The book contains practical advice on the management of both common and rare complications: when do you test thyroid antibodies and which ones do you request? Is a cervical spine X-ray needed before the child takes part in trampolining classes? What is the long-term outcome? How likely is someone with Down syndrome to become independent and what is the current life expectancy?—all essential information for clinicians guiding parents.

The phenomenon of diagnostic overshadowing (the attribution of symptoms to Down syndrome per se rather than consideration of either known associations or unrelated conditions) is highlighted and this should prompt reflection of one's own practice and assumptions. Importantly, the book contains a chapter from the Down's Syndrome Association of the UK outlining the practical day-to-day issues that families may experience and this will be an invaluable source of information for clinicians.

Having Down syndrome does not make an individual unhealthy, but there are particular conditions that are seen more commonly and clinicians need to be aware of the best evidence-based management. This comprehensive overview condenses that knowledge into one source.

It is written with authority and credibility by experts in the field. I predict it will become the main reference text for clinicians working with children with Down syndrome. I hope it will spearhead an advance in the quality and consistency of care delivered to children. Good health is the foundation of participation, fulfilment and achievement of full potential. This book is the clinicians' guide to helping individuals with Down syndrome achieve those ideals.

Dr Neil A Harrower
Consultant Paediatrician,
Ryegate Children's Centre,
Sheffield Children's NHS Foundation Trust;
and Honorary Senior Lecturer,
University of Sheffield, UK.

ACKNOWLEDGEMENTS

A project of this size requires help and support from many quarters. Knowledge about Down syndrome is advancing very fast. We had to ensure up-to-date advice on molecular genetics, clinical practice and then, of course, the application of science into practice. We are therefore indebted to all our authors and to Carol Boys, Chief Executive of the Down's Syndrome Association for mobilizing resources so that the useful perspective of the lives of people with Down syndrome of all ages could be depicted in Chapter 4. This allows practitioners important insight into the context in which we apply our medical knowledge.

All members of the Down Syndrome Medical Interest Group (DSMIG) UK and Ireland deserve mention for presentations and discussion over the years that have informed many of the ideas in this book. We should give special mention to Drs Christine Jenkins, Rebecca Ferris and Jill Ellis who laid down important groundwork to enable the chapters on Dermatology, Respiratory disorders and Intervention to take off; and Joyce Judson and Lynn Nixon, Information Officers at the Child Development Centre, City Hospital Campus, Nottingham, supported many authors by providing background information. We are grateful to Mr Antonino Morabito and Dr Nick Webb for guidance on the chapters on gastroenterology and renal abnormalities.

Gratitude should also be paid to all the children with Down syndrome and their families for all they have taught us and the motivation for writing this book. We should mention Dr Jennifer Dennis who taught many of us much about working with families with children with Down syndrome and whose painstaking work was a foundation for the DSMIG. We would like to thank scientists everywhere who through their painstaking work continue to establish the facts about Down syndrome and dispense with unhelpful myths. In this context, special acknowledgement needs to be given to our friend and colleague Professor Cliff Cunningham who sadly died at the advent of this project. He advised on its shape and a number of central themes. His experience, wisdom, scholarship and foresight, along with the establishment of the Manchester cohort, laid a solid foundation for applied psychology and medical research in the area. He was a friend to many families. His keen sense of fun is greatly missed.

Finally, we would like to thank Mac Keith Press for commissioning the project and in particular Ann-Marie Halligan and Hilary Hart for help, guidance and support.

Richard Newton, Shiela Puri and Liz Marder
December 2014

PROLOGUE

My 17-year-old son was diagnosed with PH+ ALL in November 2012. When any parent hears those words, it is normal for a rampage of fear to run through them.

For me, the fear was complicated and compounded by the fact my son has Down syndrome. Along with the normal fears of seeing your child sick, suffering, in pain, or God forbid, not surviving at all, I have the extra fears.

Will the doctors treat my son? Seventeen years ago, I had to fight for life-saving cardiac surgery to be done. Would I have to fight again? Would his human rights be respected, acknowledged or even recognized?

What will the doctors and nurses think of my son's behaviour? Being completely non-verbal, he can act out his fears, anger or frustrations with behaviours not commonly seen on a teen oncology ward. Those same behaviours can be an indication of pain or sickness. I would hate for my son to be judged as a naughty, unmanageable, learning disabled teen, when all he is trying to convey is that he feels sick or is in pain. I fear telling people in case I hear the dreaded 'maybe it is for the best'. The best for whom? Certainly not the best for my son, definitely not for his sister or I nor the best for his friends or anyone who loves him.

I fear seeing the look of the others on the ward (patients, their parents, family or visitors) looking at us as if we do not quite belong. None of the other parents can relate to us, as we share stories over a cuppa because my son is different. It is as if we are a piece of a puzzle that just does not quite fit anywhere.

I fear that his extra chromosome might breakdown his chemotherapy so differently. I fear not being able to explain to my son about his own illness. He looks at me with tear-filled almond eyes pleading, 'Why are you doing this to me?'

I fear the heavy burden of having to make life choices for him. I hope and pray I am making choices he wants and choices not just for my own selfish reasons.

I fear people looking at my son and only seeing a waste of resources. No, my son may never pay taxes, but he can and does contribute to society. He educates people, he teaches love and acceptance, he also spreads laughter and joy.

But mostly, I fear they will not see the Person, the Person we love very dearly.

Thankfully I have not had to face any of those fears here on Ward 33. My son has been welcomed, accepted and yes, even loved. I have every confidence that his consultant and her amazing staff have nothing but my son's and family's best interest at heart. They are, rightly, along with us, for us.

Thank you all eternally.

1
INTRODUCTION

The scene is a school leavers' assembly at a 1500-pupil comprehensive school. The assembled pupils have a wide range of prospects: ranging from aspirant lawyers and teachers to those with antisocial behaviour orders. One of them was asked to make a short speech. The 16-year-old begins hesitantly but the 300 gathered listen respectfully. The address is short, clear and poignant, 'I would like to thank everybody for helping me and being my friend'. There is rapturous applause. The boy leaves the stage, a little self-consciously but with a look of satisfaction. The gathering offers genuine warmth and delight in response to the lad's words.

The young person in question has Down syndrome and has just passed through mainstream education. One teacher remarked that this pupil had offered more to this school than they had been able to give him. This reflects a sea change in societal attitude to children with Down syndrome over the past 40 years (only after the 1970 Education Act [UK] where children with intellectual disability entitled to an education at all). By the 1980s, 'Mongol' was only just leaving common parlance and a prejudicial view often entered medical decision-making processes: suboptimal treatments were reported for heart disease and leukaemia. Fortunately this has changed, reflecting a view that young people with Down syndrome have prospects, can contribute to society, and deserve respect, love and emotional support along with access to appropriate medical care.

Down syndrome is not a medical condition but represents a common recognizable variation of the human form created through a random biological event. Nonetheless, as we will see, people with Down syndrome present with many common medical conditions and some that are more specific to the condition. Doctors have an important part to play in the lives of the people concerned. They help parents readjust to a new set of expectations following the birth of an affected child. They can help with the early identification and treatment of conditions attendant on the syndrome.

We will illustrate through a number of case scenarios that, unfortunately, too often medical symptoms are attributed to the 'syndrome'. This is termed 'diagnostic overshadowing' and results in a delay in the delivery of appropriate medical care. We hope this book will strengthen the knowledge of doctors and other health professionals who have this responsibility. Our book incorporates anecdotes and experiences, some good some bad, of service providers and users which illustrate good and bad practice, and missed opportunities. We hope these vignettes will help the readers reflect on their own attitudes and practice in our shared constant quest for professional development and improvement.

We begin with an overview of our current knowledge of the biology of Down syndrome. It is followed by an important contribution from the UK Down's Syndrome Association which explores the lives, experiences and at times frustrations of service users and how we might improve our practice. We then take a systematic approach to Down syndrome and its attendant medical problems—the biology, presentation and diagnostic formulations; and how we might intervene in a timely fashion. Presentations can be different in Down syndrome; the important thing is to recognize this so that opportunities to help are not missed.

An underlying theme is how we might initially set the scene for a loving and nurturing environment at home and then develop this into opportunity and encouragement outside the home as the children get older. We believe professionals will best be able to fulfil their part in this task by first examining and reflecting on their own views of disability in general and Down syndrome in particular. An increased understanding of Down syndrome should allow us as professionals to support the person at the centre and their families; and to present information and interventions clearly and positively enabling them to lead a fulfilling life.

2
ADVANCES IN MOLECULAR GENETICS

Arjan Bouman and Raoul Hennekam

Introduction

In 1959, Lejeune et al. (Lejeune et al. 1959) identified the cause of Down syndrome as an additional chromosome 21 in the human cell (since we have learnt the discovery was actually made by his colleague Dr Marthe Gautier [Harper 2006]). The trisomy of chromosome 21 influences almost every body tissue, resulting in a broad and distinct phenotype. Despite many years of intensive research, the mechanisms involved remain unclear. Everyone with Down syndrome has an intellectual disability (Nadel 2003). From the fourth decade of life, they have a significantly increased risk of developing Alzheimer disease (Zigman et al. 2008). Alterations in neurogenesis, neuronal differentiation, myelination, dendritogenesis, synaptogenesis and other mechanisms are suggested to underlie the cognitive impairment. However, the exact mechanisms responsible remain little understood (Rachidi and Lopes 2010). It is assumed that chromosome 21 gene overdosage plays a major role in Down syndrome-related neurodegeneration. Yet, the wide range of variation in the degree of intellectual disability in Down syndrome is difficult to explain with a gene overdose hypothesis.

This chapter will explore our current knowledge of the molecular mechanisms and pathways which contribute to the phenotypic features and suggest areas for future research. This growth in understanding should eventually serve as a basis to develop personalized medicine strategies for each individual with Down syndrome.

To help understand this chapter it may be helpful to look at Box 2.1 that shows the relevant biological terms.

General hypotheses

It is hypothesized that there are two pathophysiological mechanisms which may cause the Down syndrome phenotype (see Fig 2). Both hypotheses involve several mechanisms which may be acting through altered gene transcription, tissue-specific gene transcription, genetic interaction, DNA methylation, altered microRNA activity, posttranscriptional mechanisms (e.g. RNA editing) and altered chromosome territories. Many more mechanisms, currently undetected, may be present. Neither hypothesis rules out the other, and they may well influence one another. For example, overexpression of some of the chromosome 21 genes may directly influence the phenotype, but it may also disturb genetic cell homeostasis in a more general way.

BOX 2.1 A synopsis of molecular biology terms

The **genome** is the genetic material of any organism, which in humans is encoded in DNA.

The essence of life is that **Deoxyribonucleic acid (DNA)** can make **Ribonucleic acid (RNA)** which then assembles **protein**.

Messenger RNA (mRNA) is a large family of molecules that convey genetic information from DNA to ribosomes where protein is assembled. mRNA specifies the amino acid sequence of the protein.

An **exon** is a sequence of nucleotides encoded by a gene that remains in the final RNA product of that gene after introns have been removed by RNA splicing. The term *exon* refers to both the DNA sequence within a gene and its RNA transcripts.

Introns are regions inside a gene and the corresponding RNA transcript sequence not included in the final protein gene product.

RNA splicing is the process by which introns are removed and exons are joined in order to make mature messenger RNA.

The **exome** is the part of the genome formed by exons, the sequences which when transcribed remain within the final RNA sequence after introns are removed by RNA splicing.

The **transcriptome** is the set of all RNA molecules, including messenger RNA, ribosomal RNA, transfer RNA and other non-coding RNA produced in one cell or a population of cells, i.e., all the different forms of RNA required in the process of transcribing DNA into protein assembly.

The **proteome** is the entire set of proteins expressed by the genome, be it in a cell or specific tissue at a given time.

The **metabolome** is the complete set of small molecules found in a biological sample, be it a cell, organelle, organ or tissue. It would exclude macromolecules such as proteins, DNA or RNA but includes metabolites and other molecules such as drugs.

The **interactome** is the whole set of molecular interactions in a particular cell. It may refer to physical interactions among molecules or indirect interactions among genes.

Hypothesis 1: Dosage effect

The unifying simplified description of this theory is that a 1.5-fold increase of dosage results in a 1.5-fold increase of chromosome 21 gene expression causing (specific aspects of) the Down syndrome phenotype (Korenberg et al. 1990, Patterson 2007, Rachidi and Lopes 2010). Several studies on mRNA expression in Down syndrome have shown that a significant number of genes on chromosome 21 are overexpressed to 150% (Mao et al. 2003, Prandini et al. 2007). This observation was confirmed by Aït Yahya-Graison et al. (2007) who demonstrated that 29% of chromosome 21 transcripts are overexpressed in Down syndrome. The other 71% of transcripts are either compensated (e.g. with an anti-sense transcript) or highly variable. Lockstone et al. (2007) found a similar 27% of chromosome 21 genes are upregulated in the adult brain with Down syndrome. Korbel et al. (2009) constructed a phenotype map for various specific manifestations of Down syndrome by using clinical information from 30 individuals carrying a segmental trisomy of chromosome 21. This map identified candidate genes on chromosome 21 that may be involved in pathways causing particular phenotypic Down syndrome features such as Hirschsprung disease, leukaemia, Alzheimer disease and intellectual disability. It is assumed that these specific manifestations can be explained by an elevated expression of particular chromosome 21 genes. The dosage effect hypothesis does not describe specific genes, subsets of genes or molecular pathways which are responsible for specific Down syndrome features. Down syndrome mouse model experiments show that a trisomy of the Down syndrome critical region (DSCR) can explain some, but not all, phenotypic features of Down syndrome (Olson et al. 2007). The duplication of the DSCR is associated with many Down syndrome features (e.g. morphologic characteristics, intellectual disability) but does not explain the full Down syndrome phenotype. In addition, expression levels of chromosome 21 genes can differ between tissues (Li et al. 2006).

SELECTED GENES LOCATED ON CHROMOSOME 21

In 2011, GENCODE (release 8) identified 696 genes on chromosome 21. Proteins encoded by these genes are involved in 636 different biological processes, have 304 different molecular functions and are present in 163 cellular components (Letourneau and Antonarakis 2012). The specific function of about 50% of the genes lying on chromosome 21 remains uncertain (Kahlem 2006). The various candidate genes which could underlie parts of the neurological phenotype in Down syndrome can be listed in the following subgroups:

- Genes involved in brain development (neurogenesis, neuronal differentiation, myelinization and synaptogenesis)
- Genes involved in neuronal cell–cell communication
- Genes involved in metabolic processes influencing the brain.

The neurological Down syndrome phenotype cannot be explained by changes determined within a single pathway described by a gene from any of the subgroups listed above, but is likely to involve a complex interaction with disturbed regulation of several pathways. Fully understanding and dissecting these complex molecular networks requires full insight into the exome, transcriptome, proteome, metabolome, interactome, synergistic effects and probably more besides. Gaining insight in these molecular processes will give us the tools needed to identify candidate genes involved in Down syndrome aetiology. As genes within the DSCR play an important role in Down syndrome pathogenesis but cannot fully explain the phenotype, the focus should not be limited only to the chromosome 21 DSCR but rather should include all interactive aspects of a genome-wide view.

As the biological function of half of the genes located on chromosome 21 remains unknown (Kahlem 2006), it may be that several genes of great importance for producing the Down syndrome phenotype remain unrecognized as such. Further studies of the function of these genes are clearly important for our understanding. Selective knocking out of such genes in animal models and studying phenotypes in individuals who harbour variants in one of these genes are first-line studies needed for this.

Amyloid Precursor Protein and Beta-Site Amyloid Beta A4 Precursor Protein-Cleaving Enzyme 2

Chromosome 21 harbours at least two genes which are involved in the development of Alzheimer disease: amyloid precursor protein (APP) and beta-site amyloid beta A4 precursor protein-cleaving enzyme 2 (BACE2). APP serves as a substrate for amyloid β-peptide (Aß), a pathogenic amino acid peptide which can precipitate in extracellular plaques in the brain (see also Chapter 18c). Widespread Aß deposition is the hallmark feature in Alzheimer disease resulting in profound neurodegeneration. Brains of aged individuals with Down syndrome show approximately a 1.5-fold increase of APP mRNA levels compared with those of typically developed individuals (Oyama et al. 1994). Rovelet-Lecrux et al. (2006) reported on five families with early-onset Alzheimer disease caused by an isolated duplication of the APP locus (ranging from 0.58Mb to 6.37Mb). This study demonstrated that trisomy of APP can explain the neuropathology associated with Alzheimer disease in Down syndrome, but that it is not sufficient to cause the full Down syndrome phenotype. In addition, Salehi et al. (2006) demonstrated in a Down syndrome mouse model (Ts65Dn) that APP overexpression can cause degeneration of basal forebrain cholinergic neurons. The second gene of interest is BACE2, an aspartyl protease which has a 65% homology to BACE1. In the brain, β-Secretase (BACE1) is the rate-limiting protease in the generation of Aβ peptide from APP. BACE1 activity is further increased in Alzheimer disease (Webb and Murphy 2012). Unlike BACE1, BACE2 is more highly expressed in peripheral tissues, but also to some extent in the brain. Both its homology to BACE1 and its expression in the brain may pinpoint BACE2 as an important contributing factor in Aß accumulation in the brain (Dominguez et al. 2005). Therefore, both APP and BACE2 seem to contribute to Alzheimer disease neuropathology in Down syndrome but do not, of course, explain the full neurological Down syndrome phenotype.

Sorting Nexin 27
Wang et al. (2013) identified a signalling pathway that contributes to the neurological phenotype of Down syndrome. Overexpression of miR-155 (located on the mouse equivalent of human chromosome 21) reduces expression of *Sortin Nexin 27* (*not* located on the mouse equivalent of human chromosome 21). Sorting Nexin 27 (SNX27) is involved in hippocampal and cortical synaptic function. Knock-out mice (SNX27$^{-/-}$) have severe neuronal deficits in both the hippocampus and cortex. Complete loss of SNX27 in mice results in severe neuronal degeneration and mortality, mainly caused by diminished synaptic glutamate receptor expression. Upregulation of SNX27 in Down syndrome mice (Ts65Dn) rescued synaptic deficits. It was also demonstrated that SNX27 expression is decreased in the cortex of the human Down syndrome brain. These experiments show that the miR-155/SNX27 pathway is an important player in Down syndrome neuropathogenesis demonstrating the role of the chromosome 21 interactome (Fig. 2.2).

Hypothesis 2: Amplified developmental instability
This hypothesis indicates that there is a 'phenotypic instability due to extra genetic information' or 'amplified developmental instability'. Thus, dosage imbalances of genes located on chromosome 21 are responsible for a non-specific disturbance of overall genomic regulation and expression. Because of this global balance disruption of gene expression in developmental pathways, normal developmental processes are altered finally resulting in the establishment of the Down syndrome phenotype (Shapiro 1983, Patterson 2007, Rachidi and Lopes 2010). This hypothesis has a significant overlap with the dosage effect hypothesis

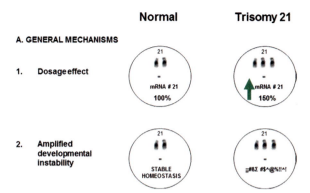

Fig. 2.1. General mechanisms: (1) Dosage effect. This hypothesis describes an upregulation of mRNA transcription of genes located on chromosome 21 to 150%. This 1.5-fold increase in chromosome 21 gene expression results in the Down syndrome phenotype. (2) Amplified developmental instability. This hypothesis describes that dosage imbalances of chromosome 21 genes are responsible for a total (non-specific) disruption of genomic regulation and expression in the cell. This results in a total disturbance of cell homeostasis leading to the Down syndrome phenotype.

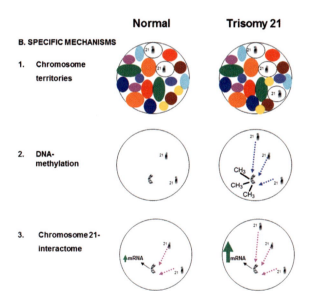

Fig. 2.2. Specific mechanisms: (1) **Chromosome territories**. The coloured areas represent the various chromosome territories within the nucleus. Territory occupied by an extra chromosome 21 causes a displacement in nuclear chromosome territory topography. As a result, expression of particular loci located anywhere in the genome can be influenced. (2) **DNA methylation**. DNA methylation of a single chromosome is depicted by the addition of CH$_3$ groups. The presence of an extra chromosome 21 causes altered DNA methylation of particular loci which subsequently influences transcription. (3) **Chromosome 21 interactome**. The extra chromosome 21 causes upregulation in mRNA transcription of a locus on a particular chromosome elsewhere on the genome. Thus, expression of genes not located at the trisomic chromosome but elsewhere in the genome is altered.

7

but describes in a broad sense that the presence of extra genetic information will result in a global cellular disturbance. It is known, however, that other autosomal trisomy syndromes (such as trisomy 13 or trisomy 18) can lead to a similar global disturbance of cellular and molecular processes but do not lead to a phenotype similar to Down syndrome. This forms an argument against a significant role for the amplified developmental instability hypothesis; though, of course, it may contribute.

Further hypotheses

The scope of these two hypotheses (dosage effect and amplified developmental instability) to explain all phenotypic variations seems too limited and non-specific. The effects of the presence of an additional chromosome 21 are likely to be much broader and complex and involve numerous molecular mechanisms (see Fig 2.2). Fortunately, molecular techniques are at present evolving rapidly and will allow us to study such mechanisms. These additional mechanisms are summarized below:

ALTERED DNA METHYLATION

DNA methylation is one of the epigenetic processes. It plays a role in silencing the expression of particular genes without changing the nucleotide sequence of the gene. This is explained by the addition of a methyl group to a DNA strand which can cause altered/decreased gene expression of this particular DNA segment (i.e. 'turning off the gene'). This molecular process, therefore, is an important regulator of gene expression (Turek-Plewa and Jagodziński 2005). Aberrant DNA methylation can influence the transcription of genes located on the chromosome itself, or loci elsewhere on the genome. DNA methylation can be tissue specific and also age specific. DNA methylation patterns have been studied in Down syndrome by using small cohorts of adults and comparing them to controls (Chango et al. 2006, Kerkel et al. 2010). A difference in DNA methylation and gene expression in adults with Down syndrome was demonstrated. One could hypothesize that the presence of an extra chromosome 21 might alter its DNA methylation or even DNA methylation on other loci or chromosomes throughout the genome. Altered DNA methylation may, therefore, influence transcription of genes located on chromosome 21 and probably elsewhere on the genome as well. Adorno et al. (2013) described ubiquitination as another epigenetic process which could be involved in Down syndrome. They demonstrated in Ts65Dn mice (the Down syndrome mouse model, sometimes referred to as the 'Down-mouse') that triplication of *Usp16*, a deubiquitination enzyme, disrupts the epigenetic state of particular genes (such as *Cdkn2a*). This results in reduced self-renewing capacity of haematopoietic stem cells, which accelerates the ageing process. Also, these mice had a defect in neural progenitor expansion, which can partly be explained by the triplication of *Usp16*.

ALTERED CHROMOSOME 21 INTERACTOME

In genetics, the interactome describes the interactions between genes located at different positions in the genome. This concept explains how altered expression of gene X can influence protein expression of gene Y, where X and Y are not necessarily located on the same chromosome. It underlies the basis of (genetic) pathway thinking and can be studied, for instance, by evaluating mRNA levels or alternative mRNA transcripts. The study from Wang et al. (2013) can serve as an example. As we have seen, miR-155 overexpression results in reduced SNX27 expression leading to neuronal degeneration. They identified the miR-155-C/EBPß-SNX27 pathway as an important player in the neuropathogenesis of Down syndrome. Billingsley et al. (2013) demonstrated that 155 non-trisomic genes are differentially expressed in the mandible of the E13.5 Ts65Dn embryo ('Down-mouse'). They showed that the presence of a trisomy can alter the expression of non-trisomic genes during development leading to structural changes associated with Down syndrome. By identifying genetic pathways that are disrupted by the presence of trisomy chromosome 21, more insight is gained into Down syndrome aetiology. This may finally serve as the basis for influencing or treating several Down syndrome manifestations (Billingsley et al. 2013). Chou et al. (2008) demonstrated that some euploid genes show a significant greater expression variance in human trisomy 21 tissues compared with controls. These studies demonstrate that the presence of trisomy chromosome 21 results in altered transcription on other genomic loci and provide the first evidence of the chromosome 21 interactome. It is likely that we will discover huge numbers of similar interactions between genes located at chromosome 21, or the proteins they encode for, and genes and proteins elsewhere in the genome explaining a significant part of the phenotype in Down syndrome.

DISTURBED CHROMOSOME TERRITORIES

Chromosomes occupy specific, non-random regions within a nucleus, called chromosome territories. Cremer and Cremer (2010) have demonstrated (by using UV-microbeam experiments and later on FISH technique) that each chromosome has its own distinct 'territory' within the nucleus of cells. Chromosome territories are specific to cell and tissue type, and can even change during differentiation and development (Meaburn and Misteli 2007). The presence of an additional copy of chromosome 21 might cause a displacement of the other two chromosome 21s as well as other chromosomes from their normal sites. Finlan et al. (2008) demonstrated that expression or transcription of some (but not all) genes can be suppressed when chromosomes are relocated to the nuclear periphery. Therefore, it is easily conceivable that the presence of an extra chromosome 21 influences the 'fixed' chromosomal territory organization and, subsequently, alters expression of genes, including genes involved in the Down syndrome phenotype. These genes could be located on chromosome 21 or on other chromosomes displaced by the additional copy 21. We are unaware of studies of chromosome territories in individuals with Down syndrome or in other chromosome abnormalities.

Genetic background as a phenotype contributor

As well as the direct effects of an additional chromosome 21 the genetic background (all the other genes present, inherited from both parents) can influence the phenotype as well. The definition of genetic background is broad and undetermined but is likely to contribute to the Down syndrome phenotype and the huge variability observed among individuals with Down syndrome (Reeves et al. 2001). The genetic background is present anyway and is not caused by the additional chromosome 21. Here, we discuss in short single nucleotide polymorphism (SNP) and copy number variations (CNVs) as part of this genetic background.

SINGLE NUCLEOTIDE POLYMORPHISMS AND COPY NUMBER VARIATIONS ON
THE BACKGROUND OF TRISOMY 21

An SNP is a variation in the DNA sequence comprehending just one single nucleotide on a particular locus in the genome. SNPs between different members of biological species are common and usually do not cause disease. Genome-wide association studies (GWAS) can identify associations between particular SNPs and a disease, that is, some SNPs can occur more frequently in individuals with a particular disease. This variation itself does not cause the disease but is likely to contribute to the phenotype. Congenital heart defects (CHDs) occur in 40% of people with Down syndrome (Patterson 2009). Therefore, trisomy 21 increases the risk for CHD but it does not necessarily cause CHD: the genetic background has to play a role. Sailani et al. performed a GWAS study comparing a group with Down syndrome and CHD to a group with Down syndrome and no CHD. Two chromosome 21 risk alleles for CHD were identified and confirmed in a replication cohort (Sailani et al. 2013).

A specific example of how polymorphisms may relate to phenotype comes from the work of Guéant et al. (2005). They investigated the influence of homocysteinaemia (t-Hcys), folate, vitamin B12 and related polymorphisms on intelligence quotient (IQ) in Down syndrome. They found an association between lower quotients and t-Hcys, carriers of the methylenetetrahydrofolate reductase 677 T allele and the transcobalamin 776 G allele. The association may be related to a defective methylation of homocysteine, affecting IQ (see more on methylation below).

CNV describes the presence of an abnormal number of copies of one or more genome segments. This form of structural variation can involve relatively large segments of the genome (either deleted or duplicated). CNVs are relatively common but despite this their contribution and meaning often remain uncertain. Sailani et al. (2013) describe three CNV regions which seem to be associated with CHD in Down syndrome. When a gene is located within a particular CNV it can be an interesting candidate gene for further (functional) studies. Both SNPs and CNVs, therefore, may well be a component of the pathological genetic background of Down syndrome contributing to particular features of the phenotype.

Key points
- Trisomy for chromosome 21 produces the Down syndrome phenotype but the mechanism is unknown.
- Gene overexpression and amplified developmental instability are likely to play a part.
- Other genetic mechanisms including altered DNA methylation, an altered chromosome interactome and disturbed chromosome territories are all likely to contribute.
- Molecular techniques currently available provide tools needed to clarify these biological processes.

- Understanding the phenotype pathogenesis is essential to developing management strategies, which can improve health and quality of life for individuals with Down syndrome and their families.

REFERENCES

Adorno M, Sikandar S, Mitra SS et al. (2013) Usp16 contributes to somatic stem-cell defects in Down's syndrome. *Nature* 501: 380–384. doi: 10.1038/nature12530. Epub 11 September 2013.

Aït Yahya-Graison E, Aubert J, Dauphinot L et al. (2007) Classification of human chromosome 21 gene-expression variations in Down syndrome: Impact on disease phenotypes. *Am J Hum Genet* 81: 475–491.

Billingsley CN, Allen JR, Baumann DD et al. (2013) Non-trisomic homeobox gene expression during craniofacial development in the Ts65Dn mouse model of Down syndrome. *Am J Med Genet* 161A: 1866–1874. doi: 10.1002/ajmg.a.36006.

Chango A, Abdennebi-Najar L, Tessier F et al. (2006) Quantitative methylation-sensitive arbitrarily primed PCR method to determine differential genomic DNA methylation in Down Syndrome. *Biochem Biophys Res Commun* 349: 492–496.

Chou CY, Liu LY, Chen CY et al. (2008) Gene expression variation increase in trisomy 21 tissues. *Mamm Genome* 19: 398–405. doi: 10.1007/s00335-008-9121-1.

Cremer T, Cremer M (2010) Chromosome territories. *Cold Spring Harb Perspect Biol* 2: a003889. doi: 10.1101/cshperspect.a003889.

Dominguez D, Tournoy J, Hartmann D et al. (2005) Phenotypic and biochemical analyses of BACE1- and BACE2-deficient mice. *J Biol Chem* 280: 30797–30806.

Finlan LE, Sproul D, Thomson I et al. (2008) Recruitment to the nuclear periphery can alter expression of genes in human cells. *PLOS Genet* 4: e.1000039. doi: 10.1371/journal.pgen.1000039.

Guéant J-L, Anello G, Bosco P et al. (2005) Homocysteine and related genetic polymorphisms in Down's syndrome IQ. *J Neurol Neurosurg Psychiatry* 76: 706–709. doi: 10.1136/jnnp.2004.039875.

Harper P (2006) *First Years of Human Chromosomes – The Beginnings of Human Cytogenetics*. Oxford shire: Scion Publishing Ltd.

Kahlem P (2006) Gene-dosage effect on chromosome 21 transcriptome in trisomy 21: Implication in Down syndrome cognitive disorders. *Behav Genet* 36: 416–428.

Kerkel K, Schupf N, Hatta K et al. (2010) Altered DNA methylation in leukocytes with trisomy 21. *PLOS Genet* 6. doi: 10.1371/journal.pgen.1001212.

Korbel JO, Tirosh-Wagner T, Urban AE et al. (2009) The genetic architecture of Down syndrome phenotypes revealed by high-resolution analysis of human segmental trisomies. *Proc Natl Acad Sci USA* 106: 12031–12036. doi: 10.1073/pnas.0813248106.

Korenberg JR, Kawashima H, Pulst SM et al. (1990) Molecular definition of a region of chromosome 21 that causes features of the Down syndrome phenotype. *Am J Hum Genet* 47: 236–246.

Lejeune J, Gauthier M, Turpin R (1959) Etudes des chromosomes somatiques de neuf enfants mongoliens. *C R Acad Sci* 248: 1721–1722.

Letourneau A, Antonarakis SE (2012) Genomic determinants in the phenotypic variability of Down syndrome. *Prog Brain Res* 197: 15–28. doi: 10.1016/B978-0-444-54299-1.00002-9.

Li CM, Guo M, Salas M et al. (2006) Cell type-specific over-expression of chromosome 21 genes in fibroblasts and fetal hearts with trisomy 21. *BMC Med Genet* 24: 1–15. doi: 10.1186/1471-2350-7-24.

Lockstone HE, Harris LW, Swatton JE, Wayland MT, Holland AJ, Bahn S (2007) Gene expression profiling in the adult Down syndrome brain. *Genomics* 90: 647–660.

Mao R, Zielke CL, Zielke HR, Pevsner J (2003) Global up-regulation of chromosome 21 gene expression in the developing Down syndrome brain. *Genomics* 81: 457–467.

Meaburn KJ, Misteli T (2007) Cell biology: Chromosome territories. *Nature* 445: 379–381.

Nadel L (2003) Down's syndrome: A genetic disorder in biobehavioral perspective. *Genes Brain Behav* 2: 156–166.

Olson LE, Roper RJ, Sengstaken CL et al. (2007) Trisomy for the Down syndrome 'critical region' is necessary but not sufficient for brain phenotypes of trisomic mice. *Hum Mol Genet* 16: 774–782.

Oyama F, Cairns NJ, Shimada H, Oyama R, Titani K, Ihara Y (1994) Down's syndrome: Up-regulation of beta-amyloid protein precursor and tau mRNAs and their defective coordination. *J Neurochem* 62: 1062–1066.

Patterson D (2007) Genetic mechanisms involved in the phenotype of Down syndrome. *Ment Retard Dev Disabil Res Rev.* 13: 199–206.

Patterson D (2009) Molecular genetic analysis of Down syndrome. *Hum Genet* 126: 195–214. doi: 10.1007/s00439-009-0696-8.

Prandini P, Deutsch S, Lyle R et al. (2007) Natural gene-expression variation in Down syndrome modulates the outcome of gene-dosage imbalance. *Am J Hum Genet* 81: 252–263.

Rachidi M, Lopes C (2010) Molecular and cellular mechanisms elucidating neurocognitive basis of functional impairments associated with intellectual disability in Down syndrome. *Am Assoc Intellect Dev Disabil* 115: 83–112. doi: 10.1352/1944-7558-115.2.83.

Reeves RH, Baxter LL, Richtsmeier JT (2001) Too much of a good thing: Mechanisms of gene action in Down syndrome. *Trends Genet* 17: 83–88.

Rovelet-Lecrux A, Hannequin D, Raux G et al. (2006) APP locus duplication causes autosomal dominant early-onset Alzheimer disease with cerebral amyloid angiopathy. *Nat Genet* 38: 24–26.

Sailani MR, Makrythanasis P, Valsesia A et al. (2013) The complex SNP and CNV genetic architecture of the increased risk of congenital heart defects in Down syndrome. *Genome Res* 23: 1410–1421. doi: 10.1101/gr.147991.112.

Salehi A, Delcroix JD, Belichenko PV et al. (2006) Increased APP expression in a mouse model of Down's syndrome disrupts NGF transport and causes cholinergic neuron degeneration. *Neuron* 51: 29–42.

Shapiro BL (1983) Down syndrome – A disruption of homeostasis. *Am J Med* 14: 241–269.

Turek-Plewa J, Jagodziński PP (2005) The role of mammalian DNA methyltransferases in the regulation of gene expression. *Cell Mol Biol Lett* 10: 631–647.

Wang X, Zhao Y, Zhang X et al. (2013) Loss of sorting nexin 27 contributes to excitatory synaptic dysfunction by modulating glutamate receptor recycling in Down's syndrome. *Nat Med* 19: 473–480. doi: 10.1038/nm.3117.

Webb RL, Murphy MP (2012) β-Secretases, Alzheimer's disease, and Down syndrome. *Curr Gerontol Geriatr Res* 2012: 362839. doi: 10.1155/2012/362839.

Zigman WB, Devenny DA, Krinsky-McHale SJ et al. (2008) Alzheimer's disease in adults with Down syndrome. *Int Rev Res Ment Retard* 36: 103–145.

3
ANTENATAL DIAGNOSIS: GIVING THE NEWS

Shiela Puri and Joan Morris

Introduction

During pregnancy, women are offered tests screening for a number of different conditions known to have an impact on a child's health and development. At the initial consultation, the midwife or doctor explains the purpose of screening and potential outcomes of the conditions involved and provides written information on the tests involved. Parents often only wish to proceed with screening tests after they have learnt more about the conditions and the potential impact the conditions may have on their family. Screening tests can create anxiety, particularly as results and their implications can be uncertain. It is therefore imperative that the professional involved at each stage of the process imparts information in a sensitive, non-judgemental fashion and is knowledgeable regarding the condition screened.

The focus of this chapter is the current approach to antenatal screening for Down syndrome. A case scenario is used to illustrate parental perspectives during each stage of the process.

Who is offered antenatal tests for Down syndrome?

In 1933, Penrose identified that older women were at an increased chance of having a baby with Down syndrome (Penrose 1933, 2009). Figure 3.1 shows how the chance increases with maternal age. The chance increases from less than 1 per 1000 for women under 30, to 4 per 1000 in women aged 35 and over, to 11 per 1000 in women aged 40. In the past as only invasive testing (amniocentesis) was available, only women who were at high risk (i.e. over 35 years old) were offered testing. Since the advent of non-invasive screening tests in England, screening is offered to all pregnant women irrespective of their age.

What tests are currently offered for the antenatal diagnosis of Down syndrome?

Two types of antenatal tests are available, screening tests and diagnostic tests. Initially non-invasive screening tests that carry no risk to the mother or fetus are offered to determine the probability of the baby having Down syndrome. If the screening tests suggest a high probability, diagnostic tests are offered; these are currently invasive and carry a 0.5–1% risk of miscarriage.

The initial screening involves taking a maternal blood sample to measure serum markers and a fetal ultrasound scan to determine nuchal translucency thickness and any other

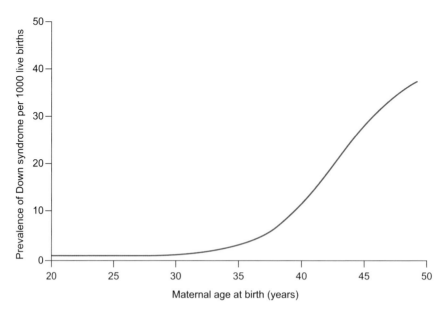

Fig. 3.1. Chance of having a baby with Down syndrome according to maternal age.

anatomical abnormalities. The probability of having a baby with Down syndrome is calculated by combining the maternal age and the results of the ultrasound findings and serum markers (Wald et al. 2003, 2004). As these markers all change during the stages of pregnancy, an initial fetal dating scan improves the accuracy of the results.

Does a previous pregnancy with Down syndrome increase the chance of having another baby with Down syndrome?

Women who have had a previous pregnancy with Down syndrome have an increased chance of having another baby with Down syndrome subsequently, this is dependent on the age of the woman at her first pregnancy. For example, if her first affected pregnancy occurred when she was 20 years old she will have an excess chance of 6.4 per 1000 above her age related chance for all subsequent pregnancies, whereas if her first affected pregnancy occurred when she was 40 years old, the excess chance is only 0.4 per 1000. In the UK women are advised to have initial screening tests rather than to proceed straight to a diagnostic test in subsequent pregnancies.

What information is available to give women regarding screening tests?

Case Scenario

Zeneb is a 33-year-old Sudanese asylum seeker, residing in the UK for 2 years. She is expecting her first child and attends her first antenatal consultation at 10 weeks' gestation with her midwife. She mainly speaks Arabic.

In the UK, women are offered a booklet 'Screening tests for you and your baby' (see Resources at the end of the chapter and Table 3.1 below). This covers all aspects of screening during pregnancy and the first few days after birth. Versions are available in 19 different languages including a video in British Sign Language.

WHAT CONSIDERATIONS NEED TO BE TAKEN AT THE TIME OF DISCUSSING SCREENING TESTS WITH ZENEB?

Is Zeneb able to understand English adequately?
Is Zeneb able to understand the concept of screening tests and their implications?
Are there any cultural and religious considerations?
Does Zeneb have access to any social support within the community to discuss her concerns?

In this case scenario, it is important for an Arabic interpreter to be available for all consultations, including when the screening ultrasound is performed. Zeneb should be strongly encouraged to attend all appointments with her partner or someone who can provide her with support at the time of the consultations. The professionals need to allow

TABLE 3.1
Overview of antenatal screening tests for Down syndrome

Screening test and timing of test during pregnancy	Test performed	Predictive value of the test
Integrated test 10 to 13 wks' gestation	Ultrasound measurement of nuchal translucency thickness (11 wks + 2 d to 14 wks +1 d) and maternal blood test PAPP-A, AFP, hCG, uE3, inhibin	90% detection rate for 1.3% false-positive rate
Combined test 10 to 14 wks' gestation	Ultrasound measurement of nuchal translucency thickness (11 wks + 2 d to 14 wks + 1 d) and maternal blood test (10–14 wks) plasma protein-A and free ß-human chorionic gonadotrophin	84% detection rate for 2.2% false-positive rate (1 in 150 cut-off)
Quad test 14 to 20 wks' gestation	Maternal blood test: alpha-fetoprotein, total human chorionic gonadotrophin, unconjugated oestriol, inhibin	80% detection rate for 3.5% false-positive rate (1 in 150 cut-off)
Cell-free fetal DNA 10 wks' gestation onwards (not routinely available 2013)	Maternal blood test karyotyping after sequencing fetal DNA in maternal blood	>98% for 0.2% false-positive rate, test failure rate is about 4%

AFP, alpha-fetoprotein; cff, cell-free fetal; free ß-hCG, free ß-human chorionic gonadotrophin; hCG, human chorionic gonadotrophin; inhibin, inhibin-A; PAPP-A, plasma protein-A; uE3, unconjugated oestriol.

themselves adequate time during the consultation to ensure that Zeneb understands the purpose and implications of screening and has an opportunity to ask questions to clarify what is involved at each stage.

Anecdotally, parents have often stated that it is difficult to understand the concept of statistics of chance and probability. Visual aids can help. It is worth asking parents what they have understood.

WHAT CONSIDERATIONS NEED TO BE TAKEN AT THE TIME OF THE SCREENING ULTRASOUND?

Zeneb attends for her screening ultrasound scan at 13 weeks; the findings showed an increased nuchal translucency thickness.

An interpreter needs to be present for all these consultations and procedures. The ultrasonographer must be trained on how to discuss results with the mother in a sensitive manner and that a senior colleague should be called to discuss results. It is important that the news is imparted to Zeneb whilst she is being supported by her partner or person of her choice.

The suspected diagnosis should be given to the mother by a health professional knowledgeable about the local process and pathways for further diagnostic testing for Down syndrome. This should be done in a quiet, private environment and face-to-face with adequate time being set aside.

Zeneb should be offered an appointment within 3 working days to discuss the probability of having a baby with Down syndrome and implications of invasive diagnostic testing. This should be clearly explained in a non-judgemental manner. If Zeneb decides to proceed to invasive diagnostic testing, it must be made clear how and when the results will be delivered to her.

What are the currently available antenatal diagnostic tests for Down syndrome?
Currently, a definitive antenatal diagnosis of Down syndrome is made by identifying the presence of an extra chromosome 21 in fetal cells obtained from the placenta, chorionic villous sampling or in a sample of amniotic fluid obtained by amniocentesis. Chorionic villous sampling can be carried out between 11 and 14 weeks' gestation, whilst amniocentesis is only possible, technically after 15 weeks' gestation. Chorionic villous sampling carries a slightly higher risk of miscarriage; however, it enables an earlier diagnosis. Current UK guidelines recommend that the screening for Down syndrome, and the consequent decision on whether to proceed with invasive diagnostic testing, should be performed before 14 completed weeks' gestation.

Are there non-invasive techniques to diagnose Down syndrome antenatally?
In 1997, cell-free fetal (CFF) DNA and RNA were discovered in maternal blood from 5 weeks' gestation. This offered the first opportunity for a non-invasive technique to identify prenatal genetic markers. A peripheral maternal blood sample with circulating free fetal DNA allows fetal karyotyping to be undertaken and hence the possibility of confirming the

diagnosis (Sifakis et al. 2012). Currently, there are limitations to this procedure; the advice in 2013 is that a positive CFF karyotyping result must be confirmed by chorionic villous sampling or amniocentesis (Benn et al. 2013). It is anticipated that in the future non-invasive antenatal diagnosis will replace the current invasive techniques of amniocentesis and chorionic villous sampling for the definitive diagnosis of aneuploidies.

What are the limitations of non-invasive testing?

The quantity of CFF DNA in maternal blood is extremely small and constitutes only 3–10% of maternal blood. Chromosome 21 is one of the smallest chromosomes and accounts for only 3% of all genetic material. To increase the sensitivity, computer-intensive methods, called massively parallel sequencing (MPS) methods, have been developed to distinguish between two copies of maternal chromosome 21 and three copies in the fetal DNA.

There are practical limitations to using the test for diagnostic purposes. The test failure rates, though not fully established, are considered to be about 4%, as the testing so far has been primarily undertaken in pregnancies where there has been a higher chance of Down syndrome and not in the general population. There is insufficient information on the accuracy of the tests in multiple gestation pregnancies or where there is an early death of a co-twin (Canick et al. 2012). The presence of placental mosaicism may also result in an incorrect diagnosis.

What are the implications of non-invasive prenatal testing?

Ethical concerns have been raised around non-invasive prenatal testing with implications of reemergence of the concept of eugenics and the burden on the woman on decision making. Natoli et al. (2012) in their systematic review of prenatal diagnosis of Down syndrome and termination rates showed evidence of a temporal reduction of termination rates in the presence of increased uptake of prenatal testing and diagnosis. They attributed this to better access to health and social care for people with Down syndrome. This is in contrast to the earlier reviews by Mansfield et al. (1999).

However, Bryant (2014) emphasizes the importance of the possible psychosocial impact of non-invasive prenatal testing and the importance for the health care professional to be trained in supporting women in making difficult decision making and maintaining neutrality. Training is available to all health professionals in the UK around counselling and life with Down syndrome through the Down's Syndrome Association, 'Tell it right, Start it right' (2014).

What is the population impact of antenatal testing?

In 1989, the National Down syndrome Cytogenetic Register began collecting information on all prenatal and postnatal diagnoses of Down syndrome in England and Wales. The top line in Figure 3.2 shows how the prevalence of Down syndrome has increased over time, mainly due to the increases in maternal age that have occurred over this time. The lower line shows how the birth prevalence of Down syndrome has remained fairly constant over the past 20 years. The difference between the two lines is due to the majority of prenatal

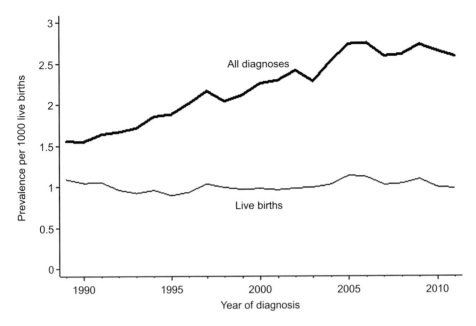

Fig. 3.2. Prevalence of diagnoses of Down syndrome and live births with Down syndrome per 1000 births in England and Wales.

diagnoses resulting in a termination and in addition a small proportion resulting in a miscarriage. A prevalence of 1 per 1000 is equivalent to 700 Down syndrome births per year.

Figure 3.3 shows how the proportion of prenatal diagnoses has increased over time, with the increases being greatest amongst women under 35 years of age. At a given cut-off level, the detection rate (and false-positive rate) is higher among older women and therefore screening tests are more sensitive for older women. This would explain why the proportion of Down syndrome pregnancies detected prenatally is higher for older mothers than younger mothers; a lower uptake of screening in younger women has not been observed and could not account for the magnitude of the difference in proportions. With the advent of more effective screening tests, the gap in proportions of Down syndrome pregnancies detected prenatally in older and younger mothers is expected to decrease even further.

WHAT CONSIDERATIONS NEED TO BE TAKEN AT THE TIME OF DISCUSSING THE RESULTS?

Zeneb has an amniocentesis at 16 weeks' gestation and the results confirm that the baby has Down syndrome.

Even though Zeneb's midwife had taken the time to explain the tests through an Arabic interpreter, the emotional impact of receiving the diagnosis of Down syndrome in her

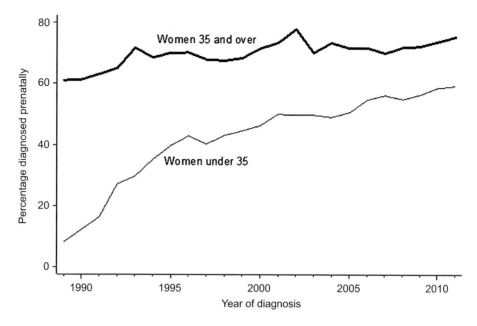

Fig. 3.3. Percentage of Newborns with Down syndrome following prenatal diagnosis according to maternal age and year of diagnosis.

unborn child can be considerable and can cause distress. The shock of any prenatal fetal abnormality makes it hard for women to take in any information, even if they are well informed prior to the testing. It is important to give parents time to understand the information, prior to making potentially life-changing decisions.

It is essential to have a well-planned and coordinated pathway in place to give the diagnosis. Professionals should be trained in giving difficult information to families, be aware of their own personal views and be non-judgemental and sensitive. The diagnosis must be given in a face-to-face consultation in a supportive environment. It is important for the information to be imparted in a sympathetic and factual manner; it must not be considered as 'bad news'. In some units, this is done jointly by the fetal medicine team including genetic counsellors with a good knowledge of the long-term outcomes.

WHAT ARE THE CONSIDERATIONS TO ENABLE THE PREGNANCY AND DELIVERY OF THE BABY TO BE A POSITIVE EXPERIENCE FOR THE FAMILY?

Zeneb and her partner decide to continue with the pregnancy.

Zeneb should be supported in her decision. It is helpful to give her the contact details of the Down Syndrome Association and the local parent support group. The booklet 'Continuing Pregnancy with a Diagnosis of Down's syndrome' (see Resources at end of chapter) is a useful resource.

It is important to ensure that the woman's needs are met in the same way as those of a typical expectant mother so that she is not excluded from universally available services. Extra effort should also be made to adapt the services to the individual as appropriate. Once the diagnosis is confirmed, a detailed fetal anomaly scan must be organized. The birth of the baby may need to be planned in a specialized unit with immediate access to specialist services, for example, paediatric surgery or cardiology. The care should be well coordinated with easy access to named health professionals throughout the pregnancy. This role is usually taken on by either the midwife or the genetic counsellor.

WHAT CONSIDERATIONS SHOULD BE MADE AT THE TIME OF THE BIRTH OF THE BABY?

Zeneb gives birth to a baby boy, Talat, at 37 weeks' gestation, weighing 2.8 kg.

As Zeneb and her partner were aware antenatally of the diagnosis of Down syndrome, every effort should be made by the midwife and obstetrician involved in her care to have a one-to-one discussion soon after birth. The parents should be congratulated on the birth of their baby boy. Staff should make every effort to approach mother and baby with sensitivity so that they are not made to feel different.

It is helpful to offer Zeneb the option of the privacy of staying in a side room if medically appropriate and allowing her partner to stay with her for support, thus enabling both parents to bond with their baby.

The diagnosis of Down syndrome should be given by a professional knowledgeable in Down syndrome with an understanding of the health and educational outcomes for people with Down syndrome, as outcomes have improved considerably over the last 25 years (Zhu et al. 2013). Many young people with Down syndrome are able to contribute positively to society.

A detailed account on the principles of imparting the diagnosis to parents after the birth of their child with Down syndrome is discussed in detail in Chapter 4.

Kathryn and John are parents to Sophie aged 6, with a diagnosis of Down syndrome, and her older sister aged 8. They kindly agreed to share an account of their experiences and want to emphasize the importance of professionals getting it right, from the start when sharing the diagnosis of Down syndrome with parents.

'I was told there were some complications during my scan, when I was on my own. John had popped out of the room for a few minutes, and he had made everyone aware it would only be a few minutes. He returned to a devastated wife. I still get incredibly upset talking about the scan and that experience and do not understand why I was told when I was on my own. It is so important, if possible, to have support when receiving unexpected news. Following further testing I was called by a doctor at the hospital who told me it was Down syndrome. I was 5 months pregnant at this time. The conversation started with, "I'm sorry, but it's bad news. . .". That phone call was so important to me and to hear my baby referred to as "bad news"

was devastating. Now 5 years on, and since Sophie's birth, I know it is not bad news. I was then asked what I wanted to do. I asked about meeting with a Genetic Counsellor. I was put in touch with one immediately. She was a wonderful support to us all and was always available if needed. The Genetic Counsellor support was not offered but was available when I asked. It would be good if it was offered routinely. After the antenatal diagnosis was established, the care given was very positive.

On having Sophie, I was taken to the transitional care ward and John was immediately told he could not stay. Why? I had just given birth. I was left alone with my new baby, no support was offered. While on the Transitional ward, both the Consultant who was there at the original scan and the Paediatrician visited us, this meant a lot to us.

Our experience of the antenatal diagnosis sounds negative, but it is such an important time for parents and how the news is delivered is vital. Making a decision following the diagnosis is of course a personal one; however I feel from my experience, it is so important to have information in order to make an informed decision'.

Key points
- In the UK, pregnant women are offered initial screening tests for Down syndrome.
- If indicated, subsequent diagnostic testing is offered.
- Diagnostic tests involve an invasive procedure with a small risk of a miscarriage.
- In the future, non-invasive diagnostic tests will be available.
- It is imperative that professionals involved in the screening and diagnostic process are trained to share information in a sensitive and non-judgemental manner.
- Information should be given to parents in an easily understood way, and they should be given the opportunity to ask questions.
- Parents who wish to proceed for diagnostic testing to prepare themselves psychologically for their baby's birth rather than for the purpose of termination should be supported in their decisions throughout the pregnancy and birth.
- Every effort should be made to ensure that the woman is supported by her partner at the time of imparting the suspected/definitive diagnosis.
- It is helpful to offer the family support from the local parents Down syndrome support group and the Down Syndrome Association.

REFERENCES

Benn P, Borell A, Chiu R et al. (2013) Position statement from the Aneuploidy Screening Committee on behalf of the Board of the International Society for Prenatal Diagnosis. *Prenat Diagn* 33: 622–629. doi: 10.1002/pd.4139. Epub 21 May 2013.

Bryant L (2014) Non-invasive prenatal testing for Down's syndrome: Psychologically speaking, what else do we need to know? *J Reprod Infant Psychol* 32: 1–4. doi: 10.1080/02646838.2014.874115.

Canick JA, Kloza EM, Lambert-Messerlian GM et al. (2012) DNA sequencing of maternal plasma to identify Down syndrome and other trisomies in multiple gestations. *Prenat Diagn* 32: 730–734. doi: 10.1002/pd.3892. Epub 14 May 2012.

Mansfield C, Hopfer S, Marteau TM (1999) Termination rates after prenatal diagnosis of Down syndrome, spina bifida, anencephaly, and Turner and Klinefelter syndromes: A systematic literature review. European

Concerted Action: DADA (Decision-making After the Diagnosis of a fetal Abnormality). *Prenat Diagn* 19: 808–812. doi: 10.1002/(SICI)1097-0223(199909)19:9<808.

Natoli JL, Ackerman DL, McDermott S, Edwards JG (2012) Prenatal diagnosis of Down syndrome: A systematic review of termination rates (1995–2011). *Prenat Diagn* 32: 142–153. doi: 10.1002/pd.2910.

Penrose LS (1933) The relative effects of paternal and maternal age in Mongolism. *J Genet* (2009) 88: 9–14.

Sifakis S, Papantoniou N, Kappou D, Antsaklis A (2012) Noninvasive prenatal diagnosis of Down syndrome: Current knowledge and novel insights. *J Perinat Med* 40: 319–327. doi: 10.1515/jpm-2011-0282.

Wald NJ, Rodeck C, Hackshaw AK, Rudnicka A (2004) SURUSS in perspective. *BJOG* 111: 521–531. PubMed PMID: 15198778.

Wald NJ, Rodeck C, Hackshaw AK, Walters J, Chitty L, Mackinson AM (2003) First and second trimester antenatal screening for Down's syndrome: The results of the Serum, Urine and Ultrasound Screening Study (SURUSS). *J Med Screen* 10: 56–104. Erratum in: *J Med Screen* (2006) 13: 51–52.

Zhu JL, Hasle H, Correa A et al. (2013) Survival among people with Down syndrome: A nationwide population-based study in Denmark. *Genet Med* 15: 64–69. doi: 10.1038/gim.2012.93. Epub August 2012.

RESOURCES

Continuing a pregnancy with a diagnosis of Down's syndrome: A guide for parents. http://www.downs-syndrome.org.uk (accessed 1 January 2015).

Kathryn White and John Edmonds, UK, Personal Communication, January 2013.

Screening tests for you and your baby. UK Screening Portal 2012. Testing for Down's syndrome. http://fetalanomaly.screening.nhs.uk/leafletsforparents (accessed 1 January 2015).

Termination of Pregnancy for Fetal Abnormality in England, Scotland and Wales: Report of a Working Party Royal College of Obstetricians and Gynaecologists, UK, May 2010. http://anr-dpn.vjf.cnrs.fr/sites/default/files/RCOGTerminationPregnancy.pdf (accessed 1 January 2015).

Tell It Right, Start It Right. Training offered by Down's Syndrome Association, UK http://www.downs-syndrome.org.uk/policy-and-campaigns/tell-it-right-start-it-right/ (accessed 30 December 2014).

4
LIFE WITH AND FOR A PERSON WITH DOWN SYNDROME

Stuart Mills, Gillian Bird, Lesley Black, Vanda Ridley, Sheila Heslam and Lou Marsden for the Down's Syndrome Association (England, Wales, Northern Ireland) with Claire McCall and Fiona Straw

Introduction

This chapter will present and explore everyday issues that families may experience when one of them has Down syndrome. It is written by Down's Syndrome Association (DSA; England, Wales and Northern Ireland) staff who regularly talk to families face to face and via the helpline. The DSA aims to create opportunity and encouragement whereby children and adults lead fulfilling, good quality and healthy lives. We hope it will enrich the lives of all health professionals and inform their practice.

New parents

WALKING IN A NEW PARENT'S SHOES

Like any new parent, parents of a baby with Down syndrome will have questions. Families need factual information (not unrealistically positive or unduly negative) about their child's condition and not unhelpful predictions about a child's future based on outdated stereotypes.

RIGHT FROM THE START—GIVING THE NEWS—GETTING IT RIGHT

Reflecting on their experiences of being told that their child has Down syndrome, parents overwhelmingly say that they would have preferred to have been told as soon as their health professionals' suspicions of Down syndrome arose.

> *I could tell the midwife was worried about something. When I asked her what it was she was very vague and dismissed me. By the time (the next day) when the consultant told us of their suspicions, I was relieved that it was only Down syndrome; I was expecting something much worse!*

But they wanted to be told when together (if both parents are involved) and at an appropriate time.

> *I was told my baby may have Down syndrome while I was still being stitched following delivery!*

> *They asked if they could have a word with me in private. I left my baby with my sister and they told me on my own in a side room. I just don't believe you should be given this news when you're on your own.*

It is important that privacy for the new parents is available at the actual time of the disclosure.

> *I was there on the ward in front of all the other mothers when they told me, and without my husband. I was very emotional and embarrassed; I didn't know what to think or feel.*

> *We were immediately whisked away to a side room and left there. I felt completely excluded, and like we were being judged because our baby wasn't 'perfect'.*

Each new family is different. After the disclosure, health professionals should talk to the family about their needs. Some parents feel much more comfortable in a private room. Some parents may feel they do not want to be treated any differently from other parents.

A good start—what does a good model of communicating the news of diagnosis of Down syndrome look like?
New parents will usually need time to readjust to the news that their baby has Down syndrome. This is probably not what they were expecting to hear. People will react in many different ways. Times are changing; people with Down syndrome are much more visible and are valued and included in their communities. It may be that the new parent already knows someone with Down syndrome. Do not assume that parents are going to react negatively. Good disclosure can go a long way towards allaying parents' fears and helping them on their journey to accepting and loving their new baby.

Are you the right person for the job?
The disclosure should be made by a paediatrician, with up-to-date knowledge about Down syndrome. This should preferably be in the presence of a midwife who has had contact with the parents. Try to keep the number of people present to the minimum; any more than two people may be overwhelming for the new parents.

Preparation
Before you to talk to parents about their baby's condition, it is vital that you have read up-to-date information about living with Down syndrome. The Down's Syndrome Association (DSA) is a useful resource; take a look at their website or call their helpline (see Resources). The DSA can send you hard copies of their new parent information. Parents generally prefer hard copies to photocopies or copies that have been downloaded and printed. Some parents may feel that being given a photocopy or printed copy is second best; that somehow a value judgement is being made about the worth of their new baby. Ensure that you have the DSA's contact details to hand and information about the local Down syndrome support group

contact. Offer to put the parents in touch with another local parent with a child with Down syndrome. If the baby has a heart condition, the Down's Heart Group (see Resources) is a good source of information and advice.

I got in touch with the DSA when I found out and they put me in touch with my local group which was a great support to know that I was not alone.

It may be the first time you have had to talk to new parents about Down syndrome or it may be a number of years since you last saw a baby with Down syndrome. It can be helpful to discuss what you are going to say with a colleague; use them as a sounding board.

It is also important, as it is before talking to any new mother, to read through the mother's maternity notes to gather any available background information regarding the mother's circumstances, for example, previous children or social situation, as this may influence the amount of additional support that the family may need.

Environment matters

Make sure the room where you intend talking to the new parents is suitable, private and that other people will not be coming and going. Ensure that there will be no phone calls or interruptions.

Telling the parents

It is really important to tell both parents together whilst the baby is present. If the mother is single or the baby's father cannot be present, try to ensure support for her through a family member or friend. If English is not the parent's first language, have an interpreter present. It is important to brief the interpreter prior to speaking to the parents.

New parents want to be congratulated and told that they have a beautiful new baby. It really helps the process of readjustment to 'normalize' the situation. Some babies with Down syndrome will have immediate presenting health problems which require intervention. For parents of babies who are unwell, their baby's health will be the overriding concern with the Down syndrome taking a back seat—thinking about their child's Down syndrome will come later. All new families need to know that first and foremost they have a baby with the same needs as any other baby. The needs of a baby with Down syndrome are similar to any baby; they need to be fed, kept warm and clean and need nappy changes, comfort and plenty of cuddles. Their baby is a unique individual who will have more in common with their family than with other people with Down syndrome. Encourage the parents to get to know and enjoy their new baby. Reassure them that they do not need to be doing anything special or different at this stage. Their baby's needs are likely to be exactly the same as any other baby.

Do's and don'ts

- Language is really important—The baby *has* Down syndrome; he or she does not suffer from it. It is not a Down syndrome child or even worse, a Down child!

- Offer a balanced view of life for people with Down syndrome.
- Be realistic about the wide range of possibilities.
- Do not recite a list of all the possible health problems that a baby with Down syndrome might have. Be positive about the fact that we know what some of the more typical health issues are and that baby will be screened for these health issues in the coming weeks.
- None of us has a crystal ball; do not attempt to predict the future!
- Do not give a list of all the things that the child won't do or achieve.

Give the parents time to absorb the information and to ask questions; it is important not to rush through disclosure.

First questions
Receiving unexpected news may mean that new parents need a little more time to process what they are being told. Some parents may have a good or basic understanding of the condition already; others may have never met anyone with Down syndrome or have vague memories from their childhood of someone with Down syndrome in their neighbourhood living with elderly parents.

What type of questions do parents ask?

- What is Down syndrome?
- Why did this happen to us?
- Do we have a greater chance of having another child with Down syndrome?
- What are we dealing with?
- Can they tell me what level of intellectual disability my baby has?
- Is there any connection between the level of physical characteristics and level of intellectual disability?
- What are some of the health issues for children with Down syndrome?
- What are the differences about living with a baby with Down syndrome?
- Will my baby be able to breastfeed?
- Do I need to be doing anything special/different?
- Do I need early intervention immediately? I am worried that my baby is missing out.
- What shall I tell my baby's siblings about Down syndrome?
- Will the confusing and negative thoughts that I have about my baby go away?
- Do children with Down syndrome go to ordinary schools?
- What difficulties do children with Down syndrome have?
- Will people stare at my child?
- Will my child have friends?
- Will my child leave home?
- What do adults with Down syndrome do? What are their lives like?
- Will my child have relationships and maybe get married?
- What will happen to my child when I am no longer here?

Many answers to these questions are covered later in this chapter. If the parents ask a question and you do not know the answer, be honest and tell them you will find out. Take the parents' lead; check as you go along that they have understood what you have told them. It is up to your judgement but it can really help some parents if you interact with the baby, call him or her by their name and show your acceptance of their new baby. Before you leave, arrange a follow-up within a few days.

Health assessment

All babies with Down syndrome should have the same health checks as any baby. In the UK, this includes a physical examination, neonatal hearing screening and a blood spot test (importantly including TSH). Additionally, they should be screened for medical conditions more commonly present in Down syndrome (Charleton et al. 2010, 2014). Although parents should not be given an extensive list of the possible medical problems, the symptoms of the commonly associated conditions, for example, congenital heart disease and gastrointestinal problems, should be discussed.

Congenital heart disorders are present in up to 40–60% of babies with Down syndrome, but signs are not always apparent at birth. An initial assessment before discharge should be made along with arrangements for specialist cardiology assessment within 6 weeks (see Chapter 8). Malformations of the gastrointestinal tract usually present clinically. The eyes should be checked for cataract. With an increased risk of blood disorders (see Chapter 12), newborns with Down syndrome should have a full blood count. Management of most health conditions in babies with Down syndrome is the same as for the general population.

Feeding

New mothers, particularly if it is their first child, can find feeding a source of worry. They should be supported to feed their child by the method of their choice. Breastfeeding as for any baby is best; however, some mothers may choose not to breastfeed or find that because of their circumstances breastfeeding is not right for them. Feeding a baby with Down syndrome can be harder and needs more time, patience and perseverance. In addition, some babies may not be allowed to feed due to medical reasons. About 10% of babies with Down Syndrome may have an associated gastrointestinal malformation that requires a surgical intervention. They may need to be given nutrition intravenously.

Babies with significant congenital heart disease may be unable to feed because they are tired or breathless. They will be fed milk by a nasogastric tube till they are well enough to be fed by the method of their mother's choice. As babies with Down syndrome commonly have low muscle tone, symptoms of gastro-oesophageal reflux are common and should be managed appropriately (see Chapter 13).

Almost all mothers who want to breastfeed or to provide breast milk for their baby with Down syndrome can, with appropriate support. Some babies are not able to breastfeed fully at first, but as they grow older their feeding usually improves and then they are able to be breastfed fully. Mothers of these babies can express breast milk by hand or pump to build up their milk supply. The DSA's New Parent booklet contains guidance about breastfeeding.

Babies with Down syndrome may be slower to regain their birthweight and this may take up to a month. It is therefore vital to use Down syndrome-specific growth charts to monitor growth (see Chapter 10).

Support in hospital after giving the news
If possible, mothers should be offered the option of moving into a single room. Partners should be offered somewhere private to make phone calls and arrangements made for them to stay overnight should they wish. If possible, encourage all relevant staff to visit the mother regularly and interact with the baby by name. It is important to talk to the parents about what will happen next to reduce any anxieties they may have. It is helpful to inform the baby's General Physician, Health Visitor or Community Midwife of the condition.

Leaving hospital
Ensure that parents know with whom and how they can make contact, if they have any concerns about their child's health. An explanation should be given about local service provision for children with Down syndrome and follow-up arrangements should be clearly discussed. Ensure that they have all the contact information that they need for the future. In the UK, the parents are provided with a copy of the Down syndrome-specific inserts for their child's personal child health record (PCHR UK), including the Down Syndrome-specific weight and growth chart inserts (see Chapter 10).

WHY IS GOOD COMMUNICATION AROUND THE DIAGNOSIS SO IMPORTANT?
UNDERSTANDING THE IMPACT OF YOUR WORDS
Some parents say that the moment that they received the diagnosis remains crystal clear in their memories for many years. It is important to think about the words that are used when delivering the diagnosis. Speculation about how a child may turn out is not helpful to parents.

> *Well, it's lucky you live by the sea, as Down syndromes make excellent deckchair attendants.*
> *If you're lucky, she'll walk by the time she's 5, and be out of nappies by 7.*
> *Don't expect him to go to university or anything.*

Parents who are told about their baby's condition in a caring way and who feel supported in the early days may find it easier to accept the diagnosis.

> *A new dad called the DSA 2 days after his partner gave birth to their first child; a baby girl with Down syndrome. He said that he felt 'a bit shocked' but he wanted to find out more and to speak to local parents. He felt that the way he and his partner had been told the news had made a big difference; he described it as 'good, honest and open'. He finished the conversation by saying that he and his partner were 'eager to enjoy their daughter and were trying not to look too far ahead'.*

The way in which a diagnosis is given may influence the manner in which a parent interacts with, and perceives, their child for many years into the future.

A mother of a 7-year-old little girl with Down syndrome child called the DSA to discuss her daughter's behaviour at mealtimes. It transpired that at every mealtime the girl was throwing food whilst her siblings were expected to sit at the table and behave appropriately. The little girl's siblings had told their mother that they had had enough. After ways of changing this behaviour were discussed, the mother said 'I have never talked to anyone about my daughter's Down syndrome'. The mother described the negative things that she had been told by the health professional who diagnosed her daughter's Down syndrome. The mother left hospital with very low expectations of her new baby daughter. The mother did not want to talk to anyone about her daughter or to meet with other families. The low expectation of the mother meant that she accepted her daughter's generally poor behaviour as normal.

Each parent will react differently on hearing the news that their baby has Down syndrome. Because of greater awareness of the condition, some new parents may not see Down syndrome as an issue. They may know people with Down syndrome in their community. Their other children may have a classmate or friend with Down syndrome. It may take some families a little longer to accept their baby with Down syndrome. Some families may react with sadness because they wanted their baby to be like most other babies. They may be scared that they will find it hard to look after their baby. They may not know anything about Down syndrome. This is where health professionals can help in providing accurate and up-to-date information about Down syndrome. Make sure that your department has an up-to-date stock of literature from the DSA. Let parents know that this literature is available if they want it. Many anxieties can be reduced with accurate information. Most parents will want this literature but some parents will feel that they cannot look at it until some time has passed after the diagnosis. Most new parents find that once the early stages are over and their baby becomes more responsive and engaging, a relationship begins to develop and the new arrival becomes an integral part of the family.

HELP PARENTS TO FOCUS ON THE HERE AND NOW, NOT A FRIGHTENING IMAGINED FUTURE

It is natural when faced with an unexpected situation for new parents to worry about the distant future. Their worries may be based on an outdated understanding of what people with Down syndrome can and do achieve. Beyond the certainty that a baby born with Down syndrome will have a degree of intellectual disability and experience some developmental delay, there is nothing further a health professional can tell a new parent about their individual child. We now know far more about the difficulties that children with Down syndrome have and how we can help them overcome some of these difficulties. The intellectual disability affects a child's ability to learn compared with other children of their age—it does not mean they cannot learn. Children with Down syndrome learn to walk, talk and meet other developmental milestones but often later than their peers. Many children with Down syndrome are being included in mainstream education where, if given the right support, they learn and thrive. The most important message to communicate to new parents is that children with Down syndrome can do and like the vast array of activities enjoyed by all children.

It is impossible to predict outcomes for any individual child when he or she is very young, but in general, children and young people with Down syndrome are achieving much more than they have ever done. In the past it was believed that there were many things that people with Down syndrome could not do, when in fact they had never been given the opportunity to try. Today the opportunities have never been greater, enabling many people with Down syndrome to lead rich and varied lives. With differing levels of support, people with Down syndrome are now leaving home, forming relationships, gaining employment and leading independent and active lives. Their quality of life, life expectancy and role in the community have been transformed as health care, education, support and opportunities have improved.

After coming to terms with the news that our son had Down syndrome we held a party—yes, that's right, a party! I knew many of my family and friends would find it difficult to approach the subject. We wanted to educate them as much as we could and let them know that we were proud of our son and we were excited about his arrival. I printed off basic information on Down syndrome, photos, a definition of trisomy 21, stories of children and adults with the condition and information about the support we had received.

It's your baby! That is the most important thing to remember. They will require everything any other baby needs and just a little more. But they will enrich your life. Our daughter is now a major driving force in our family and we are now closer and more positive than ever. She is a bundle of fun and carries a lot of the family trait for inquisitiveness! She is a constant surprise and joy—and your son or daughter will be as well!

What all children need to reach their potential—including those with Down syndrome—is Love, Opportunity and Encouragement.

Key points
- Parents should be informed that their child may have Down syndrome, as soon as the diagnosis is suspected, by an experienced paediatrician with good knowledge about Down syndrome and living with Down syndrome.
- The news should be given in a sensitive, balanced and non-judgemental manner with privacy being maintained at all times.
- At the time of giving the news, the mother should be supported by her partner/family.
- The baby should have a comprehensive health assessment, particularly looking for conditions more commonly occurring in children with Down syndrome, for example, a specialist cardiology assessment for congenital heart disease.

- The families should be provided with up-to-date written information about the condition, for example, the DSA Information leaflet for new parents. In addition, they should be provided with information about the local parents, Down syndrome support groups and health service provision including contact details.
- It is vital to support parents appropriately along their child's journey to enable them to love and enjoy their new baby.

Developmental progress: the pre-school years
WHAT IS THE DEVELOPMENTAL PROFILE IN THE FIRST 2 YEARS?
The first few months involve adjustment to the new arrival and an emerging new set of expectations. Development in the first 18 months or so has at its centre the enabling progression of motor skills. Motor skills allow infants to start to explore the world. Infants first gain truncal support and balance. This frees up the hands to reach, grasp and explore surrounding objects. Crawling or bottom shuffling will then follow allowing the ambit of operations to spread. Increased tone and control then spread caudally as the young explorer then learns to pull to stand, coast and then walk. Low muscle tone often predominates in children with Down syndrome and curtails this process. It is frustrating for the child, parents and therapists. There are ways of reducing raised tone but you cannot put tone in where it does not exist. So, if the child cannot get to the world, parents and therapists have to bring the world to the child with due attention to toys and seating. Play can involve positioning to allow the child an opportunity to feel the weight of his or her body, so enhancing resting antigravity muscle activity. The other ingredient of success is patience. Children do not learn in a linear fashion. As they pick up any new skill they will be unreliable for it for a while, until they have consolidated that learning (demonstrated well later on when potty training; we call the result of this unreliability 'accidents'). The pattern for learning is one of spurts (new skill) and plateaux (consolidation). In children with typical development, the spurts and plateaux may not be so obvious but in a child with intellectual disability, the plateaux are much more obvious. Then, just when parents are becoming disheartened and feeling their child will never learn another thing again, a new skill suddenly appears.

In the second 6 months of life, imitative gesture appears (e.g. pat-a-cake). Then children can start attributing meaning to the gesture, which represents the emergence of language (e.g. waving good-bye, shaking the head for 'no'). The very fine motor control of tongue muscles required to produce the packets of sound that are interpretable by others as spoken language is too difficult at this stage for most children with Down syndrome. Simple sign systems such as Makaton, therefore, provide the mainstay of communication for the 2 years or so that follow (see below and Chapter 19). Social and cognitive skills appear alongside language skills and, typically, children with Down syndrome will develop in the low average range in the first 2 years of life.

Social and cognitive skills develop alongside language skills. Relationships and interactions with people in the child's life affect all areas of learning and development—social emotional, cognition, play, language and communication. Adults need to be highly responsive and understand the world from the child's perspective. Being animated, accompanying communication with intonation, pointing and gesture, repeating activities the child enjoys, following the child's focus of attention and interacting on the same physical level will all promote development. Visual materials and motivating and interactive activities that incorporate modelling, copying and turn-taking encourage development in all areas. The work of Roberts et al. (2007, 2008) offers advice for speech and language therapists on interventions parents might use through a programme of daily activities to encourage receptive and expressive language and speech skills.

From the age of about 10 months, the developmental profile of a child begins to carry a broadly predictive quality. Children with higher developmental quotients will tend to keep that position, and the same applies to those with lower developmental quotients. Parents will often ask about what the future holds. Care needs to be taken in answering. If an assessment is done at the end of a plateau, it will serve to underestimate a child's ability; if done at the beginning of a plateau, it will serve to estimate ability. We have already stated that what all children need to thrive is love, opportunity and encouragement. We need to apply that knowledge to children with Down syndrome (this is considered more in Chapter 19). The information that follows is designed to inform readers about the *development of most but not all* pre-school children with Down syndrome. Figures 4.1–4.4 reflect the range of ability in children with Down syndrome in the pre-school years compared with that seen in typically developing children.

Development from 3 to 5 years

Between 3 and 5 years, most families will be enjoying seeing their children develop into active, mobile, interactive and socially engaging young people. They will see how their child with Down syndrome is progressing in a similar way to other children, albeit more slowly particularly in learning to speak. Most children will be communicating with sign language and will have begun to say some words. Families will face the same challenges as any family with a young child, with extra demands where children have additional health or developmental needs. As for any family, additional support may be required due to socioeconomic, mental health or relationship factors or where they lack a support network.

Doctors and therapists should work closely with parents to assess, support and encourage development. Most children with Down syndrome are good at learning visually and understand best by watching or being shown. They learn less easily from listening to spoken information. Interventions that enhance verbal and problem-solving environments throughout early childhood along with efforts to reduce negative, over pessimistic influences give cognitive development the best opportunity. Doctors and therapists should be sensitive to individual differences and parental concerns arising from comparisons with other children. The more difficult learning is for an individual, the more important it becomes to provide an education that takes advantage of the person's learning strengths and minimizes confrontation with learning barriers.

Communication

Between 3 and 5 years the majority of children will have developed joint attention skills, understand many single words and short sentences, be communicating in sign language and

DOWN SYNDROME—DEVELOPMENTAL MILESTONES

Finding out about moving

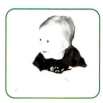

Activity	Children with Down syndrome		Typical Children	
	Average age	Range	Average age	Range
Holds head steady when sitting	5 months	3–5 months	3 months	1–4 months
Rolls over	8 months	4–12 months	5 months	2–10 months
Sits alone	9 months	6–16 months	7 months	5–9 months
Stands alone	18 months	12–38 months	11 months	9–16 months
Walks alone	23 months	13–48 months	12 months	9–17 months

Fig. 4.1. Developmental milestones in Down syndrome: Finding out about moving.
Reproduced from the Parent Held Child Record insert for babies born with Down syndrome (3rd ed, June 2011) with the kind permission of the Down Syndrome Medical Interest Group.

DOWN SYNDROME—DEVELOPMENTAL MILESTONES

Finding out about hands

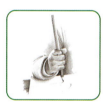

Activity	Children with Down syndrome		Typical Children	
	Average age	Range	Average age	Range
Follows objects with eyes	3 months	1.5–6 months	1.5 months	1–3 months
Reaches out and grasps objects	6 months	4–11 months	4 months	2–6 months
Passes objects hand to hand	8 months	6–12 months	5.5 months	4–8 months
Builds a tower of 2 cubes	30 months	14–32 months	15 months	10–19 months
Copies a circle	48 months	36–60 months+	30 months	24–40 months

Fig. 4.2. Developmental milestones in Down syndrome: Finding out about hands.
Reproduced from the Parent Held Child Record insert for babies born with Down syndrome (3rd ed, June 2011) with the kind permission of the Down Syndrome Medical Interest Group.

DOWN SYNDROME–DEVELOPMENTAL MILESTONES

Finding out about words

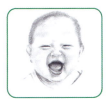

Activity	Children with Down syndrome		Typical Children	
	Average age	Range	Average age	Range
Responds to sounds	1 month	0.5–1.5 months	0 month	0–1 month
Babbles "Da-da" and "Ma-ma"	7 months	4–8 months	4 months	2–6 months
Responds to simple instructions	16 months	12–24 months	10 months	6–14 months
First words spoken with meaning	18 months	13–36 months	14 months	10–23 months
2-word phrases	30 months	18–60 months+	20 months	15–30 months

Fig. 4.3. Developmental milestones in Down syndrome: Finding out about words.
Reproduced from the Parent Held Child Record insert for babies born with Down syndrome (3rd ed, June 2011) with the kind permission of the Down Syndrome Medical Interest Group.

DOWN SYNDROME–DEVELOPMENTAL MILESTONES

Finding out about people

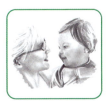

Activity	Children with Down syndrome		Typical Children	
	Average age	Range	Average age	Range
Smiles when talked to	2 months	1.5–4 months	1 months	1–2 months
Plays pat-a-cake or peek-a-boo	11 months	9–16 months	8 months	5–13 months
Drinks from an ordinary cup	20 months	12–30 months	12 months	9–17 months
Dry by day	36 months	18–50 months+	24 months	14–36 months
Bowel control	36 months	20–60 months+	24 months	16–48 months

Fig. 4.4. Developmental milestones in Down syndrome: Finding out about people.
Reproduced from the Parent Held Child Record insert for babies born with Down syndrome (3rd ed, June 2011) with the kind permission of the Down Syndrome Medical Interest Group.

be increasing their range of vocalizations and spoken words. Children may now be able to request things they want, and ask for particular people.

Some children with Down syndrome show relative weaknesses in their development of attention, communication and play skills. In this case, interventions that teach parents to become more responsive in their interactions, to understand sensory differences and manage behaviour are useful. Similarly, they can benefit from appropriate augmentative communication supports (e.g. the Picture Exchange Communication System [PECS]).

Practice through everyday play, interactive activities supplemented by focused activities will extend vocabulary. As speech skills develop spoken language begins to take over from sign language between 4 and 5 years of age. Parents may notice spoken language increases during their children's first year at school. The neurology of speech and language development is dealt with further in Chapter 18.

UNDERSTANDING AND EXPRESSION

Most children will show fairly good understanding in familiar situations and be easily engaged in social interaction. They will use non-language cues as well as their understanding of spoken language to follow instructions. The understanding of spoken language is usually less impaired than expression. They will usually be able to understand early vocabulary, including nouns for everyday items, animals, clothes, family, food, body, transport and so on; as well as verbs for daily actions; adjectives to describe colour, size, shape, quantity and personal qualities; prepositions 'in', 'on', 'under', 'up' and 'down'; and social words 'hello' and 'bye-bye'. Some children will understand many hundreds of words. Children will learn new vocabulary through daily interactions/activities as well as through targeted activities with repetition, practice and visual supports. Most children will understand/remember two key-word information but many will be less able. Remembering and understanding of sentences are affected by attention, motivation and listening environment.

SOCIAL DEVELOPMENT AND BEHAVIOUR

Most children with Down syndrome enjoy social interaction and can engage well in shared play and other activities. At preschool, they often need a high level of supervision and support for successful peer interactions and to teach new communicative behaviours as necessary. They nonetheless will develop friendships through shared activities and experiences with other children. Most pre-school infants with Down syndrome will not yet have the communication skills they need to express their feelings or to communicate about their experiences out of context.

Children with Down syndrome may develop challenging behaviours which are common behaviours for all children at a similar stage in development. However, the behaviours may continue for longer than usual and can become habitual, occasionally with longer-term consequences. Therefore, particular attention should be given to providing support for parents in behaviour management. Factors related to poor quality sleep, health issues, communication and play skills may contribute to the development of challenging behaviours in some children. There is also a risk that some children may be unintentionally rewarded for inappropriate behaviours when these behaviours are responded to with social engagement; negative or positive.

Positive behaviour management approaches applied consistently work well. These include observing and recording behaviour, analysing the functions of the behaviour and agreeing a plan for behavioural change; preventing the behaviour from occurring, teaching new skills, rewarding positive behaviours and ceasing to reward unwanted behaviours. Children benefit from clear expectations modelled to them and illustrated visually. They will learn from their successful experience of following daily routines (with support as required) for the new demands of preschool/school.

COGNITION AND PLAY

Most children between the ages of 3 and 5 years will have begun to play 'pretend' by acting out short familiar scenarios with dolls and other toys/props. Many children will probably still enjoy exploring, playing with cause and effect toys and may like moving items about from one container/place to another. Some children may be interested in playing with small world toys, particularly for known TV characters and will be able to copy a sequence of modelled play activities. Some may engage in solitary play for quite long periods in some situations, although in a busy situation, such as preschool, may go from one activity to another. Most will need a play partner to help maintain their own play, play alongside and engage with others in play.

Most will have an extensive knowledge of nursery rhymes, be able to match visually identical items (pictures, words, colours, etc.), build a small tower of bricks and have begun to hold a pen using an early tripod grip. With modelling, children may be able to draw lines up and down, make circular marks and dots. At around 5 years many children will be able to remove and replace felt pen lids, colour within a defined area (approximately) and be able to draw a face or person. Many will be able to do inset puzzles but may need help and support to do simple jigsaw puzzles.

Many children will have begun to develop 1:1 correspondence in counting tasks and count with support using a number line. Children may recite numbers out of sequence when they attempt to count objects one for one. Some children will have 'Numicon' equipment or similar visual number teaching materials at preschool and/or at home. If so, they will be learning to fill the board with shapes, match shapes, select and name shapes.

Children are likely to enjoy books and being read to. Many pre-school children will enjoy reading personal books about them and their families. Some will have been introduced to reading through word-to-word matching games and may be learning to read with published reading resources and apps.

MOTOR SKILLS

Delayed motor skill development and small stature can affect children's mobility, balance, participation with peers and self-help and independence skills. Most children will need extra help to dress and undress themselves and access the toilet. The majority of children will be eating a range of finger foods, drinking through a straw and drinking from an open cup by the age of 5. Physio- and occupational therapists can offer useful guidance but most parents will skilfully devise practical solutions. Therapists can, however, do much to improve confidence and self-esteem.

TOILET TRAINING

Between 3 and 5 years most children with Down syndrome develop toilet awareness and continence through a training programme at home and preschool, aided by wearing pants (not pull ups) and rewards. Parents and pre-school staff can choose a time for starting a toilet training programme as the date for starting school approaches.

SENSORY AND HEALTH NEEDS

All children need their sensory and health needs addressed for optimal development.

Conductive hearing loss between the ages of 2 and 4 years affects both receptive and expressive language skills of children with Down syndrome (Laws and Hall 2014; see Chapter 5 on hearing and Chapter 18 on neuropsychiatry). This finding highlights the need for audiology and speech and language therapy services to address hearing combined with speech and language interventions through a proactive service. Children with hearing loss will benefit from optimal listening environments, reduction in background noise, people speaking clearly but naturally and gaining visual attention before starting to speak. A focus on listening skills/activities is recommended.

VISION

Parents, preschools and schools are advised that children with Down syndrome do not see as clearly as children who do not have Down syndrome. At preschool and later they will be helped by using black felt pens for writing, teaching and learning materials with good contrast and by being seated near the front of the class (see Chapter 6 on visual impairment).

SENSORY DIFFERENCES

Some children experience additional sensory differences such as those involving taste, smell, touch, balance and movement (vestibular sense) and sensory information from their muscles and joints (proprioception). Sensory differences can have a significant impact on behaviour and communication. Parents, doctors and therapists, especially physio- and occupational therapists, can support children by making adjustments and providing activities that can help.

SLEEP

About 80% of children with Down syndrome are reported to show some kind of sleep problem. These can be behavioural or physical in nature (related to sleep disordered breathing-see Chapter 9) or a combination. Sleep issues can cause considerable disruption to family life and the effects may be overlooked. Poor quality sleep may lead to irritability, overactivity and impaired attention and concentration the following day.

Common behavioural patterns include difficulty in settling, repeated night-time waking with demands for parental attention, early morning waking and insisting on sleeping with parents. Commonly, the settling and night waking problems result from children never having learnt to fall asleep without their parents present. Establishing consistent bedtime routines, going to bed when tired, falling asleep without parents present and avoiding too much excitement near bedtime are some of the things that will help to improve sleep. These principles will work with persistence and a consistent approach. There are an increasing number of sleep clinics around the UK dealing with behavioural sleep problems pursuing these principles.

A physical cause may accompany a behavioural cause—or be the primary cause. Sleep-related upper airway obstruction should always be considered (see Chapter 9). Disturbed night behaviour may be part of a more general behaviour disorder or represent pain such as with an ear infection. It may be one of the very common harmless but disruptive sleep disorders. These include sleepwalking or sleep terrors, headbanging, night-time fears, nightmares and bedwetting. These events can mimic epileptic seizures which only very rarely would be the cause. Children with Down syndrome can be very restless sleepers and move around a lot during sleep.

Support for families: parents at the centre

Most parent carers will be accessing information and services to help support their child's development. They will be looking for guidance from doctors and therapists with knowledge about how Down syndrome may affect their child's development and interventions to address those specific needs. Some will be learning about ways to help their child at home and preschool by attending training events, belonging to a local parent led support group, or by being connected through Down syndrome social media networks. Many parent-led support groups provide early intervention services and speech, language and communication groups as well as social activities. Support groups provide an effective route for parents to share information. They create opportunity and encouragement. For well-informed parents, expectations for effective services and knowledgeable practitioners will be high.

Families have told us they want informed, positive practitioners who can provide relevant information and advice for their individual child. They want health practitioners to know about how people live with Down syndrome today, to have high expectations and to help them help their children. They will expect practitioners to use appropriate 'child first' terminology and be interested in their children.

Quote from parent:
I am often told what 'they' can do. I am tempted to ask, 'Who are they, are you talking about my son? Will he do that?'. I want people to talk about my child by his name, to discuss his development and his needs.

Health practitioners should be familiar with the Early Support principles, how to put children, young people and their families at the centre of coordinated and seamless service delivery; how to make informed choices; how to take the lead in decision making and become active partners in service planning, improvement and delivery (see National Children's Bureau, in Resources at the end of the chapter).

GOING TO PRESCHOOL

Most children in the UK start preschool on a part-time basis during their third year. Most parents will be anticipating progression from a mainstream preschool to a local mainstream primary school. Children usually require additional support to meet their educational needs at preschool and are likely to be receiving a variety of services including speech and language therapy, sensory impairment, physiotherapy and occupational therapy services.

SUPPORTING COMMUNICATION—HOME LINK BOOKS AND CONVERSATION DIARIES

Parents and schools may communicate through two types of home–school communication resources: (1) 'Home–school link books' are for parents and school staff to share information about the child; and (2) 'Conversation' or 'communication' books help children to share their experiences through a daily diary, a type of personal book that goes back and forth between school and home. A support assistant or teacher finds out what the child enjoyed during the day. They then draw a picture or stick a photo into the diary, accompanied by a simple, personal sentence to explain the activity. Parents can add to the diary with images and words from the weekends or evenings for their child to share with friends and teachers at school. Some parents and schools use a tablet device for this purpose.

RECOMMENDATIONS FOR PRESCHOOL

Children will continue to develop their attention skills, receptive language, play, early learning (e.g. matching, classifying, drawing) and social skills. They will be in the early stages of using language to express themselves, for both signed and spoken language.

Children will need guidance, support and tailored interventions embedded in their teaching and learning activities and daily routines at school to progress optimally. Most children will need additional support to help them succeed across the curriculum at preschool and later school.

Children will need a speech and language therapy service to provide a comprehensive programme for developing their communication skills, receptive language, expressive language and speech skills.

An occupational therapy service will advise school on seating, access to the toilet and activities to promote the development of fine motor skills, through the encouragement of daily living activities-skills that will continue to improve through enjoyable practice. A box of fine motor activities, use of large felt pens on a white board, easel activities and side-by-side modelling/copying will help most children to practise.

Children will need structured literacy teaching, including whole word and phonic activities, beginning with learning letters and their sounds, and graded book reading. Many can learn to recognize words, letters and sounds if they are taught how to do this. Children with Down syndrome can progress well in learning to read at school, so expectations should be high.

Children will benefit from a visual timetable to anticipate activities, helped by teaching them time words such as 'now' and 'next'.

In preschool and later school, making a whiteboard and pen available for an adult to draw pictures illustrating information for the child will help refocus the child's attention when required and support listening, understanding and remembering in group listening situations.

Most children with Down syndrome learn from their peers through observation and imitation. Therefore, children should be encouraged to work in pairs and groups at school, with the support to facilitate this.

The school years

The information below is as general as possible but is set within the context of families in England. Education systems in other countries may differ considerably.

Introduction

The aim for school-age children with Down syndrome should be the same as for any other child: to become happy and flourishing members of their family, their school and their local community. This is a realistic goal but can only be achieved by professionals working together with parents to ensure that the right support is put in place.

Starting school

It is important for parents to be prepared and plan ahead for their child starting school. Children in England now can start school in September after their 4th birthday, so parents should be thinking about school once their child is 3 years old. However, as children develop and change quickly in the early years, they will need to be flexible in their hopes and expectations.

Which is the right school for a child with Down syndrome?

There is no one size fits all answer to this question. The majority of young children with Down syndrome are educated in mainstream primary schools, generally in their local school alongside their brothers and sisters and children from the community where they live. Extra help is available for children with Down syndrome in mainstream schools.

Parents are always advised to visit schools, look around carefully and talk to the special needs coordinator in the school. The following are some questions they might want to ask:

- Is the atmosphere welcoming to children with different needs and backgrounds?
- What is the school's experience of children with special educational needs in general and Down syndrome in particular?
- Are school staff keen to learn and undertake training on Down syndrome?
- How involved are class teachers in teaching children with special educational needs—are children with special educational needs taught separately or with the whole class?
- Does the school focus exclusively on getting good results, or do they look at the progress made by all children?

- How do they manage behaviour—are they firm but flexible?
- How does the school communicate with parents?

The most important thing is an inclusive attitude and willingness to learn and to get to know the child as an individual.

Some parents of children with Down syndrome and more complex needs prefer them to go to a special school, as therapies and medical support are more likely to be available on site. There are no special schools specifically for children with Down syndrome, so they may attend a variety of schools for children with a learning disability. If the child has an additional disadvantage, such as autism or a visual or hearing impairment, that will need to be taken into account. For a special school, families may want to think about the following:

- What is the specialism of school?
- What sort of peer group would the child have?
- Are there good role models for behaviour?
- Are therapies and medical support available at the school?

SHOULD CHILDREN WITH DOWN SYNDROME BE HELD BACK A YEAR?

This is a frequent question from parents. Many parents of children with Down syndrome, in common with parents of summer-born children, may feel that their child is not ready to start school at the usual age and would benefit from an extra year in nursery. In England, children are assigned to year groups by chronological age. It is possible to be placed in a different year group but this is relatively rare and is generally only recommended where the child has perhaps missed out on nursery education for health reasons and would be very young for the year group. All schools have a duty to adapt the curriculum for all the children in a class, whatever stage they are working at, so children should not be held back because they have not reached a particular target. It is also important for children with Down syndrome to be with their age peers in order to have good role models of age appropriate behaviour.

LEGAL AND BUREAUCRATIC

There are certain legal and bureaucratic hoops that parents will need to jump through to get their child into school and get the right help. One of the problems faced by families is that services do not always work well together and the right people do not know about the child at the right time. The DSA would always advise parents to be proactive and not sit back and expect things to happen. The DSA and similar organizations elsewhere can help by giving parents information to make sure that the right procedures are triggered at the right time.

SOME SCHOOL ISSUES: PRIMARY SCHOOL

How are children with Down syndrome supported at school?

Children with Down syndrome in mainstream schools are likely to be supported by one or more teaching assistants (TA). However, support is not the sole responsibility of the TA, but should be a whole school matter. Ideally, all staff in the school should receive training in the learning and communication needs of children with Down syndrome. The child should take part in the life of the school along with his or her classmates. As social skills are a strength, children should be part of the normal class group, not be constantly taken out of the classroom. The curriculum will need to be differentiated according to the needs of the child.

To meet children's educational needs at primary school, schools need to have a positive attitude towards inclusion and whole school systems to support this outcome, with training for staff about the needs of children with Down syndrome and the use of evidence-based interventions. It will help schools and other practitioners to be aware of the evidence for the benefits of inclusion for children with Down syndrome who do not have additional or complex needs, following a model of full inclusion with a high level of individual support (Buckley et al. 2002; Fox et al. 2004; Turner et al. 2008). The support is likely to include the following:

- Developing self-help skills and personal care, including taking to the toilet,
- Developing play skills—using modelling and imitation strengths,
- Facilitating interaction with peers,
- Delivering differentiated activities under the guidance of the class teacher, particularly for supporting spoken information and listening activities with visual information—signs, gesture, pictures, written words, modelling and repetition,
- Providing daily speech and language activities, guided by the child's speech and language therapist,
- Providing short periods of additional, focused literacy and language activities, including a daily 'conversation diary', whole word reading and phonic programme,
- Providing focused numeracy activities, including use of visual supports,
- Providing practice for developing fine motor skills, guided by an occupational therapist,
- Modelling of drawing and handwriting activities for children to copy,
- Guidance to ensure that children follow routines at school (including using a visual timetable) and maintain positive behaviour.

Successful education will require a flexible approach with school and parents working in partnership.

Inclusion
Example of inclusion from the DSA leaflet 'Celebrating success—primary'
Conor is fully integrated into his class and participates in all activities to a level that he is comfortable with. He sits with his peers and interacts with them and his class-mates are aware of his needs as well as his limitations. Sitting alongside his class-mates allows Conor to improve his interpersonal skills and use his classmates as role models. He definitely follows their lead! There are clear expectations for on-task behaviour for all the children. Conor receives a great deal of positive attention and

his successes are celebrated both in the lesson plenaries and in the classroom displays.

Work is differentiated and personalized, and support and demands are varied. There is a good balance between Conor being unsupported as part of the whole class, working with his peers, receiving 1:1 support and being allowed to play independently.

Communication and Language

By the time they reach school age, most children with Down syndrome will have started to talk but may still be using sign language or gesture to help them communicate. Language and communication will continue to be an area where support is required. Schools should make use of visual strategies throughout the curriculum rather than relying purely on speaking and listening, as children with Down syndrome are good visual learners but often have poor auditory memory.

Most children with Down syndrome will require speech and language therapy to support their communication needs. In England, this is generally provided by the National Health Service (NHS) therapists going into school to observe and assess the child and monitor progress. A programme will then be drawn up, which may be delivered directly by the speech and language therapist in individual sessions, by school staff during the school day or a combination of the two. All speech and language goals should also be embedded into the curriculum.

Children rarely get as much speech and language therapy as parents would like. In some areas, the service is overstretched and children may only receive sporadic visits. Many parent support groups run their own speech and language sessions with an independent therapist.

Speech and language therapy
Example of the difficulties in obtaining speech and language therapy from the DSA helpline
Ella is 4 and has just started mainstream primary school and James is 12 in mainstream secondary in different parts of England. Both of their families had to go to an educational tribunal to get individual speech and language sessions as legally enforceable provision. However, in both cases, the local speech and language therapy service now wants to reduce this to termly monitoring with no individual sessions, so the families are looking at further tribunal appeals, which will be costly in terms of effort, expense and strain on the parents.

Health Issues at School

Some children with Down syndrome may have additional health issues that affect their education. Coordinating health support in mainstream schools can be difficult and families often find themselves having to liaise with different professionals. Children with Down syndrome who have additional health needs should have a health care plan drawn up in collaboration with parents, the school and relevant health professionals. Often the school nursing service can help coordinate this. Teachers in England are not obliged to administer medicines, so it should be written into the plan who will do this—this could be an appropriately trained TA. Schools may be anxious and overcautious where health needs are concerned, so it would helpful for them to be given specific medical information relevant to the particular child.

Where children are likely to miss a lot of school for health reasons, the school should be planning in advance for this by having work available to send home and thinking about how the child can keep in touch with classmates. For long-term absences, it may be possible to arrange for some home tuition.

Behaviour

Generally, positive behaviour approaches with lots of positive reinforcement when a child behaves well are most effective in supporting good behaviour. When challenges do arise it is important to remember that most behaviour problems can be addressed by parents and school working together, calling in outside help if necessary.

Behaviour problems as such are not an intrinsic part of Down syndrome. Difficult behaviour can occur for the following reasons:

- Immaturity—a child is showing behaviour that is typical of a younger child.
- Communication skills—maybe the child is not able to tell another child to go away or that he or she wants to join in or may not understand what is required of them.
- Frustration because of increased demands at school.

It is helpful if everyone works together to find out what is behind a certain behaviour. The school should carry out an ABC (antecedents, behaviour, consequences) analysis; outside professionals such as an educational psychologist or a behaviour support teacher may be able to help with this. The school can then draw up a behaviour plan with agreed strategies. These might include social stories or visual reminders to understand how to behave. Generally, positive behaviour approaches with lots of positive reinforcement when the child behaves well are most effective.

Getting inclusion right

Example from the DSA helpline

Sophie is 8 and goes to her local mainstream primary school with her brother and sister. Her mother rang the DSA as she was constantly being rung by the school complaining about Sophie's behaviour. She was a bit baffled about this as Sophie is well behaved at home and fits in well with the demands of family life. It turned out that Sophie was being taken out of her class every morning and being taught with children 3 years younger than her. When she returned to the class in the afternoon, she spent her time sitting on a separate table with a Teaching Assistant and had no interaction with her classmates. Sophie lost the friends that she had made in previous years and became very isolated. As she is a sociable child, she became frustrated and showed this by her behaviour in school.

44

FAMILY AND COMMUNITY LIFE

During the school years children with Down syndrome will, like other children, be moving from doing most things with their family to becoming more independent. They will be doing the same kind of activities as their brothers and sisters, sports, arts, dance, scouts ... Families want their children to be fully included in community life but this may need a lot of parental support. They need information about outside sources of support. It is a good idea to get the child's and family's needs assessed by the local social services or children's services department. This may open the doors to additional help such as a carer to take the child out to activities or give parents a break. This may be arranged by a 'direct payment' so that families can employ someone of their choice. As children grow, it is important to encourage independence by having someone else apart from Mum or Dad involved in some activities.

If social services know about the child when he or she is still young, there is less likely to be difficulty getting support once the young person approaches adulthood.

MOVING ON TO SECONDARY SCHOOL

Where children are moving on to secondary school at age 11, parents should start planning ahead when their child is about 9. Many children do progress to mainstream secondary and are able to sit exams and obtain qualifications. Some parents may consider a special school if they feel that their child would not manage in the large and busy environment of a main-stream school. It is important to remember at this stage that children with Down syndrome cover a whole spectrum of abilities and needs, so it is vital to keep an open mind and focus on the individual child.

Some additional questions to think about at secondary level are as follows:

- How big is the school site? How secure? How often do pupils have to move around?
- How are children with special educational needs supported? Is this by TAs in the class-room or are children taken out to a separate learning support unit?
- How does the school support friendships and social interaction?
- What happens at break and lunchtimes? Are there clubs at lunchtime or after school?
- How do they differentiate the curriculum, especially at the age when most children are doing exam courses?
- How will the child get to school? Is transport available?

Adolescent years and transition

Mood swings, pushing the boundaries, tiredness, confusion, crushes, first loves, introspec-tion and spending ages in the bathroom. These may occur a little later and last longer in some people but a teenager with Down syndrome will essentially be like any other teenager. Sexuality, a desire for greater independence, a need for more personal space, encouraging good personal hygiene, explaining and facilitating relationships and fostering self-esteem are some of the issues that need to be considered. Parents worry about the future and what will happen to their child; teenagers begin to develop a sense of self and independence and have to come to terms with their condition. The changes brought by adolescence will have a greater impact for some families than others in the difficulties they present and their intensity and timing.

What does the future hold?

As their children travel through adolescence, all parents have concerns about what the future holds. For parents of children with Down syndrome, their fears are more pronounced as they must increasingly depend upon the support of health, education and social care professionals in planning for the future of their children. Families who call the DSA helpline ask for a map to navigate the labyrinthine system called 'Transition' (the period between 14 and 25 when people move into adulthood). *Transition* is a word most first come across at the year 9 review when they are asked to begin planning for their child's adult life. Representatives from health and social care are supposed to attend along with their education colleagues; however, this frequently does not happen. The quality of such reviews is variable and the advice of one father based on his experiences is to

> *... find out as much information as you can. Especially speak to parents with an older son or daughter who is already in receipt of adult 'services'. Find out what leisure and employment opportunities are available and find out about different housing options. Start to put together a person-centred plan for your son or daughter yourself. No-one else understands them and their needs and aspirations like you do. It's a document that you can put together during the teenage years, and tweak and modify it as you go.*

The onset of adolescence raises a number of questions for parents:

- Can they go to college?
- Will they be able to work?
- Where will they live?
- Who will look after them when we are not there?
- Will they have relationships and maybe get married?
- Can they have children?

The answers will be determined by a vast number of variables:

- The degree of support necessary for an individual to be independent
- Is there a suitable college or work placement?
- Are social care and health services supportive in planning for the future?
- What are the local housing options like?
- What leisure activities are available in the community?

Many young people with Down syndrome have similar questions as they grow into adulthood and become more aware of themselves, their abilities and the abilities of those around them. Those attending mainstream school see their peers achieve a level of freedom and independence in their lives which is denied them and this can cause friction at home.

> *Churchill School has taken on board the broader view of secondary schooling and asked the question, 'What are the long term goals for Tom?' If Tom is to become a successful adult, happy about who he is and optimistic about his future, then he needs to become as independent as possible, and it is understood that it will be the years spent at Churchill that will help him get there.*
>
> *Churchill staff have viewed Tom as an individual with needs like any other student and have developed an insightful means of empowering him and allowing him the autonomy that will serve him well in future life. They have not stunted his development by erecting a safety boundary around him to protect him. Tom is a shining example of the successful transfer of a student with Down syndrome to a large mainstream secondary school. His placement is supported by a strong partnership with his family and the local Down syndrome group.*

Most young people with Down syndrome become increasingly aware during this time of the differences between themselves and their mainstream peers who they see achieve greater independence. As with all children, positive experiences during this time will strengthen their ability to cope in adulthood. The case of Tom shows how the impact of collaborative working, timely planning and the ability to be flexible can support a young person to gain skills that will support him or her in adult life.

GETTING THE ASSESSMENT RIGHT

Perhaps the most important question of all for a teenager and his or her family experiencing the 'Transition Process' is the Adult Care Assessment which provides the gateway to support from adult social care. This assessment looks at whether a person needs support, what that support should be and how it is to be provided. It should cover all areas where a person needs help—for example, daily living, health, work and/or education and leisure. People with Down's syndrome can often be underestimated in their abilities because of their poor communication skills but some young people who appear articulate can have their abilities overestimated because of their language skills. In either case, a poor assessment of needs can result if there is not sufficient evidence gathering and time set aside to plan collaboratively. Calls to the DSA helpline highlight poor practice in this area. Parents are often ill-informed and unprepared to support their child in getting a robust assessment of their needs, and social workers fail to gather sufficient information to support the assessment or fail to carry it out in a timely fashion. As a result, young people leave school at 16 or 19 years of age and say goodbye to a structured day and a network of friends and after-school activities and step into the unknown. Parents have to support their child's social life and depend upon there being suitable local activities available.

> *A lot of Jack's activities in the evenings and weekends are geared to making him as independent as possible, for example, going to the dry ski slope every week means*

that he keeps his skills ready for the next skiing holiday. Jack also attends a fantastic youth club, run by dedicated volunteers for typically developing teenagers, which is split into age groups. Here he can dance, play pool and go on trips. Jack also plays football and wants to have drumming lessons. He was doing regular gymnastics but is just starting a new football club run at a local community college for students with additional needs.

It is vital that all the people involved in a young person's life in both a caring and professional capacity work together to support him or her in planning the future. Agencies have a duty to collaborate. Parents speak of this time as *stepping off the edge of a cliff* or *staring into a black hole* and have negative experiences of the information and support provided.

Mrs. S' son has complex needs requiring a high level of support from education, health and social care. He had been placed in an independent specialist provision for 11 years but this was coming to an end. The establishment was able to support him post 19 but funding needed to be arranged for the following September. Mrs S was concerned that a local mainstream college had stated it could meet her son's needs despite not having seen the young man for over a year. The Learning Difficulty Assessment carried out by a representative of the authority stated that he would be at risk in a mainstream college. Mrs. S had waited patiently for 3 months, following the assessment in February to hear about a decision regarding her son's future. She approached the DSA for help in a state of anxiety in May, requiring support in discovering what her local authority had in mind for her son. She was not aware of the transition process or the individual responsibilities of the agencies involved in her son's care. She did not feel meaningfully involved in the decision making process and had no one she could trust to guide her through the current situation.

The situation causes stress and frustration for families and can impact upon their mental health and financial status. Some parents give up work to care for their child as they are not aware of their rights as carers and those of their adult child. Information is available from charities like the DSA and DS Scotland in addition to that which local authorities must provide by law on their website. The problem can often be knowing the right questions to ask. Parents need to be tenacious.

WHAT ARE THE BARRIERS?
In 2011, National Foundation for Educational Research (NFER)[1] carried out a study into the experiences of young people with special educational needs/intellectual disabilities and disabilities: research into planning for adult life and services. The findings were not a surprise to people with Down syndrome and their families and indicated the following:

• Transition planning usually begins too late and is too focussed on short-term goals.

- There are low expectations of what people with an intellectual disability can achieve, which can limit their options.
- There is a focus on education provision rather than planning for independent living beyond college.
- There is a lack of suitable opportunities for young people with Down syndrome in accessing meaningful college courses, community activities and work.
- There is concern about the lack of capacity in services, in terms of levels of staffing, staff expertise and workload.

The solution seems simple:

- Involve young people and families in planning the future.
- Ensure agencies work collaboratively to support families.
- Improve the assessment process for adult care support so that young people are able to live, socialize and be actively involved in their community.
- Provide adequate staff and training levels.
- Provide meaningful college courses to prepare people for adult life with appropriate levels of support.
- Provide employment opportunities for those who want to work.

Achieving them is a much greater challenge as success will be in part determined by the pattern of government spending.

WHAT ARE THE POSSIBILITIES?

As people come to the DSA, for the most part, when they need help and support, it is easy to paint a negative picture, but there are also positive stories from people with Down syndrome, their families and employers about what happens when things go well. It is very important to remember that teenagers with Down syndrome have hopes and dreams like anyone else and some are able to realize them. The following are some of the success stories.

Nathan
Nathan Walker has ambitions—he has a girlfriend who he likes to take out, he hopes to live in his own place, he looks forward to holidays abroad and he wants a job so that he can afford to pay for all of this.

Andrew
Andrew is 16 and is always on the go—he flips on the trampoline, plays cricket, football and does the most amazingly perfect cartwheels—he is very flexible—but the thing he enjoys most is dancing. He dances before he goes to school, at school and most of the time at home—in fact—he hardly stops dancing—our own little Billy Elliot. Andrew says he wants to be famous too because dancing makes him feel happy and great.

Path and Peter
Path and Peter, both born with Down syndrome, have been in a relationship for more than 20 years. Fifty-seven-year-old Path and sixty-six-year-old Peter live with three other people with special needs, in a house managed by a few caregivers. Ever optimistic Peter is the joker in the relationship; Path is more calm and measured. The pair enjoy strolls in their garden and the company of each other.

Prem
Eighteen-year-old Prem works for 6 hours a day for 2 days a week at Brown's Hairdressing Salon. He needs more support than some others from the DSA's WorkFit programme, but this reality has not stopped him thriving in his role or from becoming a valued member of the workforce. He feels included and understands the routines necessary for the world of work.

Sara
Sara is a young woman who has Down syndrome. Sara has held a number of volunteering positions including an administrative role at the Down's Syndrome Association's Wales Office, as a community councillor and on an oversees visit to Lesotho with Mencap. Sara now works for Mencap in Wales as a 'Partner in Politics Officer' and has established herself as an actress who has recently toured with Hi Jinx Theatre Company, Wales.

Andrew
Tyre fitter Andrew is a first rate employee. He started here not long after I was put in charge of staff training and to begin with I was Andrew's mentor. He was quick to learn and has incredible attention to detail. He is so fastidious and that's important in a workshop environment. Many of the other guys here could learn a thing or two from Andrew. We were first approached by a local intellectual disability training and employment organization called Gabalfa Community Workshop (now Vision 21). Andrew had gained a lot of practical skills by being involved with their training projects and the next step for him was some work experience. We were happy to offer that and we've never looked back.

At first we had regular input from the employment agency who assigned Andrew a 'job coach', but we soon realized that Andrew was coping well and that hands-on support phased-out, with us taking over this responsibility. When discussions took place about whether we could offer Andrew a paid job, we did so without hesitation—he is a valued employee.

Guy and Esme
Guy and Esme were married in 2010. They live independently with Guy's best friend whom he has known since early childhood. They rent a small house and share duties such as shopping, cooking and housekeeping. A small team of carers go in (one at a time) for approximately an hour each morning, 2 hours each evening and 3 hours

for each adult once a week for their personal care and house duties. They met at Foxes Academy College where they completed a 3 year course in catering and life skills. This prepared them both for their independent living skills and their personal development, so that when they returned home, they immediately moved into their own home with their friend who also went to college at Foxes.

Puberty and some sexual health issues

'Sexual health is a state of physical, mental and social well-being in relation to sexuality. It requires a positive and respectful approach to sexuality and sexual relationships, as well as the possibility of having pleasurable and safe sexual experiences, free of coercion, discrimination and violence' (World Health Organization definition).

The timing and sequence of puberty is broadly similar to that of all adolescents. People with Down syndrome experience the same feelings of human sexuality as the general population. Sexuality influences an individual's self-worth, interpersonal relationships and social experiences. People with Down syndrome have sexual feelings and the need for intimacy. These issues require sensitive handling and good practical advice and consideration of health issues.

HOW WILL MY CHILD AND I COPE WITH MANAGING HER PERIODS?

The majority of women with Down syndrome do not require help with menstrual hygiene, although at times 20% need help changing pads and a minority may consider medical treatment to alter their menstrual pattern. As with all women, many women with Down syndrome experience some kind of menstrual disorder—heavy, painful, scanty, non-existent or irregular menstrual flow—at some point in their lives. In Down syndrome, it usually takes 6–18 months to establish a regular menstrual cycle. There are conflicting reports but the age of the menarche in Down syndrome is similar to that in the general population and similarly seems to be falling. Girls start menstruating towards the end of puberty, though occasionally it can be the first sign of puberty. The average duration of menstrual flow is 4 days (3–6 d) occurring every 25–30 days.

Menorrhagia (prolonged/excessive periods) and metrorrhagia (frequent/irregular periods) are the most common complaints in women with Down syndrome. Any menstrual disturbance should be fully investigated, bearing in mind that thyroid dysfunction can cause menstrual irregularities. Once treatable medical disorders have been excluded, treatment options can be discussed. These include mefenamic acid or tranexamic acid for dysmenorrhoea; and progesterone and oestrogen hormones, for example, depo-provera injection, progesterone-only pill, combined oral contraceptive pill and implant for irregular or heavy periods. Caution is necessary in women with a medical history of congenital heart disease, venous thromboembolism, migraine with aura, obesity and immobility when using oestrogen-containing medication.

Kirsty was 12 years old when she started her periods; she was anxious and unable to attend school during her next three periods. They were heavy, painful and irregular. She is independent for toileting when she is not menstruating. She has regular support at home and school to help establish a routine and independence for managing her periods. After 12 months, her periods are now regular and less painful.

She is confident and is able to manage herself at period times. However, her periods are heavy for the first 2 days and restrict her physical activity. Kirsty's parents are now considering whether using hormonal treatment to reduce or stop her menstrual flow would be in her best interest.

DO CHILDREN AND YOUNG PEOPLE WITH DOWN SYNDROME NEED THE HUMAN PAPILLOMA VIRUS VACCINATION?

The risk of cervical cancer is very low if a woman has never been sexually active. So when deciding whether to vaccinate against the Human Papilloma Virus (HPV), it is important to remember that it is difficult to predict future sexual behaviour. Cervical cancer may also be diagnosed late when symptoms are not reported or cervical smear tests are not tolerated well. The HPV vaccine has been offered to all 12–13-year-olds since 2008 in the UK. In the UK, it is given by the school nursing service, three injections, preferably over a 6-month period. It is well tolerated. Common side effects are mild, such as redness at the injection site and headaches. HPV vaccines protect against a number of HPV types, offering protection against genital warts, premalignant genital lesions and cervical cancer (see Resources for UK government guidance).

Claire is 13 years old; she brings home a consent form for the HPV vaccine from school. Her mother is unsure whether it is in her best interest to have the vaccine. Claire expressed a wish that she would like to have children in the future. On further discussion with Claire, her parents, school nurse and paediatrician, it was felt that it would be beneficial for Claire to have the HPV vaccine as it is difficult to predict future sexual behaviour.

IS CONTRACEPTION NEEDED?

There have been many pregnancies in women with Down syndrome. Most women with Down syndrome ovulate and approximately 50–70% are fertile. Men with Down syndrome have lower fertility than the general population; however, there have been at least two reported proven cases of men with Down syndrome becoming fathers (Pradhan et al. 2006). Women with Down syndrome who become pregnant have a much higher risk of miscarriage, and having a child with a chromosomal abnormality. There is an increased risk of low birthweight, congenital abnormalities in the infant and pulmonary hypertension in the mother (see Chapter 8).

Young people and adults with Down syndrome have a right to express emotions and sexuality and develop relationships as an important part of a full and equal life based on a right to independence, control and life choices.

People with Down syndrome have a right to

- fulfil personal and sexual relationships;
- marry or cohabit;
- make an informed choice about whether or not to have children;

- take risks and make mistakes in personal relationships;
- privacy and freedom from exploitation;
- receive sex education, including counselling on personal relationships, and the social rules of sexuality, sex and sexuality, contraceptive advice and sexual health support services which should be taught at a developmentally appropriate level. These lessons are compulsory in England from age 11 onwards.

Young people and adults with Down syndrome may wish to form relationships and may be able to manage all aspects of their relationship but some will need extra support when considering contraception and pregnancy.

Women with Down syndrome who are sexually active or planning to become sexually active need to be supported in considering and choosing appropriate contraception. All hormonal and barrier methods of contraception should be considered ensuring that the most appropriate choice is made, taking into account the medical history and level of ability. A medical history and examination needs to rule out any contraindications to the use of oestrogen-containing contraceptives (see above). Progesterone-only methods, for example, progesterone-only pill, depo-provera injection or a progesterone implant may be preferable in the presence of oestrogen contraindications. Long-acting reversible contraceptive (LARC) methods, for example, implant, depo injection or an intra-uterine device, should be considered to reduce the failure rate if there are concerns about compliance issues.

Barrier methods such as the condom and diaphragm can be very effective at preventing pregnancy but need much practice to use safely. These are probably not practical for those with an intellectual disability who lack dexterity.

Helen is 19 years old and lives with her mother and sister. Helen has epilepsy and takes carbamazepine. Helen is becoming increasingly independent and would like to have children in the future. Her partner attends the same College course. Her periods are very heavy and she needs support during menstruation, but otherwise toilets independently. Helen meets regularly with a doctor and nurse at her local Contraception and Sexual Health Clinic. It is clear that Helen has capacity to consent to treatment; she receives appropriate sexual health advice and decides to start on the progesterone depo injection. Helen is pleased with the subsequent reduction in her periods and is also aware of its contraceptive effect should she become sexually active in the future.

MALE SEXUAL HEALTH

There is no doubt that men with Down syndrome have the same array of sexual feelings as any man. However, impairment in social skills both in them and women in their peer group along with limited social opportunity usually restricts the number of sexual encounters. Sexually transmitted disease is, therefore, very rare. Personal hygiene, especially cleaning under the foreskin, may require some prompting. Occasionally, and usually in those with more severe social impairment, masturbation in an inappropriate setting requires behavioural management intervention. We have found no reports of erectile dysfunction. They must exist and would need standard management adapted to the personality and ability of the affected person. Yearly testicular examination should be encouraged as men with Down syndrome are at higher risk of testicular cancers (see Chapter 14).

Adult life with Down syndrome

INTRODUCTION

Adults with Down syndrome are likely to have the same aims and aspirations as others: to be happy and flourishing members of their family and their local community. This is a realistic goal but is generally achieved only with some level of support from parents and professionals. Increasingly, people with Down syndrome are living in their own homes with support, finding employment and getting married.

However, for some young people, once they reach the age of 25, much of the support they have enjoyed through their school life and at college is reduced or disappears completely; families are left having to work hard to find the right help to continue appropriate inclusion within the local community.

This section aims to provide an overview of the variety of situations that people with Down syndrome encounter in their adult life.

A PLACE TO LIVE

Many adults with Down syndrome aspire to leave the parental home and set up in a place of their own. The UK government policy endorses this aspiration and allows for the provision of support to enable people to live independent lives.

However, 60% of adults with Down syndrome at the age of 30 still live at home with their parents/families (Carr 2008).

Kirsty lives at home with her mum and dad. She is in her mid-thirties and has a very active social life. She has two brothers, and a sister who lives in Canada. Kirsty has been to see her sister several times with her mum and on the last visit took advantage of assisted flights and visited her sister by herself. She was delighted (and a little bit scared) that she was able to do this by herself. Kirsty has no support from the local authority currently, as the family supports Kirsty in all her needs. Her parents worry about what will happen to Kirsty when they are no longer around to care for her, and other than staying at her sister's house, Kirsty has little experience of being away from home.

Most people with Down syndrome can live independently from their parents when adequately supported.

Jane lived at home with her parents until she was 19, and then attended a residential college to study on a catering course. At the end of her course, she returned to her local town and worked with her parents and the local authority to find a place to live. There were several opportunities available to Jane, but with advice from her family, she decided to rent a flat from a housing association. She now lives with a friend who also has a learning disability. Jane uses direct payments to buy the 24 hours of support she needs each week to help with some of the tasks she finds difficult. Jane's parents live close by and provide support in other areas. Jane is helped to manage her money, is helped to look after her health and her home and has support to maintain her employment. Jane enjoys a similar lifestyle as her brothers do, going to the cinema and bowling, out for meals when her budget allows and meeting up with her family for Sunday lunch. Jane belongs to an amateur dramatics society and performs in a variety of locations. She also loves gardening.

Other people have particular needs that are currently not being met under the social model of care.

At 23 only recently received any support having lived in county for almost 15 years. Very few available adult services—**Parent**

This includes a range of medical needs as well as support for specific cognitive difficulties. Indeed, the recognition of medical need and specific difficulties is essential to an optimum level of support. Some people with Down syndrome get good levels of support, and others have to fight hard to get any support at all. Families often need help to challenge various agencies to provide adequate support.

GOOD HEALTH

It has been known for some time that adults with Down syndrome experience poorer health than the general population and are less likely than others to access regular health checks or routine screening.

As well as being predisposed to certain medical conditions such as cardiac disease, thyroid disorders, hearing impairment, visual problems and coeliac disease, people with Down syndrome may be more prone to depression, and dementia can occur earlier than in the general population (see Chapter 18 on neuropsychiatry).

In England and Wales, annual health checks have been introduced for people with intellectual disabilities to address the inequalities in health care, but uptake has been slow. People with Down syndrome now have access to a user-held health book to encourage general practitioners (GPs) to pay attention to the specific health problems that occur more commonly in people with Down syndrome. For more detail you can visit the Royal College of General Practitioner's website and download the document 'Annual Health Checks for People with a Learning Disability'. The UK Down's Syndrome Association website offers more detail on the DSA Health book for adults and advice on adult health check content (see Appendix 1 at the end of the book for links).

It's good to keep a record of your health and start to improve on any issues. It helps me remember, having it written down. My key worker and parents can share the info. I can keep an eye on my weight. I understand better which medicines help me with different things—**Matthew**

This is a first step towards people taking care of their own health, but carers still need to provide significant support in this area. Where appropriate support is not available, significant issues can arise. Guidance for care staff on specific health issues is very important, and health professionals can help to inform social care assessments to ensure adequate support is provided to maintain health and well-being.

> *Mary attended mainstream school, attaining several Certificates of Achievement. She was a confident, happy, well-adjusted and sociable outgoing young woman. At the age of 23, Mary was funded by her local authority to live in supported accommodation. Two years later, after consistently being left to make uninformed choices about her diet, clothing, health care, medication and hygiene, her parents observed a drastic deterioration in her mental, emotional and physical health. Feeling out of control, she took refuge in routine to the point where normal day-to-day activity became severely compromised. She suffered constipation, overflow and incontinence of urine due to her poor diet and lack of compliance regarding medication for slow gut motility. She had poor hygiene and was continually feeling anxious about her situation. Mary finally received psychological assessment followed by some psychology support, leading to some improvement in her emotional state as well as her toileting issues.*

MENOPAUSE OR OTHER TREATABLE HEALTH CONDITIONS

Women with Down syndrome on average reach the menopause earlier than the general population at the median age of 46 years. Hypothyroidism does not influence this age. Hot flushes, mood swings and night sweats are commonly experienced but symptoms can vary. The menopause should not be blamed for a change in function or new symptoms in a woman in this age group. A medical assessment is always important to rule out other medical causes such as hypothyroidism or depression (Seltzer et al. 2001, Schupf et al. 2003).

> *Joy is a 44-year-old woman who has lived in supported housing since her mum died when she was 30. She has developed irregular periods, become socially withdrawn and her hygiene levels have deteriorated; she has been gaining weight and is reluctant to eat. Her sister wonders if she is going through the menopause. At her annual GP assessment, it was clear that she needed further investigation as hypothyroidism could explain her symptoms. A blood test later confirmed hypothyroidism and her symptoms improved with treatment with levo-thyroxine.*

CHOICE AND AUTONOMY

Making choices is something that we all do every day; some choices appear minor but are important, for example choosing the colour of the paint in your bedroom, whilst others are fairly major, for example, moving house or getting married, but they all help us to form our identity and contribute to our feelings of independence and self-esteem.

It is important to recognize that people with Down syndrome have the same rights as other adults—they should have the autonomy to do what they can and should expect to receive help and support when this is needed.

People with Down syndrome can often perform certain tasks very well, for example cleaning the home or preparing food. However, some people may make poor decisions, particularly where these require motivation or organizational skills. Getting it wrong with sleeping, eating and leisure activities can be harmful to health, well-being and self-esteem, with many families reporting poor self-management of diet and physical activity.

Sarah lives with two other people with learning disabilities in a house on the out-skirts of town, with support. She is overweight and spends no time doing physical activity, because the carers do not have enough time allocated to go with her for swimming sessions, which have been recommended by her GP. Her carers will agree readily to providing a poor diet, based on the premise that Sarah asks for burger and chips for her evening meal most days. However, Sarah's friend will eat with her once a fortnight, and on those evenings, Sarah is helped to choose between two alternatives (neither of which is burger and chips)—and Sarah has no difficulty in finding a healthier option. She can explain which foods are healthy and which are not, but this is never discussed with her care team. She is also happy to be involved in the preparation of food, but her care team tend to do this for her.

Where Sarah is supported to make good decisions which are appropriate to her skills and abilities, she is able to do this. Visual recipes and cooking with others can reinforce good eating habits, as well as taking an active role in menu planning and shopping for food.

A different problem that people with Down syndrome frequently have to face is others making decisions on their behalf, when this is not only unnecessary, but completely inappropriate.

Sam and Jo have been in a relationship for some years. They had decided to get married and were busy making the arrangements for their wedding. They had seen the registrar and the vicar of the local church and a date had been set. Out of the blue, Jo's family received a visit from the local authority, advising the family that the wedding could not take place as Jo did not have capacity to consent to the marriage. They insisted that Jo had an appointment with a psychologist to be assessed for her capacity to make this decision. The psychologist refused as she did not consider the local authority had grounds to insist on this. Social services even-tually dropped the issue, and the couple went ahead with the wedding.

Choice and autonomy should be encouraged, but it is important to ensure people are not put under undue stress, with too many options too soon; this can lead to feelings of anxiety. However, people sometimes have to take risks in life to achieve their aspirations.

*My daughter was depressed and wanted to leave home as there was nothing here in the outskirts of the town. She wanted a chance to participate in life. 'Life's not worth living for disabled people'. 'It's boring living opposite a field'. We have irregular bus and taxi services and the walk to town is 1.5 miles. The Social Worker was very apprehensive about our daughter's move and even got the community Nurse involved to state reservations when a placement was offered at the Housing Scheme (neither had visited). Our daughter did us all proud when she read from a list she had written, 'My reasons for wanting to move'. This clinched the decision and all were in agreement for the move. A year on, she is a different young woman. She has got her bubble back, is more confident, happy and has an aura of self-importance. Eventually, she is her own person. I am so relieved and happy for her—***Parent***

LEISURE AND WORK

Some people with Down syndrome may find it difficult to attend social or recreational activities if they are responsible for organizing them, leading to isolation and a risk of depression. People should be supported to maintain their current friendships as well as making new friends.

People with Down syndrome need opportunities to participate in the life of their community through personal hobbies and interests, community events and employment, as this will boost their self-esteem and help develop and improve social skills. Interaction with others through a range of activities can provide the social connection necessary for well-being.

After attending college, many young people with Down syndrome find it difficult to find appropriate activities to stay occupied during the day. Sometimes, they will attend specific activities aimed at people with intellectual disabilities, but many would like to work. There are a number of schemes available that help people with disabilities find employment, sometimes voluntary, sometimes paid.

*Will has been working as a volunteer ranger and horticulturist at Hardwick Hall National Trust since October 2012. He has developed within the role and the staff know that if needed William can be left to get on with a task once the requirements of that task are established. Some people might have preconceptions, but they are unfounded as far as I am concerned... Will is one the team—***Head Ranger Steve***

However, people with Down syndrome are often not well supported by these programmes, and in the UK the DSA developed a specific project—WorkFit. This has improved access to mainstream employment and other meaningful activities for people with Down syndrome.

Jenny is 24 years old, who in her spare time is a keen actor, having appeared in films alongside famous actors like John Hurt and Elijah Wood. She was also in the opening and closing ceremonies of the Paralympics. Via the WorkFit program she has found a paid work placement with a specialist insurance broker in Billericay Essex, where she has been working for the last 12 months.

Jenny's duties include managing the post, including updating the post-log, franking, shredding and sending out quotes. Jenny is a productive and valued member of the team. She is closely supported by her supervisor, who has made some adaptations to work practices to ensure success. For Jenny, the placement has allowed her to achieve her goals; she has more self-confidence and this has opened up more opportunities for her. Being paid for her work not only makes her feel great but allowed her to 'invest' in a holiday later. Jenny is thoroughly enjoying the job and the people; the benefits are seen at home too where Jenny is now motivated to get up in the morning; she happily tells her family, friends and particularly her boyfriend about the job and encourages her friends to sign up for WorkFit.

Jenny is not a stranger to work and has experienced a variety of jobs. Prior to her current role, Jenny had attended a training centre run by the Salvation Army where she worked as a waitress in their tea rooms and also learnt some office skills. Jenny had previously undertaken voluntary front of house work with a theatre for 3 years, which she loved but which unfortunately was unable to survive the economic downturn. Whilst Jenny had clearly been active and had experience of a work environment, she had not had a 'proper' regular paid job.

Travel to work training can be accessed on an individual basis, developing independent travel and problem-solving skills, as well as providing general support for those who need it.

Joe can catch a bus from his home to the railway station, get the train and then a tube to work; he can also return home. However, as yet he is unable to catch a bus to an adjoining town, as he does not know the route and is unable to transfer the skills he has learnt from the one journey to another. Joe does know how to contact a member of his support team by mobile under any circumstances if his phone is switched on—he has not learnt, however, to keep his phone switched on, making it problematic when someone needs to contact him. Joe is working with his support team to develop his independent travel training skills.

The common theme here is working out how to create opportunity and encouragement for people with Down syndrome so that they can fulfil their aspirations, at least the realistic ones). Even after the age of 25 when many support networks melt away, the opportunity and encouragement can be achieved through good liaison between parents, care staff, church groups and other community support networks, college (there are many suitable courses for non-disabled), the DSA, social services and so on. The key ingredients for success are energy, time, persistence and creativity.

Down syndrome and dementia

The link between Down syndrome and dementia has been recognized for many years; however, it is still very distressing for family and carers when a person they know is suspected of having or has dementia. The real-life situations in this section will help to inform health care professionals of some of the attendant feelings experienced by affected people with Down syndrome and the relatives who offer them care. They will inform practice and how best to help.

In the world of intellectual disability, the emphasis is on supporting people to be as self-sufficient as they possibly can be. When dementia occurs, the focus of care changes so that the individual can be reassured and kept as safe and calm as possible, whilst receiving increasing amounts of physical and nursing care as the condition progresses. This change can be difficult for all concerned and it is important that relatives and staff understand how dementia affects the individual so that they can offer the best support. The diagnosis of dementia is the starting point; accepting the changes that will happen, beginning to collect stories and information about the individual to share later on, thinking about life experiences and noting things that mattered to them will all help in the later stages. Celebrating the person as they are at that point is key to creating the optimal environment.

How do we get a diagnosis?

> *My brother is 51 and over the last few months he has been slowing down and losing skills—the community nurse has mentioned dementia and we need to know what will happen next.*

The starting point is a psychological assessment. The first point of contact for most families is their GP, particularly if a relative does not have contact with the local Community Learning Disability Team (CLDT). The GP will make the referral to the psychologist, although in many areas families can self-refer. The assessment will define how well the individual manages in daily life and should involve someone who knows the person really well and who can discuss what changes have been observed.

In some areas, people have a baseline assessment of abilities done by the CLDT and this will be used as a benchmark to help identify any changes. It is recommended that all people with Down syndrome aged over 30 have such an assessment. It is worth family and professionals checking whether one has already been done.

> *My sister had a query of dementia but recently when she was in hospital, the nurse said she thought it was all down to the menopause.*
>   *Our brother was being assessed for dementia, they mentioned depression and that made sense since it's not long since we lost our mum.*

There are many other health issues that can present the same signs and symptoms initially as dementia and it is important that these are considered and eliminated rather than jumping to the wrong conclusion. Women going through the menopause may experience symptoms which could be mistaken for dementia such as forgetfulness and lethargy. Depression causes people to become sad and withdrawn, less interested in the things they used to enjoy and altered sleep patterns—all of which could be mistaken for dementia.

It is really important that the GP considers these alternative diagnoses so that appropriate treatment is given (see Chapter 18).

DOES THE PERSON WITH DOWN SYNDROME KNOW THAT THEY HAVE DEMENTIA?

My brother is still living at home with our mum; he is getting very reluctant to do things and is happy just to sit around all day. It's not like him; he used to be very sociable and outgoing.

Although people with Down syndrome may not understand the word *dementia* or its implications for their life, they are usually aware that something is happening to them. This can make the world feel scary and unsafe and the individual may choose to stay in the place where they feel most secure.

It is important to acknowledge that something is happening and to provide reassurance them that it is okay; that parents and carers will be there for them. You do not have to mention dementia, which could be meaningless anyway, but perhaps saying something like, 'it's your memory that's changing, it happens to lots of people' can help them feel better and less unsure. Remember that even people with Down syndrome who have lived with someone with dementia may not recognize that the same thing is happening to them.

With gentle reassurance and by making the world feel as safe as possible, the individual can be supported and encouraged to continue to participate in the activities and interests they have always enjoyed.

GETTING THE RIGHT SUPPORT

My brother lives with us and has just been diagnosed with dementia, what can we do to help him and where can we go for support?

It is important that when a person with Down syndrome is diagnosed with dementia, as far as possible, he or she maintains the same her routine, daily activities and social lives, for as long as possible. However, adaptations to the environment and the individual's care package will have to be made as the dementia progresses.

Social services should be informed of the recent diagnosis and altering circumstances. A new community care reassessment should be requested to identify changing needs and additional support within the home. This should include long-term planning so that changes can be accommodated later on. There should be continuing contact with the CLDT psychologists, nurses, speech and language therapists, physiotherapists and occupational therapists who will all have important roles to play as the dementia progresses.

THE ONSET OF EPILEPSY

> *My sister has started having seizures, they are horrible to watch and I didn't know that they are very common with dementia, I am quite angry that none of the professionals we see told me about this possibility.*

Sadly, the majority of people with Down syndrome who have dementia also develop epilepsy after a couple of years. This should be seen as a treatable consequence of the disease. It is important that appropriate antiepileptic medication is prescribed to reduce and control the seizures as much as possible. The hospital epilepsy clinic, specialist epilepsy nurse, GP or intellectual disability nurse can all be useful sources of advice on medication and monitoring.

CREATING A SUPPORTIVE ENVIRONMENT

> *My son isn't walking around like he used to, he sometimes totally refuses to go outside.*
> *We are really concerned about his safety on the stairs, he has started turning the landing light off and coming down the stairs in the pitch black.*

One of the first things that happens with dementia is that people lose their 3D vision, which makes getting around very difficult, especially coming downstairs, negotiating steps and moving from one type of floor covering to another. Typically, the person will toe-tap the edge of the stair, kerb or carpet before they take a step.

In the home, floor coverings should be kept as similar as possible. Stairs can be highlighted using brightly coloured strips at their edges to help the individual know where the step ends.

Colour is very important—dark colours (black, navy, dark brown, etc.) can look like holes or something to be stepped over, bright colours (red, yellow, orange) can help the person to identify objects more easily. Red toilet seats can help the person identify and use the toilet.

> *My daughter used to like sitting with us at the dining table but won't do that at the moment, it's a shame as she isn't eating properly anymore.*

Having clearly identified areas can help the person with dementia to understand what is happening. Sitting at a dining table is a great clue that food is about to arrive. It is also a social event. A check should be made whether the person can sit on a chair with his feet on the floor—if he can't, it makes him feel very unsteady as he may rock to and fro whilst trying to eat. Placing a footstool underfoot is a simple, but effective, way of helping someone to remain stable.

> *I hadn't thought about why she never left the living room, I did think it was odd that she kept talking about the hammer stuck in the wall.*

Doors should be visible; white doors next to pale cream or white walls can disguise exits and mean that people remain in one room all day because they cannot see the way out. The hammer in the wall was actually the door handle.

What can I do to keep him to keep calm when it's starting to go dark, he gets very upset when the light starts to fade?

Many people with dementia struggle with the change in light as afternoon becomes night and it can affect their behaviour during the evening. A good idea is to turn on lamps whilst it is still light and close the curtains before it goes dark outside. This will reduce reflections in the window and any agitation caused because there is a 'man in the garden'.

[We had] *5 burnt out electric kettles before it dawned on us that we needed to get one that goes on the gas cooker! Sometimes, it's the simple things that make the most difference.*

As the person begins to roll back in time, it is important to have objects and mementoes around, which will help them to feel 'at home'. Photographs of family members, ornaments from years gone by, family heirlooms like clocks and pieces of furniture can be very comforting when someone is losing the ability to recognize more modern items. Making the environment feel homely and safe can have a massive impact on the individual.

CHANGES IN BEHAVIOUR

Changes in behaviour are very common when people have dementia. There is always a reason for behaviour and it is important to remember that all behaviour is a form of communication. It might not immediately make sense, but with some observation and a bit of detective work, the cause is usually identifiable.

It's hard you know, trying to figure out what's going on, it's like he's had a whole personality change.

As the memory rolls back, being in the here and now becomes much more difficult. The person may revert to old habits and routines, which might seem strange but will be meaningful to the individual. Unless they are potentially harmful behaviours, it is best to go with them. Many people can be distracted after a few moments.

She would spend ages rooting in the cupboard for a carrier bag, then when she found it, she'd scrunch it up and put it back in there, but she would be very annoyed if you tried to stop her.
One night after tea, he came into the kitchen and insisted on washing up—he hadn't done that for years.

> *Every night, he packs a bag and puts it under his bed—it took a while before his brother told us that he used to stay in a residential unit from Monday until Friday morning so on Thursday night he used to pack his bag for his weekend at home.*

Sometimes behaviours are more difficult to deal with but using a calm and reassuring approach, using clues to help the person understand what is happening and going with that person's reality can all help to maintain the person's equilibrium.

GETTING OUT AND ABOUT

Enjoying being out and about is an intrinsic part of living well with dementia. No one should be cooped up inside all day, some activity and being in the fresh air may even help the affected person to sleep better at night.

> *Sometimes, she takes a bit of cajoling but when we do get out she usually loves it and doesn't want to come back in once we get home.*

One of the issues can be that the person does not know what to expect, giving them lots of different clues can help. For example, a trip to the shops could be achieved by giving the person a shopping bag and his/her purse or wallet and perhaps a list of things to buy. It does not matter if he or she can no longer read the list, it is simply a visible and tangible clue about the activity that is going to happen.

> *He loved going to the local football matches but had become very resistant to it and would say no, stay here when we talked about it. We got round it by having the sports programme on TV in the morning, listening to the radio in the car, making sure he was wearing his team shirt and scarf and giving him an old match programme to carry. That seemed to help him tune in to where we were going. Once we were in the ground, he responded really well to the noise and joined in the chants and football songs.*

MIXING UP DAY AND NIGHT

Night time waking is very common for people with dementia and can be the first cause of difficulty in maintaining a placement if the cost of waking night staff cannot be met. Trying to establish a good bedtime preparation routine can be beneficial.

> *We used to make sure that he was dressed in his clothes during the day and distracted him from putting his pyjamas in until a reasonable time in the evening. Nearer to bedtime, we would encourage him to have a bath, help him make a hot chocolate and turn the telly volume down. He liked to sing along to nursery rhymes so we bought him a CD and we would have that playing when he got into bed. It didn't work every night but more often than not it did.*

LIVING IN SUPPORTED ACCOMMODATION

Many people with Down syndrome live in supported accommodation and may have been in their home for many years before the dementia onset. Often, there is a willingness to continue to support an individual and adaptations are made to assist this. Training staff teams to understand how dementia affects a person is paramount. This will reduce any fear and anxiety they may have. It will also give an opportunity to share ideas and highlight any issues currently being faced so that strategies can be agreed.

Sadly, as the individual's support needs become more intense there can be problems with securing additional support packages such as the need for waking night staff.

There are some intellectual disability organizations that recognize the continuing and increasing needs of their tenants with Down syndrome and dementia and are now setting up dementia-friendly services. This is to be commended.

Unfortunately, it is still very common for people to have to move from their home into a Nursing Care Home or Elderly Mentally Ill setting as the dementia progresses. This move is often very difficult for relatives and intellectual disability staff teams to accept and cope with, causing a great deal of stress and anxiety.

As time has gone on, they have made adaptations and increased staffing levels but the nature of the building is just not conducive to catering for her longerterm needs. The increased care package is more expensive and we have been asked to look at alternative placements.

My sister is in hospital as her seizures have increased and I need to find a new care home, I don't know where to start looking.

We have a brother who is 53 and who has lived very happily in an 'assisted living' home with three other men with intellectual disabilities. Unfortunately his condition has deteriorated quite severely in the last month and we have been advised that the home feels that his needs are now beyond those which they can accommodate.

A lady who has lived here for 26 years has just been moved because of her increased care package. There was nothing we could do. We have four other people with Down syndrome living here, they are very concerned.

Even with the best will in the world, finances often play the decisive role in deciding where someone with Down syndrome will be placed in the later stages of dementia. It is important that relatives are part of this process and are involved in locating the most suitable place available.

As of today social services have informed us that a place has been reserved at a residential Care home with an EMI unit and we have no option but to go with this since they say that his assisted living residence can no longer cater for his needs. There does not seem to be any targeted provision for such people in his area. As for everyone in this situation, it is a particularly difficult time, but my sister and I did go and visit this place today, and it did seem to have a good caring feel.

For those who do remain in place, relatives and staff teams report some satisfaction in being able to look after the person until the end of their life. Recognizing that support from other intellectual disability and palliative care professionals is an intrinsic part of ensuring that the individual remains comfortable in the late stages of dementia and can reassure carers that they are doing the best for their loved one or person they are looking after.

> *It was very hard, quite exhausting to be honest but we wouldn't have had it any other way. She seemed to know us right until the very end and we just knew that she felt safe and comfortable in familiar surroundings. It was very peaceful at the end and we've all agreed that we will do the same if it happens to anyone else.*

LIFE EXPECTANCY IN DOWN SYNDROME

Several studies have shown substantially longer survival for people with Down syndrome in recent decades (Zhu et al. 2013). Presson et al. (2013) comment that median life expectancy increased from 25 to 50 years in the US population between 1983 and 2000 and from 24 to 52 years in European studies. This is due primarily to a dramatic decline in infant and child mortality, especially in children with congenital heart disease (CHD). As we will see in Chapter 8, early identification and intervention in CHD significantly improves outlook.

The life expectancy of older people with Down syndrome has improved over a similar period but far less markedly. Zhu et al. (2013) report a mortality of 5–11 times that of the general population, similar to other studies. There is better survival for people with mosaicism than for people with standard trisomy 21 or translocation Down syndrome. Day et al. (2005) reported that leukaemia (standardized mortality ration [SMR] = 17), respiratory

Table 4.1
Age distribution prevalence of people in 2011
with Down syndrome in England and Wales

Age in years	Number of people with Down syndrome (%)
0–9	6145 (16.57)
10–19	5480 (14.77)
20–29	5803 (13.70)
30–39	5829 (15.71)
40–49	7862 (21.20)
50–59	4475 (12.07)
60–69	1403 (3.80)
70+	93 (0.25)
Total	37090

illnesses (SMR = 27), congenital anomalies (SMR = 72) and circulatory diseases (SMR = 5.3) accounted for most of the excess mortality not attributable to CHD. With the exception of leukaemia, cancer mortality was not different from that of the general population. Despite the improvements in medical care conferring significant benefit to younger people, brain degeneration continues to limit longevity. Alzheimer disease brain degeneration leads to a gradual decline in intellectual and physical function and the great majority of people with Down syndrome do not survive beyond age 70.

This is shown in Table 4.1 that displays data adapted from Wu and Morris (2013). The sharp fall in the population prevalence of people with Down syndrome after the age of 60 can readily be seen. So, the picture is changing and improving with survival into the late 50s and 60s to be expected for most, but the life-limiting influence of Alzheimer disease is yet to be overcome.

Note
1. NFER: Young people with special educational needs/learning difficulties and disabilities: Research into planning for adult life and services, Kerry Martin, Ruth Hart, Richard White and Caroline Sharp Research Report, September 2011, http://www.nfer.ac.uk/publications/SENT01

REFERENCES

New parents
Charleton PM, Dennis J, Marder E (2010) Medical management of children with Down syndrome. *Paediatr Child Health* 20: 331–337.
Charleton PM, Dennis J, Marder E (2014) Medical management of children with Down syndrome. *Paediatr Child Health* 24: 362–369. http://dx.doi.org/10.1016/j.paed.2013.12.004.

Developmental progress preschool and school years—some references for further reading
Abbeduto L, Warren SF, Conners FA (2007) Language development in Down syndrome from the pre-lin-guistic period to the acquisition of literacy. *Ment Retard Dev Disabil Res Rev* 13: 247–261. doi: 10.1002/mrdd.20158.
Buckley S, Bird G, Sacks B, Archer T (2002) A comparison of mainstream and special education for teenag-ers with Down syndrome: Implications for parents and teachers. www.dseinternational.org.
Fidler DJ (2005) The emerging Down syndrome behavioural phenotype in early childhood: Implications for practice. *Infants Young Child* 18: 86–103.
Fidler DJ, Philofsky A, Hepburn S (2007) Language phenotypes and intervention planning: Bridging research and practice. *Ment Retard Dev Disabil Res* 13: 47–57. doi: 10.1002/mrdd.20132.
Fox S, Farrell P, Davis P (2004) Factors associated with the effective inclusion of primary-aged pupils with Down syndrome. *Br J Spec Educ* 31: 184–190. doi: 10.1111/j.0952-3383.2004.00353.x.
Laws, G, Hall, A (2014) Early hearing loss and language abilities in children with Down syndrome. *Int J Lang and Commun Disord,* Early View. DOI: 10.1111/1460-6984.12077.
Roberts JE, Chapman R, Warren SF (2008) *Speech and Language Development and Interventions in Down Syndrome and Fragile X Syndrome.* Baltimore, MD: Paul H. Brookes Publishing.
Roberts JE, Price J, Malking CI (2007) Language and communication development in Down syndrome. *Ment Retard Dev Disabil Res* 13: 26–35. doi: 10.1002/mrdd.20136.
Turner S, Alborz A, Gayle V (2008) Predictors of academic attainments of young people with Down syn-drome. *J Intellect Disabil Res* 52: 380–392. doi: 10.1111/j.1365-Turner2788.2007.01038.x.

Some sexual health issues
https://www.gov.uk/government/publications/human-papillomavirus-hpv-the-green-book-chapter-18a.
Burke LM, Kalpakjian CZ, Smith YR, Quint EH (2010) Gynecologic issues of adolescents with Down syndrome, autism, and cerebral palsy. *J Pediatr Adolesc Gynecol* 23: 11–15. doi: 10.1016/j.jpag.2009.04.005. Epub 29 July 2009.

Elkins T (1995) Medical issues related to sexuality and reproduction. In: Van Dyke DC, Mattheis P, Eberly
S, Williams J, editors. *Medical and Surgical Care for Children with Down Syndrome: A Guide for
Parents*. Bethesda, MD: Woodbine House, 253–266.

Pradhan M, Dalal A, Khan F, Agrawal S (2006) Fertility in men with Down syndrome: A case report. *Fertil
Steril* 86: 1785.

Ranganath P, Rajangam S (2004) Menstrual history in women with Down syndrome – A review. *Indian J
Hum Genet* 10: 18–21.

Adult life with Down syndrome

Carr J (2008) The everyday life of adults with Down syndrome. *J Appl Res Intellect Disabil* 21: 389–397.

Schupf N, Pang D, Patel BN et al. (2003) Reduction of oestrogen levels after menopause contributes to the
pathological processes leading to Alzheimer's disease. *Ann Neurol* 54: 433–438.

Seltzer GB, Schupf N, Wu HS (2001) A prospective study of menopause in women with Downs syndrome.
J Intellect Disabil Res 45: 1–7.

Life expectancy

Day SM, Strauss DJ, Shavelle RM, Reynolds RJ (2005) Mortality and causes of death in persons with Down
syndrome in California. *Dev Med Child Neurol* 47: 171–176.

Wu J, Morris JK (2013) The population prevalence of Down's syndrome in England and Wales in 2011. *Eur
J Hum Genet* 21: 1033–1034. doi: 10.1038/ejhg.2013.104.

Zhu JL, Hasle H, Correa A et al. (2013) Survival among people with Down syndrome: A nationwide population-based study in Denmark. *Genet Med* 15: 64–69. doi: 10.1038/gim.2012.93.

RESOURCES

New parents

Down's Heart Group: http://www.dhg.org.uk/.
UK Down's Syndrome Association Helpline: http://www.downs-syndrome.org.uk/information.html.

Developmental progress preschool and school years

Many parents and practitioners use Early Support information and development resources to help them
understand children's development, share successes and inform next steps in development.

Early Support information resources help practitioners to answer the questions parents are most likely
to ask either at the time of diagnosis, soon after or as the child grows and matures. http://www.ncb.org.uk/
early-support/resources/information-resources.

Early Support developmental journals are designed to help families and practitioners improve their
encouragement of development with easy to use tools to help with observing, recording and celebrating
progress, and to identify areas where extra help and support may be needed. The main body of each journal
consists of milestones that parents and practitioners can easily observe in the course of everyday life. The
journals provide information on development and allow families to build a record of achievement for their
child. http://www.ncb.org.uk/early-support/resources/developmental-journals.

The developmental journal for babies and children with Down syndrome has eleven steps, each of which
describe typical patterns of development in five main areas: communication, social-emotional, cognition and
play, motor and sensory and self-help. http://www.ncb.org.uk/early-support/resources/developmental-journals/
developmental-journal-for-babies-and-children-with-down-syndrome.

The developmental journal for children and young people with multiple needs can help families and
practitioners support the development of children who have Down syndrome and additional needs. http://
www.ncb.org.uk/early-support/resources/developmental-journals/developmental-journal-for-children-
and-young-people-with-multiple-needs.

There are also developmental journals for deaf infants and infants and children who have visual
impairment.

Adolescence and transition

Terri Couwenhoven (2007) *Teaching children with Down's syndrome about their bodies, boundaries and
sexuality: A guide for parents and professionals. Topics in Down's syndrome* (Bethesda MD, Woodbine

House). A useful, thorough guide to helping children and young people with Down syndrome understand about puberty, sexuality, relationships and every other aspect of growing up. Has a useful section on self-talk.

Dennis McGuire, Brian Chicoine (2006) *Mental wellness in adults with Down syndrome* (Bethesda MD, Woodbine House). An easy-to-read guide on what the common behavioural characteristics of Down's syndrome are, how some could be mistaken for mental illness and what actual mental health problems occur more commonly in people with Down's syndrome.

Brian Chicoine MD (2010) *Guide to good health: For teens & adults with Down syndrome* (Woodbine House 2010). An excellent guide to health, healthy living and nutrition for parents and carers of young people and adults with Down's syndrome.

Asking for a Community Care Assessment, Preparing for a Community Care Assessment and Getting the Care Plan Right. DSA Community Care Assessment Guides: http://www.downs-syndrome.org.uk/.

Some sexual health issues
Sexual health (a guide for parents and carers) available to download from DSA website. http://www.downs-syndrome.org.uk/download-package/14-sexual-health/

Adult life with Down syndrome
DSA Annual Health Check Information for GPs
http://www.downs-syndrome.org.uk/for-professionals/health-information-for-medical-professionals/annual-health-check-information-for-gps/

DSA Health Book for People with Down Syndrome
http://www.downs-syndrome.org.uk/for-families-and-carers/health-and-well-being/annual-health-checks/

Royal College of General Practitioners (2010) A Step by Step Guide for GP Practices: Annual Health Checks for People with a Learning Disability, http://www.rcgp.org.uk/learningdisabilities/

5
HEARING ISSUES

Emma McNeill, Patrick Sheehan and Liz Marder

Introduction

The majority of individuals with Down syndrome will experience impaired hearing at some point in their life. Hearing losses may be conductive, sensorineural or mixed in nature. They can be temporary or permanent. Hearing is very important for development, and particularly language development. Young people with an intellectual disability are less able than others to recognize hearing difficulties and take measures to minimize the impact. Health care professionals need to have a heightened awareness of this possibility, identify impairment early and provide appropriate treatment to maximize the educational and social development of children and independence and quality of life for adults.

How common are hearing problems in people with Down syndrome?

The type of hearing loss likely to occur in Down syndrome changes through life. Conductive loss is by far the most common in childhood, with sensorineural deafness being the most common type of hearing loss in adults. The incidence of sensorineural hearing loss discovered on newborn screening is approximately 6% (Barr et al. 2007, Park et al. 2012). This increases to around 20% in adolescence and early adult life. Sensorineural loss may be unilateral (around 60% of losses) or bilateral (Davies 1998, Park et al. 2012). Presbyacusis or age-related hearing loss occurs more commonly in Down syndrome than in the general population, and at a younger age, occurring approximately 20–30 years earlier. This may be a manifestation of the precocious ageing that occurs in Down syndrome. Evenhuis et al. (1992) found that 57% of those aged 35–62 years old with Down syndrome had a bilateral hearing loss greater than 40dB. In 68% of those, the hearing loss was sensorineural. Prior to their study, hearing loss had been diagnosed in only around 25% of those considered to have a disabling loss.

Otitis media with effusion (OME), which is commonly termed 'glue ear', has been shown to affect as many as 35% of children with Down syndrome at birth, 93% at the age of 1 year, while reducing to 68% by the age of 5 years (Barr et al. 2007, Austeng et al. 2013).

Why are people with Down syndrome at a higher risk of developing a hearing impairment?

There are a number of anatomical and physiological reasons why those with Down syndrome are at a higher risk of developing a hearing impairment. Stenosis and the exaggerated curvature of the external auditory canal predispose to wax impaction, which can make examination difficult, as well as potentially reducing hearing. OME has been shown to affect as many as 93% of children with Down syndrome at the age of 1 year, reducing to 68% by the age of 5 (Barr et al. 2011). The cause is multifactorial. Mid-face hypoplasia with an associated reduction in postnasal space volume, adenoid hypertrophy, reduced muscle tone and Eustachian tube dysfunction are all contributing factors. Reduced immune response to bacterial colonization can contribute to repeated ear infections (Loh et al. 1990). Significant laryngopharyngeal reflux has also been shown to predispose to OME in children, which may be exaggerated in Down syndrome secondary to hypotonia (Miura 2012). The relative shortening and patulous nature of the Eustachian tube, in combination with mucus pooling and stagnation, also predispose to infection. As the child grows, Eustachian tube function improves but the incidence of OME is still higher than in other adults. A sensorineural component to a hearing loss may be a feature from birth and progress with age.

How can a hearing loss be detected?

Where there is a good hearing screening programme in place, hearing loss is likely to be identified early, rather than presenting later with signs and symptoms. The Newborn Hearing Screening Programme in the UK is very effective and as a result a number of children will come to the attention of audiology services in infancy. Guidelines (DSMIG 2007) suggest a full audiological assessment at 6–10 months of age to establish by 10 months of age whether there is a hearing loss, with annual surveillance until school age and at least two yearly thereafter. So, a hearing loss that is not presenting with obvious behavioural clues can be detected.

For others, hearing loss will be suspected by parents or carers, or in older children and adults may be noticed by the affected individual themselves. Even when it is not suspected, a careful history should focus on questions that may indicate a hearing loss. Delayed speech and language development may be a manifestation of hearing impairment, although it can often be multifactorial and may be a reflection of the associated intellectual disability. The progression of listening and concentration skills should be assessed, and general development can be established from discussion with parents/carers. Hearing loss should be considered if a child develops problems with behaviour and socializing, often manifesting as frustration and reduced communication. Enquiries should also be made about previous ear surgery, hearing aid use and recurrent ear infections. There is a higher incidence of obstructive sleep apnoea, chronic rhinosinusitis and adenoid hypertrophy in children with Down syndrome, and related symptoms may become apparent during the consultation.

In adults, those with hearing problems may present with decreased responsiveness, social withdrawal, loss of independence, low mood and change in behaviour or apparent loss of cognitive ability. A misdiagnosis of depression or dementia can be made. Assessment of hearing is therefore an essential part of assessment for these conditions.

How is hearing loss assessed?

EXAMINATION

Good rapport with the child or adult and their parents or carers during the examination is essential. Consideration of extended and appropriately timed appointments, for example, first or last appointment slots, will be appreciated by carers. Observation of behaviour and social interactions is a useful tool in assessing hearing and general development.

If the tympanic membrane is difficult to visualize due to wax or discharge, or the child has difficulty cooperating, examination under general anaesthetic may be required. Previous ear surgery may be evident by the presence of an endaural or postauricular scar. Examination of the tympanic membranes may reveal middle ear effusions and evidence of chronic Eustachian tube dysfunction (such as retraction of the tympanic membrane or a cholesteatoma). Ears with discharge should be fully examined as this may be due to otitis externa or otitis media, which can be managed conservatively, or conditions requiring surgical intervention, for example, chronic perforation of the tympanic membrane, or cholesteatoma. The nasal airway should be assessed for patency and the presence of discharge. Examination of the oral cavity may reveal crowding due to tonsillar hypertrophy, or a relatively large tongue, which may predispose to obstructive sleep apnoea.

INVESTIGATIONS

Audiological assessment should be carried out by clinicians with experience in evaluating the hearing of those with special needs. The hearing assessment tools used should be appropriate to the child's developmental stage, rather than chronological age. Pure tone audiometry (either visual response audiometry, where the child's response to detecting various frequencies of sound is reinforced by the use of visual stimuli, or play audiometry, where the response to detecting sound is reinforced by the use of games) can be used in children who are able to comprehend and follow instructions, but there should be a low threshold for using objective audiometry (e.g. brainstem evoked response audiometry) if the hearing level cannot be established reliably. Tympanometry should be carried out in all children at each assessment to assess for middle ear effusion (Lewis et al. 2011). Radiological investigations are not commonly used, but may be required for specific indications, for example, MRI if cochlear implantation is being considered.

How should hearing loss be managed in people with Down syndrome?

A multidisciplinary team approach should be used in the management of children with hearing loss and Down syndrome, and may involve an otolaryngologist, paediatric audiologist and paediatrician, with strong associations with speech and language therapists and teachers for the deaf. Correspondence should be shared with all members of the team and parents.

Communication with the whole team is as important in adults where carers and health professionals are frequently unaware of the hearing loss in those they care for. It is also important to ensure that the individual is fully involved in the discussion and decision making about his or her treatment, with appropriate modification taking into account cognitive and communication difficulties.

REGULAR DEWAXING

Some children and adults may need regular dewaxing of the external auditory canals to prevent hearing loss and reduce interference from their hearing aids. The facility for regular ear care should be made as accessible as possible. Some will require a general anaesthetic for the procedure. Consideration should be given to coordinating with other specialties to include other evaluations and procedures, for example, venepuncture for thyroid function tests, dental examination or procedures.

MANAGEMENT OF OTITIS MEDIA WITH EFFUSION

OME (glue ear) can be managed conservatively with hearing aids or with the insertion of ventilation tubes. If a child is coping well with a mild conductive hearing loss due to a middle ear effusion, then a watch-and-wait policy is perfectly acceptable. Many other treatments have been proposed including antibiotics, intranasal steroids, antihistamines or decongestants, autoinsufflation, cranial osteopathy and homeopathy. There is little or no evidence to support any of these. There is evidence that a milk-free diet may reduce the amount of mucus production, with a consequent reduction in OME (Failla et al. 1998). Diagnosis and treatment of reflux, where present, may help. The mainstay of treatment, however, is either hearing aids or insertion of ventilation tubes (grommets).

Hearing aids are the recommended first-line treatment for hearing loss associated with OME in children with Down syndrome in the current NICE guidelines (NICE 2008). However, the use of hearing aids can be difficult because of behavioural issues and difficulty fitting hearing aids in the presence of narrow ear canals. Fitting and keeping on hearing aids alongside glasses is an additional challenge for many. The support of an experienced teacher of the deaf can be invaluable in encouraging acceptance and use of hearing aids.

The use of the BAHA Softband (Cochlear Ltd., Australia) has reduced some of the difficulties associated with behind-the-ear hearing aid use. The BAHA Softband is designed to fit comfortably around the head with a sound processor attached to a connector on a metal spring. It has particular benefits if standard hearing aids have not been tolerated in the presence of persistent ear discharge or in those where grommet insertion is not possible or no longer appropriate (Sheehan and Hans 2006). The BAHA Softband is an alternative to a traditional bone-anchored aid in those where it is felt surgery should be avoided or in young children where the skull bone is not yet thick enough to hold the fixture for a sound processor. A significant improvement in quality of life has been demonstrated in children using the osseointegrated BAHA with no excess of complications (McDermott et al. 2008).

Grommet (ventilation tube) insertion into the tympanic membrane has an important role in the management of OME, the advantages being the improvement in hearing without the need for external amplification and the reduction in acute otitis media. Grommet insertion needs to be carried out under a general anaesthetic, often at the same time as objective audiometry or adenotonsillar surgery. As children with Down syndrome often have narrow ear canals, smaller grommets may need to be used, with the associated disadvantage of earlier extrusion. Children can be managed very successfully with grommets, with studies suggesting that early and aggressive treatment of OME from birth, including the use of grommets, can significantly improve hearing levels (Pappas et al. 1994, Shott et al. 2001). Grommets usually extrude spontaneously within 6–8 months of insertion, and about one in five children with Down syndrome will go on to develop further episodes of OME. Children should therefore be followed up regularly and their parents made aware of the possible need for further grommet insertion, with some studies showing the need for two or more ventila-tion tube insertions. A higher risk of complications, including infection and permanent perforation of the tympanic membrane, has been reported (Paulson et al. 2014). The pres-ence of ear discharge in a child with grommets should always be reviewed and infections treated with topical antibiotic ear drops. Keeping the ears dry when swimming and bathing may be helpful in those who have problems with repeated ear infections.

Adenoidectomy should be considered in the management of recurrent OME, recurrent acute otitis media and also as part of the management of chronic nasal obstruction and obstructive sleep apnoea. The aim of adenoidectomy is to improve Eustachian tube function and to reduce the presence of bacteria within biofilms in the adenoidal pad, with an associ-ated reduction in acute middle ear infections.

Each child's case should be considered on its own merits with regard to the use of hearing aids or grommets. Watchful waiting or active observation before determining definite need for intervention is now accepted to be good practice. In some cases a period of using a hearing aid before having grommets is helpful, and others elect for hearing aids following grommet surgery.

MANAGEMENT OF SENSORINEURAL HEARING LOSS

Sensorineural hearing loss may be present at birth or develop later. This is typically a high frequency loss, which can present during school years, becoming increasingly common in adult life. The use of hearing aids should be actively encouraged. Cochlear implantation has proved to be successful in the management of severe to profound sensorineural hearing loss in children with Down syndrome, without excessive complications, even in the pres-ence of middle ear disease (Hans et al. 2010). This suggests that referral for cochlear implantation should be considered in children with severe hearing loss, based on the same audiological criteria as for a child with typical development.

For adults, consideration of hearing loss either as a cause or an exacerbating factor is an important part of any assessment of mental health or cognitive decline. Treatment of identified hearing impairment with encouragement to use hearing aids, where appropriate, is likely to have a significant impact on functioning even where the hearing loss is only part of a wider picture.

Kathy had been living semi-independently in a small group home since she was 25 years old. She was a lively member of the group who enjoyed shopping and helping prepare meals. She had a part-time job in a noisy local café. When she was 35, she started to struggle at work, making mistakes with orders and became so anxious about this that she had to leave. She stopped doing the shopping and spent increasing amounts of time alone in her room. Her parents started to worry that she was depressed and her carers arranged a mental health assessment. During the course of this assessment, she had a hearing test which showed her to have moder-ate to severe bilateral hearing loss. A behind-the-ear hearing aid was prescribed, and the care staff encouraged her to use this. Within weeks, Kathy was back to her usual lively self and able to return to work at the café.

ADDITIONAL TOOLS FOR MANAGING HEARING LOSS

Sign language such as Makaton has become increasingly established as a means of aiding communication, and its use should be encouraged. Children with Down syndrome are strong visual learners and the use of visual learning aids assists in language processing. Surround sound amplification systems can also help in the classroom environment. Specialized speech and language therapists and teachers of the deaf have an important role in the development of communication and learning skills and should be involved in the multidisciplinary management.

How often should people with Down syndrome have their hearing reviewed?

Guidelines for management of children and adults with Down syndrome recommend hearing surveillance (see Appendix 1). Current UK Guidelines (DSMIG 2007) are that hearing evaluation should be carried out at birth, at 6–10 months and then at least yearly until school age. Audiometry every 2 years is recommended beyond school age and throughout adult life. Regular otolaryngology review may also be required for the management of wax impaction, ear infections, associated ear problems, for example, cholesteatoma and other ENT problems including adenotonsillar hypertrophy, obstructive sleep apnoea and rhinosinusitis.

Parental perspective

Useful advice for parents on hearing assessment and management of hearing loss can be found in the leaflet Down's Syndrome and Childhood Deafness (NDCS 2011). This includes practical information with tips on managing grommets, getting children to wear hearing aids and communication with a child with hearing loss.

Key points

- Hearing loss is extremely common in Down syndrome.
- Poor hearing can have a major impact on development of language, and behaviour and social functioning.
- It is essential that all people with Down syndrome have regular screening for hearing loss.
- Conductive hearing loss, due to OME, is most frequently encountered in children but may persist into adulthood.
- Age-related hearing loss is more common in those with Down syndrome and occurs more frequently and at a younger age than in the general population.
- Grommets play a part in management of OME in Down syndrome, but benefit may be short-lived.
- Hearing aids can be very effectively used by children and adults with Down syndrome.

REFERENCES

Austeng ME, Akre H, Overland B, Abdelnoor M, Falkenberg E-S, Kvaerner KJ (2013) Otitis media with effusion in children with Down syndrome. *Int J Pediatr Otorhinolaryngol* 77: 1329–1332. doi: 1016/j. ijporl.2013.05.027.

Barr E, Dungworth J, Hunter K, McFarlane M, Kubba H (2007) The prevalence of ear, nose and throat disorders in preschool children with Down' syndrome Glasgow. *Scott Med J* 56: 98–103. doi: 10.1258/ smj.2011.011036.

Davies B (1998) Auditory disorders in Down's syndrome. *Scand Audiol Suppl* 30: 65–68.

DSMIG (2007) Guidelines on hearing. Basic medical surveillance essentials for people with Down's syndrome – Hearing impairment. http://www.downs-syndrome.org.uk/for-families-and-carers/health-and-well-being (accessed 2 January 2015)

Evenhuis HM, van Zanten GA, Brocnar MP, Roerdinkholder WHM (1992) Hearing loss in middle-age persons with Down syndrome. *Am J Ment Retard* 97: 47–56.

Failla P, Barone C, Pettinato R, Romano C (1998) IgG antibodies to beta-lactoglobulin and cow's milk protein intolerance in Down syndrome. *Down Synd Res Pract* 5: 120–122. doi: 10.3104/reports.86.

Hans PS, England R, Prowse S, Young E, Sheehan PZ (2010) UK and Ireland experience of cochlear implants in children with Down syndrome. *Int J Pediatr Otorhinolaryngol* 74: 260–264. doi: 10.1016/j.ijporl.2009.11.018.

Lewis MP, Bradford Bell E, Evans AK. (2011) A comparison of tympanometry with 226 Hz and 1000 Hz probe tones in children with Down syndrome. *Int J Pediatr Otorhinolaryngol* 75: 1492–1495. doi: 10.1016/j.ijporl.2011.06.008.

Loh RK, Harth SC, Thong YH, Ferrante A (1990) Immunoglobulin G subclass deficiency and predisposition to infection in Down's syndrome. *Pediatr Infect Dis J* 9: 547–551.

McDermott AL, Williams J, Kuo MJ, Reid AP, Proops DW (2008) The role of bone anchored hearing aids in children with Down syndrome. *Int J Pediatr Otorhinolaryngol* 72: 751–757. doi: 10.1016/j.ijporl.2008.01.035.

Miura MS, Mascaro M, Rosenfeld RM (2012) Association between otitis media and gastroesophageal reflux: A systematic review. *Otolaryngol Head Neck Surg* 146: 345–352. doi: 10.1177/0194599811430809.

NDCS (2011) National Deaf Children's Society, with DSA, UK and DSMIG, UK. http://www.downs-syndrome.org.uk/for-families-and-carers/health-and-well-being (accessed 2 January 2015)

NICE (2008) National Institute for Health and Clinical Excellence Clinical guideline 60: Surgical Management of Otitis Media with effusion in Children. February 2008. http://publications.nice.org.uk/surgical-management-of-otitis-media-with-effusion-in-children-cg60 (accessed 1 January 2015).

Pappas DG, Flexer C, Shackelford L (1994) Otological and habilitative management of children with Down syndrome. *Laryngoscope* 104: 1065–1070.

Park AH, Wilson MA, Stevens PT, Harward R, Hohler N (2012) Identification of hearing loss in pediatric patients with Down syndrome. *Otolaryngol Head Neck Surg* 146: 135–140. doi: 10.1177/0194599811425156.

Paulson LM, Weaver TS, Macarthur CJ (2014) Outcomes of tympanostomy tube placement in children with Down syndrome – A retrospective review. *Int J Pediatr Otorhinolaryngol* 78: 223–226. doi: 10.1016/j.ijporl.2013.10.062.

Sheehan PZ, Hans PS (2006) UK and Ireland experience of bone anchored hearing aids (BAHA) in individuals with Down syndrome. *Int J Pediatr Otorhinolaryngol* 70: 981–986.

Shott SR, Joseph A, Heithaus D (2001) Hearing loss in children with Down syndrome. *Int J Pediatr Otorhinolaryngol* 61: 199–205.

6
VISION AND EYE DISORDERS

Pat Charleton and Maggie Woodhouse

Introduction

Ocular abnormalities are found in up to 60% of people with Down syndrome, presenting as a wide variety of eye conditions that have an impact on visual functioning. As children and young people with Down syndrome are visual learners, screening for visual impairment is essential to prevent a secondary disadvantage and maximize independent living and learning. Accurate visual assessments can be a challenge because of underlying learning and behavioural difficulties.

How do eyes in individuals with Down syndrome differ from eyes in the general population?

In general, the eyes in Down syndrome are different in only minor ways. The palpebral apertures usually slant upwards, and the upper eyelids often show a marked nasal epicanthic fold. This is of no visual consequence but can give rise to 'pseudostrabismus', giving a false appearance of a convergent squint. However, since children with Down syndrome are at a high risk of squint (strabismus), all children should have an assessment of their vision. The cornea is a different shape, being steeper and thinner and subject to greater aberrations than the typical cornea (which may in part explain the poorer visual acuity in people with Down syndrome) (Haugen et al. 2001, McCullough et al. 2013).

Pale coloured spots at the junction of the middle and outer thirds of the iris (Brushfield's spots) occur commonly, though they are more noticeable in blue than brown eyes. They have no functional significance or impact on vision. Typically, the retina has more blood vessels leaving the optic disc and vessels radiate out in many more directions than in the typical retina (in which vessels are largely confined to inferior and superior bundles). Peripapillary atrophy or retinal thinning around the optic nerve head is quite common and can give the retina a myopic appearance even when the refraction is not myopic (see Fig. 6.1). The optic disc can appear raised or smaller than normal. However, any unexpected disc appearance should be investigated. It is not known whether these changes have any functional consequences.

How do eye conditions commonly present?

NASOLACRIMAL DUCT OBSTRUCTION

Nasolacrimal duct obstruction presents clinically in 10–36% of infants with Down syndrome compared with 2–4% of typical infants. It usually presents as watery eyes or

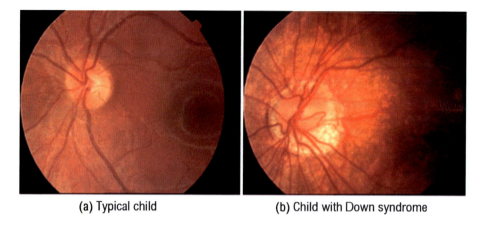

(a) Typical child   (b) Child with Down syndrome

Fig. 6.1. Retinal appearance of a typical child (a) and a child with Down syndrome (b) matched for refractive error (low hypermetrope) and axial length.

recurrent sticky eyes. In the general population, spontaneous resolution usually occurs by 1 year of age; in children with Down syndrome, it can take a bit longer but in the majority canalization occurs by 3 years.

Frequent daily massaging over the lacrimal sac to clear any build-up of mucus is advisable to prevent infections and aid resolution. Stubborn cases require surgery: a syringing and probing procedure is usually successful, but some may require a dacryocystorhinostomy. Acute conjunctival infections can occur and are treated with short courses of topical antibiotics.

BLEPHARITIS

Blepharitis has been reported in up to 30% of children and elderly adults with Down syndrome and around 10% of young adults. Blepharitis is the inflammation of the eyelids; it is usually a recurring condition. The increased incidence of blepharitis in Down syndrome is probably due to the presence of an increased tendency to dry skin resulting in seborrhoeic blepharitis, whilst an underlying immune dysfunction and susceptibility to infection results in staphylococcal blepharitis and meibomian gland dysfunction. Eyelids can feel itchy and inflamed if untreated, which can lead to distortion of the follicles and abnormal lash growth towards the cornea (trichiasis).

Blepharitis responds well, in most cases, to practising regular 'lid hygiene' measures. Only the most stubborn cases need a referral to an ophthalmology service.

CONGENITAL CATARACT

The prevalence of congenital cataract in Down syndrome is 1.4% (Haargaard and Fledelius 2006), whereas in the general population it is estimated at 0.03% (Rahi and Dezateux 2000). As infants with Down syndrome have a higher incidence of cataracts, it is recommended that they are examined for cataract as newborns and again aged 6 weeks by a trained person. Rahi and Dezateux (1999) reported that less than half of all congenital cataracts were detected by 6 weeks.

Management is the same as for typical infants, with early surgical extraction in sight-threatening cases, followed by contact lens and/or spectacle correction or intra-ocular implants. The visual outcome of cataract surgery can be good, with age at surgery as the most important predictor of outcome. In some infants with Down syndrome, early surgery may be complicated by heart and/or respiratory problems.

DEVELOPMENTAL CATARACT

Cataract developing in childhood or adulthood is more common in Down syndrome, but prevalence reports are complicated by the age of the research participants and by the disparate definition of 'cataract'. Many lens opacities in childhood are sparse and peripheral (e.g. blue-dot cataracts) and do not affect vision but visually significant cataract development is possible even in this age group. All professionals should be alert to the possibility of vision loss as a result of developmental cataract.

A recent study from the USA of 455 adults with Down syndrome reported an increase in cataract prevalence with advancing age. The risk increases rapidly from 40 years of age, and individuals with Down syndrome are significantly younger than those in the general population at diagnosis (e.g. over 40% of people with Down syndrome in their 50s compared with 6.8% in the general population; other values for Down syndrome are 13% in their 30s and almost 80% in those living into their 70s) (Krinsky-McHale et al. 2012). This is consistent with accelerated biological ageing in Down syndrome (see Chapters 2 and 18).

At diagnosis, many people do not need treatment and cataracts should be monitored over time. However, if as cataracts develop they cause significant visual impairment that will have a negative effect on aspects of cognitive functioning, adaptive behaviour and ability to perform activities of daily living (Krinsky-McHale et al. 2012). The possibility of impaired vision should always be investigated if there is a decline in functional ability in adults with Down syndrome. Vision assessment is recommended at least every 2 years throughout adult life and more frequently if cataracts are detected.

Treatment options typically depend upon the degree of visual loss caused by the cataract and include management of the environment to minimize visual problems and ultimately surgery with intraocular lens implantation. There are no studies comparing the treatment of cataracts in the general population with that in Down syndrome, but the same options apply.

NYSTAGMUS

Nystagmus is defined as the involuntary oscillatory movement of the eyes; it can occur in association with congenital visually impairing conditions (e.g. cataract) or in isolation. In Down syndrome, the prevalence is over 10% and in almost all cases is not associated with another eye condition, except for strabismus, which is a common association (Wagner et al. 2000). Nystagmus is usually noticeable within the first few weeks or months of life.

Most children with nystagmus have a 'null point', an eye or head position in which the nystagmus is lessened, so the condition can be associated with a head tilt or head turn, which is the child's own automatic and unconscious strategy to stabilize the eyes and improve vision. Nystagmus often improves (in terms of the extent of the eye movement) over time, although it rarely disappears altogether. Nystagmus itself causes visual impairment, which will be life-long.

It is important that nystagmus in a child or adult with Down syndrome is recognized as a separate visually impairing condition and not considered as part of the syndrome; referral to the local Visual Impairment Education Service is recommended for children, and the local association of the visually impaired can help adults.

There is currently no treatment for nystagmus in children, although surgery to move the null point has been reported as being beneficial in rare cases of extreme head posture. There are many strategies and support services, particularly within education, that can help a child cope with poor vision.

GLAUCOMA

Congenital glaucoma is slightly more prevalent in infants with Down syndrome than in typical infants, but it is very rare. Age-related glaucoma has been reported to occur with an increased prevalence in adults with Down syndrome, possibly related to the increased production of β-amyloid (Yokoyama et al. 2006).

How do refractive errors differ in Down syndrome?

Refractive errors (sufficient to require spectacle correction) are about 10 times more common in children with Down syndrome than among children with typical development; about 60% of children with Down syndrome will need spectacles by the time they start school (Woodhouse et al. 1997). The reason appears to be a failure in emmetropization, a process which eliminates refractive error. In typical newborn infants, the distribution of refraction is wide, with many neonates being hypermetropic and some being myopic. Over the first 2 years of life, the distribution markedly narrows with the majority of children clustering around low hypermetropia or emmetropia (zero error). The mechanism by which the eyes outgrow infantile errors, emmetropization, is not fully understood, but appears to be visually guided. Young infants with Down syndrome have the same distribution of refraction as typical infants at 6 months of age, but their distribution widens over the next 2 years, with refractive errors in individual children remaining or worsening. The result is that most children with Down syndrome are hypermetropic at school age, with a few being myopic (Fig. 6.2).

Acknowledgement of this failure in emmetropization means that most eye clinics will now prescribe spectacle corrections earlier for children with Down syndrome than for children with typical development. The 'watching and waiting' approach appropriate for typical children with refractive errors, who are likely to outgrow them, is not appropriate. Beyond the age of 4 years, refractive errors in Down syndrome tend to stabilize, with possibly a slight reduction in hypermetropia at adolescence (Al-Bagdady et al. 2011). The onset of myopia at adolescence that typifies the general population does not seem to occur in Down syndrome.

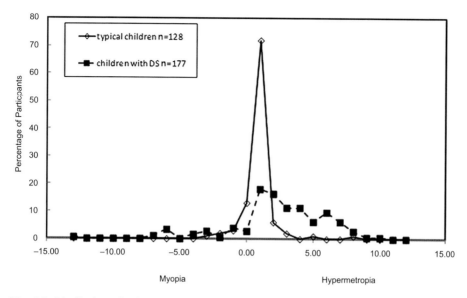

Fig. 6.2. Distribution of refractive error among school-age children (age 4–18 years) with Down syndrome (DS; filled markers) and without (open markers).

Astigmatism is also subject to the emmetropization process in typical children, disappearing in most children over the first 2 years of life. Children with Down syndrome tend to retain infantile astigmatism. Moreover, the axis of astigmatism shows a marked shift towards oblique orientations in later childhood, so oblique astigmatism is the most common form at adolescence (Al-Bagdady et al. 2011).

Refractive errors that appear in childhood will persist into adulthood and anyone with Down syndrome should have regular eye examinations throughout life.

ACCOMMODATION DEFICITS

Accommodation is the ability of the eye to change its power to focus objects at different distances by changing eye lens shape. Generally, children (whose lenses are very flexible) are assumed to have large reserves of accommodation and can focus accurately on very close objects. The flexibility of the lens reduces with age, so adults experience increasing difficulty in focusing at near with age. Studies show that the majority (reportedly 75%) of children with Down syndrome cannot focus accurately at distances that typical age-matched children can manage easily (Cregg et al. 2001) (see Fig. 6.3). This has important implications for their vision in school, where most of their learning takes place at near.

The accommodation deficit is successfully corrected with bifocals, and the children attain accurate accommodation when wearing them (Stewart et al. 2005). This is reflected in improved visual acuity at near and in significantly improved performance in literacy and visual perceptual tasks (Nandakumar and Leat 2010). It is therefore important that a measure of accommodation is included in all sight tests for children with Down syndrome.

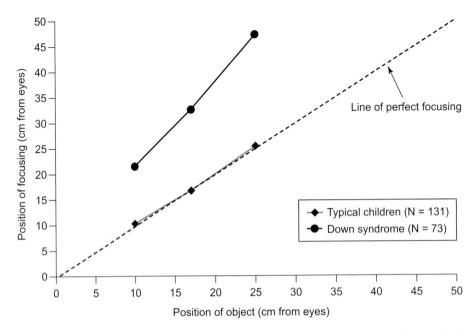

Fig. 6.3. The focusing response to near targets for children with Down syndrome (filled markers) and without (open markers).

All adults, including those with Down syndrome, will experience presbyopia (the loss of accommodation with age). In the general population, this starts at around the age of 45 years. There are no studies reporting the age at presbyopia in Down syndrome and it may be that it manifests earlier, in line with accelerated ageing.

STRABISMUS

Strabismus (squint) occurs in 2–4% of children with typical development and is highly associated with hypermetropia. In children with Down syndrome the prevalence is much higher, at around 25–30% and can occur with any refractive error (Haugen and Hovding 2001). Most cases are of esotropia (convergent or inward turn). As with typical children, in some cases, the strabismus is completely or partially corrected with spectacles. In other cases, spectacles make little difference (although bifocals can be successful in reducing strabismus for near). Surgery is an option, although parents should be aware that the benefit is likely to be cosmetic rather than visual.

Strabismus that is mainly confined to one eye may result in amblyopia (reduced visual acuity in the squinting eye), and occlusion therapy is the usual approach to improve acuity. However, alternating squint, in which the child can fix with either eye and freely change between the two, is much more common in Down syndrome than in typical children and is much less likely to give rise to amblyopia.

KERATOCONUS

This condition is a degenerative disease of the cornea, which thins and protrudes into a more conical shape. The condition can be associated with allergic conditions and may be associated with eye-rubbing. The result is visual distortion that cannot be satisfactorily corrected with spectacles. Contact lenses provide a good optical correction and are successfully worn by a number of people with Down syndrome, although they require specialist fitting and significant ocular allergy can cause difficulty with wear. The prevalence of keratoconus in Down syndrome is about 15% (in the general population about 1 per 1000) with an onset at adolescence to late teens. The condition often stabilizes in the mid-20s. In some cases, the condition progresses and vision worsens due to increasing irregular astigmatism and central corneal scarring causing severe visual impairment. Corneal transplant is required where the condition continues to progress and is usually highly successful, although in Down syndrome extremely careful surgical aftercare is required.

There are new therapies becoming available, most notably collagen cross-linkage that can halt the progression and even reverse some of the distortions. The therapy is only viable in the early stages, while the thickness of the central cornea is greater than 400μ. Therein lies a challenge for eye care practitioners because the non-keratoconic cornea in Down syndrome is, on average, 475μ, compared with 575μ in the general population (Haugen et al. 2001). Thus, keratoconus needs to be diagnosed early in adolescents with Down syndrome if this particular therapy is to be possible. However, another characteristic of the Down syndrome cornea is its curvature; the cornea is steeper in Down syndrome and therefore can appear slightly keratoconic even when quite healthy. Recognizing keratoconus in Down syndrome in its early stages is therefore challenging and the key to detection at its earliest stage is regular monitoring to pick up progression in corneal shape. This emphasizes the importance of awareness that regular eye examinations should include corneal topography.

VISUAL ACUITY

Studies have shown, over many years, that children and adults with Down syndrome have poorer visual acuity than age-matched peers (Courage et al. 1994, Woodhouse et al. 1996). In many cases, it could be assumed to be due to any number of the conditions described above, many of which, if untreated, can reduce visual performance. Alternatively, poor acuity scores may be considered as due to low motivation, lack of cooperation, limited understanding and processing difficulties, all associated with the intellectual disability. Recent work has shown that none of these factors fully explain the poor results. Even when refractive errors are fully corrected, ocular pathologies are excluded and when entirely objective techniques are used, children with Down syndrome (aged 2y and older) have poorer visual acuity than typical children (John et al. 2004) (Fig. 6.4).

However, when the optics of the eye are bypassed (by laser diffraction techniques), visual acuity in children with Down syndrome improves to a standard almost equal to typical children (Little et al. 2007). The major factor in poor acuity is the low-quality optics of the eyes in Down syndrome, as shown by measures of ocular aberrations.

Even when eye-care practitioners do everything in their power to ensure that children with Down syndrome have the best vision of which they are capable, the children are still

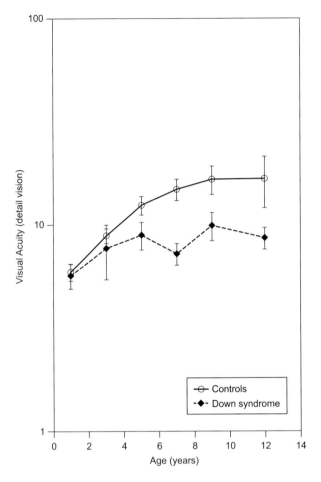

Fig. 6.4. Visual acuity recorded with objective techniques for children with Down syndrome (filled markers) and without (open markers).

at considerable disadvantage in terms of vision. Considering that children and adults with Down syndrome are categorized as 'visual learners', this uncorrectable and largely unrecognized deficit must have a negative impact on their development. It is vitally important that parents, educators and health professionals are aware that people with Down syndrome do not see the world as clearly as the typical population. Learning materials in schools that are easily seen by typical children may prove an obstacle for children with Down syndrome. Modification of materials, such as writing in black pen and emboldening faint lines, can make the difference between success and failure in a school task.

In adults with Down syndrome, significant visual impairment compounds their intellectual disability and has a detrimental effect on independent living skills, communication and language skills, social skills and initiative and persistence.

Eye conditions such as nystagmus and squint are usually quite visible to parents and usually trigger a concern and a referral to specialists. Refractive errors and poor accommodation are much less obvious to family and friends. Children's toys are usually big and bright, and children bring smaller things very close, thus enlarging the image, so any difficulty in focusing is not apparent in a young child. A very young child's sphere of interest is at near. If a child becomes myopic (short-sighted), he or she may not develop an interest in far objects; in a child with Down syndrome, this may be considered an example of developmental impairment rather than an eye-sight issue.

For many years, teachers and parents have been aware that children with Down syndrome have difficulty writing on the lines; this has always been considered as due to 'poor fine motor control'. It is only recently that we have become aware that this, too, is an eye-sight issue:

> *A quote from a parent after information from Down syndrome research on vision was passed to her son's school:*
>
> *I know what a difference this will make to Ben as one of his targets at school was to write on the line which he couldn't do. It turned out the line was in pencil so I suggested that perhaps he couldn't see it and showed his TA's your information, they then drew the lines in pen and instantly he could write on the lines!!*

Most children with Down syndrome can learn to read. All children learn with big print; the visual deficit resulting from poor accommodation may not stop them learning with large print. But as the child progresses through the reading scheme, the print becomes smaller, and the time may come that the child cannot make the next step in reading. This may be considered 'plateauing development' whereas, once again, it is an eye-sight issue:

> *An excerpt from Minnie's parents:*
>
> *Minnie (aged 12) in secondary school started to find reading really tedious and started displaying difficult behaviour to avoid reading altogether; at times the teachers and support staff would have to exclude her from class. In year 8, she was fitted with bifocals and within 2 weeks the change was remarkable; not only did she take part willingly in reading at school but started to undertake independent reading for pleasure, reading the Radio Times and magazines. She started actively to seek out reading material on topics that interested her. This was also the point in time when she started taking a real interest in independent writing. Her behaviour and attitude improved immensely. Minnie was so much more engaged by everything that involved reading, including her transition planning and college work when she finished school.*

Parents worry that their child may not be able to cope with spectacles. It does take time for a child to become used to the new experience and there are challenges if a child has to get used to spectacles and hearing aids at the same time, as many do. But a correction for the eye sight problem can make a very positive impact on a child's quality of life and learning:

> *From mother of Ethan, who was prescribed bifocals at aged 3.*
>
> *Just thought I'd let you know that he took to the bifocals straight away and hasn't put his old glasses back on since wearing them.*
>
> *Just this morning his key worker at preschool asked me if I'd noticed a difference in Ethan since he's been wearing his bifocals—they noted he was steadier on his feet, better communication and attention when looking at flash cards and so on. It's nice that someone else has noticed too.*
>
> *Also, I know I mentioned to you that I was worried about his peripheral vision when we visited because he only seemed to look at 1 out of 4 words on a matching board when we were practising reading. I think it's because he had to try so hard to focus that he could only look at one word at a time. Now he looks at the whole board and understands better what I'm asking him to do!*

In summary, parents may not be able to tell whether their child has a visual difficulty. So parents should ensure that they arrange for regular eye examinations, which include accommodation measurement for all ages and thorough corneal assessment for adolescents. Even when there are no problems, the children will have poorer vision than their classroom peers and teachers should be informed of this. Parents should ask their eye care practitioner for a full report on their child's eye sight, along with the values expected for a typical child of the same age.

Key points
- Regular surveillance throughout childhood by an orthoptist and ophthalmologist/optometrist is strongly recommended to detect the many conditions that affect vision in Down syndrome.
- All infants with Down syndrome should be examined for congenital cataract and other eye anomalies by a trained person at birth and age 6 weeks.
- Paediatricians should monitor visual behaviour at every review and refer any children who have abnormal visual behaviour for full ophthalmological assessment.
- Formal ocular/visual assessment, including orthoptic assessment and refraction with ophthalmoscopic examination for cataract, is recommended between the ages of 18 months and 2 years and again at 4 years.
- At least 50% of children will have refractive errors requiring spectacles by age 4 years. Early correction for hypermetropia and the use of bifocals can be beneficial in many children, to help with accommodative errors.
- After the age of 4, eye checks should be at least every two years throughout life by professionals with expertise in managing this client group.
- In adulthood, screening should continue at least every two years for keratoconus and cataract.

REFERENCES

Al-Bagdady M, Murphy P, Woodhouse JM (2011) Development and distribution of refractive error in children with Down's syndrome. *Brit J Ophthalmol* 95: 1091–1097. doi: 10.1136/bjo.2010.185827.

Courage ML, Adams RJ, Reyno S, Kwa Pg (1994) Visual acuity in infants and children with Down syndrome. *Dev Med Child Neurol* 36: 586–593.

Cregg M, Woodhouse JM, Pakeman VH et al. (2001) Accommodation and refractive error in children with Down syndrome: Cross-sectional and longitudinal studies. *Invest Ophthalmol Vis Sci* 42: 55–63. PubMed PMID: 11133848.

Haargaard B, Fledelius HC (2006) Down's syndrome and early cataract. *Brit J Ophthalmol* 90: 1024–1027.

Haugen OH, Hovding G (2001) Strabismus and binocular function in children with Down syndrome: A population-based, longitudinal study. *Acta Ophthalmol Scan* 79: 133–139.

Haugen OH, Hovding G, Eide GE (2001) Biometric measurements of the eyes in teenagers and young adults with Down syndrome. *Acta Ophthalmol Scan* 79: 616–625.

John FM, Bromham NR, Woodhouse JM, Candy TR (2004) Spatial vision deficits in infants and children with Down syndrome. *Invest Ophthalmol Vis Sci* 45: 1566–1572.

Krinsky-Mchale SJ, Jenkins EC, Zigman WB, Silverman W (2012) Ophthalmic disorders in adults with Down syndrome. *Curr Gerontol Geriatr Res* 2012: 9. doi: 10.1155/2012/974253.

Little JA, Woodhouse JM, Lauritzen JS, Saunders KJ (2007) The impact of optical factors on resolution acuity in children with Down syndrome. *Invest Ophthalmol Vis Sci* 48: 3995–4001.

Mccullough SJ, Little JA, Saunders KJ (2013) Higher order aberrations in children with Down syndrome. *Invest Ophthalmol Vis Sci* 54: 1527–1535. doi: 10.1167/iovs.12-10597.

Nandakumar K, Leat SJ (2010) Bifocals in children with Down syndrome (BiDS) – visual acuity, accommodation and early literacy skills. *Acta Ophthalmol* 88: 196–204. doi: 10.1111/j.1755-3768.2010.01944.x.

Rahi JS, Dezateux C (1999) National cross sectional study of detection of congenital and infantile cataract in the United Kingdom: Role of childhood screening and surveillance. The British Congenital Cataract Interest Group. *Brit Med J* 318: 362–365.

Rahi JS, Dezateux C (2000) Congenital and infantile cataract in the United Kingdom: Underlying or associated factors. British Congenital Cataract Interest Group. *Invest Ophthalmol Vis Sci* 41: 2108–2114.

Stewart RE, Woodhouse JM, Trojanowska LD (2005) In focus: The use of bifocals for children with Down's syndrome. *Ophthal Physiol Opt* 25: 514–522.

Wagner RS, Caputo AR, Reynolds RD (2000) Nystagmus in Down's syndrome. *Brit J Ophthalmol* 90: 1024–1027.

Woodhouse JM, Pakeman VH, Cregg M et al. (1997) Refractive errors in young children with Down syndrome. *Optometry Vision Sci* 74: 844–851.

Woodhouse JM, Pakeman VH, Saunders KJ et al. (1996) Visual acuity and accommodation in infants and young children with Down syndrome. *J Intellect Disabil Res* 40: 49–55.

Yokoyama T, Tamura H, Tsukamoto H, YamaneK, Mishima HK (2006) Prevalence of glaucoma in adults with Down's syndrome. *Jpn J Ophthalmol* 50: 274–276.

7
IMMUNE FUNCTION, INFECTION AND AUTOIMMUNITY

Peter Arkwright and Liz McDermott

This chapter explores the differences between the immune response in people with Down syndrome and the general population. It discusses the reasons for their propensity to infection and autoimmunity.

What proportion of people with Down syndrome have problems with infections?

Infections, particularly respiratory, are the most common cause of hospitalization and death in people with Down syndrome. Tenenbaum et al. (2012) found that in a cohort of 120 adults with Down syndrome, hospitalizations were not only 2.5 times more frequent, but also more prolonged than in the general population with a median stay of 8 days compared with 5. More than a quarter of hospitalizations were due to respiratory infections. One-third of all people with Down syndrome have had at least one episode of pneumonia, with 18% having repeated episodes. Middle ear infections are also very common, particularly in the under 30s (52%), compared with older adults (20%) (Määttä et al. 2011). Ten percent of children under the age of 2 years with Down syndrome will be hospitalized for respiratory syncytial virus (RSV) bronchiolitis compared with 0.5% of the general population (Zachariah et al. 2012). However, other viral infections such as chickenpox and shingles, herpes stomatitis, infectious mononucleosis, molluscum, warts and rotavirus gastroenteritis are not more common or severe in Down syndrome. There is little published information to suggest that Down syndrome per se is associated with more frequent fungal infections, although anecdotally parents commonly report athlete's foot and candidal groin infections.

Why are individuals with Down syndrome susceptible to infection?

The cause of the increased incidence of infection is multifactorial. Non-immune factors such as preterm birth, congenital heart disease and other anatomical and neuromuscular abnormalities are just as, if not more, important than immunological factors in increasing the risk of respiratory infections in Down syndrome.

What abnormalities in immune function have been found in Down syndrome?

T-cell immunity has been most extensively studied. Sixty percent of children with Down syndrome have absolute T-cell numbers below the 5th centile with subsequent improvement and normalization by adulthood. Early T-cell development is abnormal. Using ultrasound, De Leon-Luis et al. (2011) found that 10 out of 12 fetuses with Down syndrome had a thymic perimeter less than the 5th centile for gestational age. Histology consistently shows reduced cortical thymocytes, cystic changes and fibrosis. Naïve, rather than memory or effector, T-cells are low in Down syndrome suggesting peripheral expansion compensates for reduced thymic output. A greater than two-fold reduction in T-cell receptor excision circles, a marker of early T-cell differentiation, provides further supportive evidence for these observations. Apoptosis of T-cells in Down syndrome is no different to the general population (Bloemers et al. 2011). Possible mechanisms explaining the relative lack of naïve T-cells are discussed below in the section on autoimmunity. Even healthy children with Down syndrome demonstrate impaired maturation of T lymphocytes (Guazzarotti et al. 2009), decreased lymphocyte markers (de Hingh et al. 2005) and decreased mitogen stimulation responses (Mahmoud et al. 2005).

Regulatory T-cells (Treg) are a subset of T-cells that can suppress other immune cells and hence modulate overstimulation of the immune system particularly in endocrine organs and the gastrointestinal tract (Long and Buckner 2011). Treg numbers are normal or high in Down syndrome, but functional activity may be impaired (Pellegrini et al. 2012). Further research is required to determine whether impaired Treg function explains the higher prevalence of autoimmune diseases in Down syndrome.

Although it was previously thought that only T-cells are affected in Down syndrome, there is growing evidence for similar abnormalities in B-cells. B-cell numbers, particularly naïve B-cells, are also significantly lower in Down syndrome (Verstegen et al. 2010). In keeping with these findings, serum immunoglobulin (Ig) M concentrations are classically low, whereas IgG and IgA tend to be higher than quoted normal ranges (Joshi et al. 2011). As with T-cell studies, low naïve B-cell output seems to be offset by peripheral B-cell and plasma cell expansion. Vaccine responses in Down syndrome tend to be preserved (Troisi et al. 1985, Ferreira et al. 2004, Joshi et al. 2011).

Other immune abnormalities described in Down syndrome include neutrophil defects (Yamato et al. 2009), mannan-binding lectin deficiency (Nisihara et al. 2010) and early lymphocyte apoptosis (Elsayed and Elsayed 2009). However, phagocytic function is also preserved in people with Down syndrome (Ram and Chinen 2011).

What non-immune factors should be considered in people with Down syndrome with infections?

Abnormal anatomy of the respiratory tract plays a role in predisposing to respiratory infections. Stenotic ear canals and mid-face hypoplasia causing abnormal Eustachian tubes and small sinuses result in poor drainage of fluid from the middle ear and sinuses (see Chapter 5). This predisposes to upper respiratory infections such as otitis media, pharyngitis and sinusitis. Drainage may be further affected by increased production of mucus. Hypotonia and lower respiratory abnormalities such as tracheomalacia may predispose to lower respiratory tract infections, as may increased pulmonary vascular reactivity. Silent aspiration from swallowing difficulties and gastro-oesophageal reflux can also result in lower respiratory tract infection.

Concurrent medical problems such as congenital cardiac disease are additional factors predisposing to infection (Bloemers et al. 2010). Chemotherapy used for leukaemia or other malignancies may lead to profound secondary immune deficiency. This should be taken into account when choosing the chemotherapy regime (Bruwier and Chantrain 2012).

Ben's first hospital admission was with RSV bronchiolitis at the age of 3 months. He required ventilation in the paediatric intensive care unit for 7 days. From then on, he was admitted to the general paediatric ward every 2–3 months with upper and lower respiratory infections. He had a constant purulent nasal discharge during the winter months. Following an atrial septal defect (ASD) repair at age 3 years, his infections became less frequent. When reviewed at 4 years, he had had a total of 20 admissions for respiratory infection. Immunology tests showed low IgM but normal IgG and IgA. Specific antibodies to tetanus were normal but he only had protective levels to 2/12 serotype-specific antibody titres to Streptococcus pneumoniae despite routine immunization with Prevenar 7 on two occasions and a subsequent booster dose of Pneumovax II after 2 years of age. He was commenced on regular oral prophylactic antibiotics and did much better only occasionally requiring additional antibiotics for an acute infection. He remained on prophylactic antibiotics during the winter until age 11. He responded well to a recent Prevenar 13 booster with protective pneumococcal antibodies to 12/12 serotypes tested.

Ben's respiratory infections improved following ASD repair and were kept under control with prophylactic antibiotics. Growth of his facial bone and thus better drainage of his upper airways contributed to his spontaneous recovery. In later childhood, he managed a response to the Prevenar vaccine suggesting maturation of his immune system. Vaccine responses often wane during the pre-school years, even in children with typical development and will usually improve after pre-school boosters. Polysaccharide vaccines may not lead to sustained antibody responses and poor responses to Pneumovax II should not be interpreted as indicating an antibody immunodeficiency.

Approach to management

ACUTE AND CHRONIC INFECTIONS

All infections should be assessed and treated promptly. People with Down syndrome tend to have infections with the same bacterial pathogens as the general population. Respiratory syncytial virus and influenza A virus cause more severe disease in Down syndrome, and infants with Down syndrome have a higher risk of being hospitalized with severe RSV-related lower respiratory tract infections, independent of other risk factors (Zachariah et al. 2012). In general, standard courses of antibiotics based on local guidelines should be used.

In children with Down syndrome who have recurrent or persistent respiratory infections, prophylactic antibiotics are often helpful, particularly over the winter months. In a small minority, immunoglobulin (antibody) replacement significantly improves quality of life, although these infusions are rarely needed life long. Immunoglobulin therapy should only be considered and prescribed by physicians with experience in investigating and treating people with recurrent infections and antibody immunodeficiency disorders.

Advice should be provided to carers and susceptible individuals about when to seek medical attention, for example, if there is a fever and productive cough, or chronic green nasal discharge.

GENERAL MEASURES

Calorie intake and any feeding problems should also be reviewed. Aspiration from uncoordinated feeding should be managed with specialist speech and language therapy advice. Gastro-oesophageal reflux should be treated aggressively. Management of respiratory comorbidities such as asthma should be optimized. Nutrition should also be optimized with supplements, where appropriate, and specific deficiencies such as iron and vitamin D should be investigated and treated.

IMMUNE INVESTIGATIONS

Immune abnormalities vary between individuals. Immune tests should be requested according to clinical need. Lymphopaenia is common and does not generally indicate that regular follow-up is required unless there are problems with recurrent viral infections or thrush. Low serum IgM and raised IgG and IgA are present in many people with Down syndrome who do not have recurrent infections. Over the last few years, more extensive and extended childhood vaccination programmes have been introduced against, particularly, *Streptococcus pneumoniae*, but in countries where this is not the case, additional booster vaccines may be required. Rather than immune testing, it is important that a referral to a specialist is made if infections are frequent or troublesome. Autoimmune screening is discussed in a separate section below.

VACCINATION

All children with Down syndrome should follow the childhood immunization schedule for the country in which they live. This may include seasonal influenza vaccine for certain ages but it is advised that annual influenza vaccine should be considered in all those with Down syndrome. Live vaccines such as MMR, BCG and chickenpox may also be included. There is no evidence that immune abnormalities in people with Down syndrome put them at risk from the live-attenuated vaccines except for those receiving chemotherapy or immunosuppressants. Wild-type measles can however pose a significant risk to children with Down syndrome, particularly if they have other comorbidities.

Additional polysaccharide pneumococcal vaccination after 2 years of age might be considered in those with recurrent lower respiratory infections, but may not result in sustained protective antibody titres. Repeated polysaccharide vaccination should be avoided because of the potential risk of poorer responses (hyporesponsiveness) (Poolman and Borrow 2011).

Some high-risk infants, such as those with complex congenital heart disease, or who are oxygen dependant are particularly at risk of severe RSV bronchiolitis (10-fold increase in the risk of hospitalization) (Bloemers et al. 2010). Passive immunization with anti-RSV immunoglobulin in the RSV season should be considered based on local guidelines.

Published literature, albeit from 30 years ago, found an 18-fold higher prevalence of chronic hepatitis B infection in Down syndrome over that seen in others living in residential accommodation (Clarke et al. 1984). With modern screening of blood products, the transmission risk of hepatitis viruses for instance during cardiac surgery is negligible in developed countries. However, close daily living contact and the possibility of behavioural problems may lead to residents being at increased risk of infection. In the UK, hepatitis B vaccination is therefore recommended in this setting. Similar considerations may apply to children and adults in day care, schools and centres for those with severe intellectual disability. Decisions on immunization should be made on the basis of a local risk assessment. Particularly, in settings where the individual's behaviour is likely to lead to significant exposure (e.g. biting or being bitten) on a regular basis, immunization should be offered even in the absence of documented hepatitis B transmission (Salisbury et al. 2013).

Commonly asked questions on immunization

Do regular antibiotics weaken the immune system?

Regular or prophylactic antibiotics should only be prescribed when the benefits outweigh the risks. The antibiotics do not stop the immune system working, but if used for prolonged periods may lead to the development of resistant bacterial infections, in which case the doctor may choose an alternative.

Should my child have the MMR vaccine?

Measles is a serious infection and can cause pneumonia and encephalitis. MMR is a 'live vaccine', which not only protects against measles, but also mumps and rubella. The vaccine should not be given to children with very poor immunity, for example, children on chemotherapy or immunosuppressive drugs. It is safe to give the MMR to children with Down syndrome unless they are receiving these medicines.

Autoimmunity

Are autoimmune disorders more prevalent in Down syndrome?

Compared with the general population, people with Down syndrome have a 10-fold or even higher prevalence of certain autoimmune disorders, particularly organ-specific diseases of endocrine glands (e.g. Hashimoto thyroiditis, Graves disease and type 1 diabetes mellitus), as well as of the gut (coeliac disease) and skin (alopecia areata, vitiligo) (Karlsson et al. 1998, Bonamico et al. 2001, Book et al. 2001, De Luca et al. 2010) (see Table 7.1).

The autoimmune diseases detailed in Table 7.1 more commonly occur together, even in the general population (Ban 2012). Indeed, the combination of type 1 diabetes mellitus (T1DM) and autoimmune thyroid disease is sometimes referred to as autoimmune polyglandular syndrome type 3 variant (APS3v; Villano et al. 2009). In view of this known association, any person with T1DM is routinely screened for both autoimmune thyroid disease (which occurs in up to a third) and coeliac disease (which occurs in up to a fifth). Autoimmune thyroid diseases occur in up to 12% of those with vitiligo. The association between these autoimmune diseases is just as strong in Down syndrome.

TABLE 7.1
**Prevalence of common autoimmune diseases in people with Down syndrome (trisomy 21)
compared with the general population and people with Turner (XO) syndrome**

	General population (%)	Down syndrome (%)	Turner syndrome (%)
Hashimoto thyroiditis	0.3	3–33	33
Graves disease	0.5	2–6	4
T1DM	0.1	1–11	<0.5
Coeliac disease	0.5–1	7–43	5
Alopecia areata	0.1	6	<0.5

T1DM, type 1 diabetes mellitus.

Systemic autoimmune diseases such as idiopathic inflammatory arthritis, systemic lupus erythematosus (SLE) and dermatomyositis may occur in people with Down syndrome. Large comparative population studies are needed to determine to what extent these conditions may be more prevalent in those with Down syndrome than in the general population.

The increased prevalence in autoimmune diseases in chromosomal disorders is not unique to Down syndrome. People with Turner syndrome (females with XO) are also 10 times more likely to have both autoimmune thyroid disease (clinical disease occurs in one-third) and coeliac disease, but not T1DM or alopecia areata (Mortensen et al. 2009). Thus, the genetic predisposition to autoimmune diseases cannot be solely linked to disordered gene expression on chromosome 21.

WHY MIGHT SOME AUTOIMMUNE DISEASES BE MORE COMMON IN DOWN SYNDROME?

The reason why people with Down syndrome are more prone to organ-specific autoimmune diseases is currently unknown. There is some evidence in Europeans, but not other racial groups, that specific HLA genotypes are more likely to present cross-reacting peptide antigens to potentially autoreactive helper T-lymphocytes. Environmental exposure to potentially cross-reacting antigens, for example, certain microbes in a predisposed individual, might lead to the development of autoimmunity (Menconi et al. 2010). One example is a child with a HLA-DP genotype who develops T1DM after exposure to a Coxsackie virus infection. The gene coding HLA is not on chromosome 21 but rather on chromosome 6 and thus the logarithmic increase in autoimmunity in Down syndrome and Turner syndrome cannot be directly due to HLA (Aitken et al. 2012).

The autoimmune phenotype of Down syndrome does not fit with that of currently defined monogenetic autoimmune disorders such as ALPS, IPEX, IL-10R deficiency, SPENCDI, AGS or APS1 (Cheng and Anderson 2012). APS1 is the only one of these disorders to have its gene coded on chromosome 21 (21q22.3) (Lima et al. 2011). The triad of mucocutaneous candidiasis, hypoparathyroidism and Addison's disease that characterizes APS1 (Akirav et al. 2011) are not present in Down syndrome and therefore other explanations need to be sought. The 21q22 region of chromosome 21 is critical in determining the

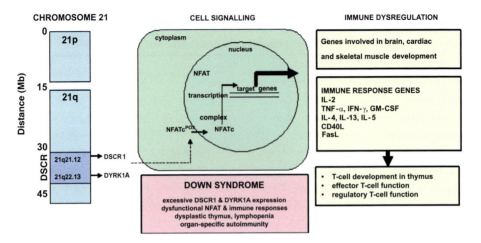

Fig. 7.1. Putative mechanisms by which overexpression of dual specificity tyrosine-phosphorylation-regulated kinase 1A (*DYRK1A*) and Down syndrome critical region 1 (*DSCR1*) genes in the Down syndrome critical region contributes to immune dysfunction in Down syndrome. (1) Inheritance of an extra chromosome 21 in Down syndrome results in increased activity of genes coded by this chromosome including *DSCR1* and *DYRK1A* in the Down syndrome critical region (DSCR). (2) *DSCR1* and *DYRK1A* regulate nuclear factor of activated T-cells—cytoplasmic components (NFATc) translocation of NFATc into the nucleus. (3) Dysregulation of NFAT activity results in aberrant immune responses of effector and regulatory T-lymphocytes—thymic dysplasia, lymphopenia and propensity to organ-specific autoimmune diseases.

clinical phenotype of Down syndrome and also codes for *DYRK1A* and *DSCR1*. These two related genes are involved in the regulation of nuclear factor of activated T-cells (NFAT) activity (Arron et al. 2006). NFAT is particularly important in guiding naïve T-cells into distinct effector T-cell subsets, and is also involved in the control of regulatory T-cell activity (Crabtree and Olson 2002, Ghosh et al. 2010, Pellegrini et al. 2012). Further research is required to determine if overexpression of *DYRK1A* or *DSCR1* might explain the immune basis of Down syndrome-associated autoimmune diseases as summarized in Figure 7.1, and thus provide a therapeutic target for the prevention or alleviation of these Down syndrome-associated complications.

Is the clinical presentation of autoimmune disease the same in Down syndrome as in the general population?

The onset of autoimmune disorders in Down syndrome is typically at a younger age (De Luca et al. 2010) than both the general population and in females with Turner syndrome. For instance, in children with Down syndrome who develop hypothyroidism, the disease starts before the age of 8 years, while in the general population it typically commences in adulthood. The average age at onset of T1DM in Down syndrome is also less at 7–8 years compared with 10–14 years in the general population (Graber et al. 2012).

The prevalence of thyroid disease in Down syndrome is equal between the two sexes, in contrast to the general population where it is more common in women in their 20s to 40s, and often commences postpartum.

WHY MEASURE AUTOANTIBODIES IN DOWN SYNDROME?

Laboratory tests should help with the diagnosis and treatment of disease. Measurement of some autoantibodies is helpful in the diagnosis. Anti-transglutaminase antibodies are specific and useful in the diagnosis of coeliac disease in both the general population and people with Down syndrome. Antithyroid receptor antibodies are also specific and present in over 95% of people with Graves disease. In contrast, other antithyroid antibodies such as antithyroid peroxidase (TPO) and thyroglobulin are often absent in children under the age of 8 years with biochemical evidence of thyroid dysfunction, although they are present in more than half of older children and adults (Karlsson et al. 1998). These antibodies may support the diagnosis of an autoimmune aetiology, but treatment is determined by measurement of thyroid function tests (see Chapter 11 for more detailed discussion of these issues).

The reason for the incomplete correlation between autoantibodies and autoimmune hypothyroidism is that the immune mechanism leading to Hashimoto disease is both T-cell and antibody mediated. T-cell mediated destruction can trigger clinical hypothyroidism in the absence of detectable autoantibodies. TPO can be expressed on the cell surface, but much of it is on intracellular organelles (ER and Golgi), which are more difficult for damaging autoantibodies to reach (Ruf and Carayon 2006).

Key points
- Respiratory infections are the most common cause of death and hospitalization in people with Down syndrome.
- Non-respiratory viral, bacterial and fungal infections are generally not more common or severe in Down syndrome.
- Although people with Down syndrome tend to have lower B and T-lymphocytes, particularly naïve lymphocytes, as well as low IgM concentrations, their immune response to infection is usually adequate.
- Non-immune causes for recurrent or persistent respiratory infections should be considered.
- Where these have been excluded and there are still concerns, specialist referral may be required.
- It is essential that clinicians are aware of the higher prevalence of autoimmune thyroid disease, type 1 diabetes mellitus, coeliac disease and some autoimmune skin conditions in Down syndrome, particularly as thyroid disease and coeliac disease may have an insidious onset.
- Physicians should also be aware that in contrast to the general population, autoimmune disorders can occur earlier in childhood with equal sex prevalence.
- Physicians should enquire about symptoms relevant to these autoimmune diseases at each consultation.

- In view of the high prevalence, in particular of thyroid disease and coeliac disease, there should be a low threshold for testing.
- Parents should also be aware of common presentations of these diseases so that they can alert their doctor if there are concerns between clinic appointments.

REFERENCES

Aitken RJ, Mehers KL, Williams AJ et al. (2013) Early-onset, co-existing autoimmunity and decreased HLA-mediated susceptibility are the characteristics of diabetes in Down syndrome. *Diabetes Care* 36: 1181–5.

Akirav EM, Ruddle NH, Herold KC (2011) The role of AIRE in human autoimmune disease. *Nat Rev Endocrinol* 7: 25–33.

Arron JR, Winslow MM, Polleri A et al. (2006) NFAT dysregulation by increased dosage of DSCR1 and DYRK1A on chromosome 21. *Nature* 441: 595–600.

Ban Y (2012) Genetic factors of autoimmune thyroid diseases in Japanese. *Autoimmune Dis* 2012: 236981.

Bloemers BL, Bont L, de Weger RA, Otto SA, Borghans JA, Tesselaar K (2011) Decreased thymic output accounts for decreased naïve T cell numbers in children with Down syndrome. *J Immunol* 186: 4500–4507.

Bloemers BLP, Broers CJM, Bont L, Weijerman ME, Gemke RJBJ, van Furth AM (2010) Increased risk of respiratory tract infections in children with Down syndrome: The consequence of an altered immune system. *Microbes Infect* 12: 799–808.

Bonamico M, Mariani P, Danesi HM et al. (2001) Prevalence and clinical picture of celiac disease in Italian Down syndrome patients: A multicenter study. *J Pediatr Gastroenterol Nutr* 33: 139–143.

Book L, Hart A, Black J, Feolo M, Zone JJ, Neuhausen SL (2001) Prevalence and clinical characteristics of celiac disease in Downs syndrome in a US study. *Am J Med Genet* 98: 70–74.

Bruwier A, Chantrain CF (2012) Hematologicial disorders and leukemia in children with Down syndrome. *Eur J Pediatr* 171: 1301–1307.

Cheng MH, Anderson MS (2012) Monogenic autoimmunity. *Annu Rev Immunol* 30: 393–427.

Clarke SK, Caul EO, Jancar J, Gordan-Russell JB (1984) Hepatitis B in seven hospitals for the mentally handicapped. *J Infect* 8: 34–43.

Crabtree GR, Olson EN (2002) NFAT signaling: Choreographing the social lives of cells. *Cell* 109: S67–S79.

de Hingh YC, van der Vossen PW, Gemen EF et al. (2005) Intrinsic abnormalities of lymphocyte counts in children with Down syndrome. *J Pediatr* 147: 744–747.

De Leon-Luis J, Santolaya J, Gamez F, Pintado P, Perez R, Ortiz-Quintana L (2011) Sonographic thymic measurements in Down syndrome fetuses. *Prenat Diagn* 31: 841–845.

De Luca F, Corrias A, Salerno M et al. (2010) Peculiarities of Graves' disease in children and adolescents with Down's syndrome. *Eur J Endocrinol* 162: 591–595.

Elsayed SM, Elsayed GM (2009) Phenotype of apoptotic lymphocytes in children with Down syndrome. *Immun Ageing* 6: 2–6.

Ferreira CT, Leite JC, Taniguchi A, Vieira SM, Pereira-Lima J, da Silveira TR (2004) Immunogenicity and safety of an inactivated hepatitis A vaccine in children with Down syndrome. *Pediatr Gastroenterol Nutr* 39: 337–340.

Ghosh S, Koralov SB, Stevanovic I et al. (2010) Hyperactivation of nuclear factor of activated T cells 1 (NFAT1) in T cells attenuates severity of murine autoimmune encephalomyelitis. *Proc Natl Acad Sci U S A* 107: 15169–15174.

Graber E, Chacko E, Regelmann MO, Costin G, Rapaport R (2012) Down syndrome and thyroid function. *Endocrinol Metab Clin North Am* 41: 735–745.

Guazzarotti L, Trabattoni D, Castelletti E et al. (2009) T lymphocyte maturation is impaired in healthy young individuals carrying trisomy 21 (Down syndrome). *Am J Intellect Dev Disabil* 114: 100–109.

Joshi AY, Abraham RS, Synder MR, Boyce TG (2011) Immune evaluation and vaccine response in Down syndrome: Evidence of immunodeficiency? *Vaccine* 29: 5040–5046.

Karlsson B, Gustafsson J, Hedov G, Ivarsson SA, Annerén G (1998) Thyroid dysfunction in Down's syndrome: Relation to age and thyroid autoimmunity. *Arch Dis Child* 79: 242–245.

Lima FA, Moreira-Filho CA, Ramos PL et al. (2011) Decreased AIRE expression and global thymic hypofunction in Down syndrome. *J Immunol* 187: 3422–3430.

Long SA, Buckner JH (2011) CD4+FOXP3+ T regulatory cells in human autoimmunity: More than a numbers game. *J Immunol* 187: 2061–2066.

Määttä T, Määttä J, Tervo-Määttä T, Taanila A, Kaski M, Iivanainen M (2011) Healthcare and guidelines: A population-based survey of recorded medical problems and health surveillance for people with Down syndrome. *J Intellect Dev Disabil* 36: 118–126.

Mahmoud SA, Lowery-Nordberg M, Chen H, Thurmon T, Ursin S, Bahna SL (2005) Immune defects in subjects with dysmorphic disorders. *Allergy Asthma Proc* 26: 373–381.

Menconi F, Osman R, Monti MC, Greenberg DA, Concepcion ES, Tomer Y (2010) Shared molecular amino acid signature in the HLA-DR peptide binding pocket predisposes to both autoimmune diabetes and thyroiditis. *Proc Natl Acad Sci U S A* 107: 16899–16903.

Mortensen KH, Cleemann L, Hjerrild BEet al. (2009) Increased prevalence of autoimmunity in Turner syndrome—influence of age. *Clin Exp Immunol* 156: 205–210.

Nisihara RM, Utiyama SR, Oliveira NP, Messias-Reason IJ (2010) Mannan-binding lectin deficiency increases the risk of recurrent infections in children with Down's syndrome. *Hum Immunol* 71: 63–66.

Pellegrini FP, Marinoni M, Frangione Vet al. (2012) Down syndrome, autoimmunity and T regulatory cells. *Clin Exp Immunol* 169: 238–243.

Poolman J, Borrow R (2011) Hyporesponsiveness and its clinical implications after vaccination with polysaccharide or glycoconjugate vaccines. *Expert Rev Vaccines* 10: 307–322.

Ram G, Chinen J (2011) Infections and immunodeficiency in Down syndrome. *Clin Exp Immunol* 164: 9–16.

Ruf J, Carayon P (2006) Structural and functional aspects of thyroid peroxidase. *Arch Biochem Biophys* 445: 269–277.

Salisbury D, Ramsay M, Noakes K (2013) *Immunisation against Infectious Disease: The Green Book.* England: Public Health, Hepatitis B, Chapter 18, 161–184.

Tenenbaum A, Chavkin M, Wexler ID, Korem M, Merrick J (2012) Morbidity and hospitalizations of adults with Down syndrome. *Res Dev Disabil* 33: 435–441.

Troisi CL, Heiberg DA, Hollinger FB (1985) Normal immune response to hepatitis B vaccine in patients with Down's syndrome. A basis for immunization guidelines. *JAMA* 254: 3196–3199.

Verstegen RH, Kusters MA, Gemen EF, De Vries E (2010) Down syndrome B-lymphocyte subpopulations, intrinsic defect or decreased T-lymphocyte help. *Pediatr Res* 67: 563–569.

Villano MJ, Huber AK, Greenberg DA, Golden BK, Concepcion E, Tomer Y (2009) Autoimmune thyroiditis and diabetes: Dissecting the joint genetic susceptibility in a large cohort of multiplex families. *J Clin Endocrinol Metab* 94: 1458–1466.

Yamato F, Takaya J, Yasuhara A, Teraguchi M, Ikemoto Y, Kaneko K (2009) Elevated intracellular calcium in neutrophils in patients with Down syndrome. *Pediatr Int* 51: 474–477.

Zachariah P, Ruttenber M, Simoes ES (2012) Down syndrome and hospitalizations due to respiratory syncytial virus: A population-based study. *J Pediatr* 160: 827–831.

8
CARDIOVASCULAR DISEASE

Robert Tulloh, Emma Pascall and Natali Chung

Introduction

People with Down syndrome have a unique range of cardiac and circulatory issues. Historically, these issues were not well-recognized or treated and resulted in significant morbidity and mortality. With early recognition and prompt treatment, outcomes are good. It is mandatory that guidelines are followed to achieve a high standard of care.

The congenital heart diseases (CHDs) seen in Down syndrome are not particularly unusual, although their frequency of distribution is not straightforward. Typical signs and symptoms of congenital and acquired heart disease may not be present in Down syndrome and hence the clinician or parent might not be aware of conditions that need treatment. Changes in the management of children over the last two decades are likely to affect the future long-term management as they reach and progress through adulthood. Moreover, as in the general population, CHD may not be diagnosed until after adulthood is reached. There is also a risk of acquired cardiovascular disease, which may be exacerbated by medical conditions that are more common in the syndrome.

Congenital heart disease

WHAT CONGENITAL HEART DISORDERS OCCUR IN DOWN SYNDROME, AND HOW COMMON ARE THEY?

CHD is present in approximately 40–60% of children with Down syndrome (Weijerman et al. 2010). The classic lesion is the atrioventricular septal defect (AVSD), present in approximately 45% of newborn infants with Down syndrome (Greenwood and Nadas 1976) but which only occurs in less than 0.05% of the general population. Other lesions include ventricular septal defect (VSD, 35%), secundum atrial septal defect (ASD, 8%), persistent ductus arteriosus (PDA, 7%) and Tetralogy of Fallot (4%), as well as a variety of mixed lesions (Roizen and Patterson 2003). Some children with Down syndrome may develop further cardiovascular complications in adolescence, including mitral valve prolapse (46%) and aortic regurgitation (17%; Baraona et al. 2013). It is very rare for children with Down syndrome to have coarctation of the aorta, aortic valve stenosis or transposition of the great arteries.

HOW DOES THE GENETICS OF DOWN SYNDROME RELATE TO CONGENITAL HEART DISEASE?

Although it is known that trisomy 21 is a risk factor for CHD, it is not a sufficient requirement (about 60% of people with trisomy 21 do not have CHD). Sailani et al. (2013) studied single-nucleotide polymorphisms (SNPs) and copy number variations (CNVs) in people with Down syndrome compared with the general population. The study showed that the genetic architecture of the CHD risk in Down syndrome is complex. It includes not only trisomy 21 and chromosome 21 SNP and CNV variations but also as yet-unidentified genetic variation in the rest of the genome.

WHAT IS THE ROLE OF FETAL SCREENING?

In the UK, it is routine practice for women to have a detailed ultrasound scan at around 20 weeks' gestation. In some cases, CHD picked up at this stage prompts further assessment leading to a diagnosis of Down syndrome (see Chapter 3). If Down syndrome is diagnosed antenatally fetal echocardiography by a recognized expert should be offered. This achieves accurate diagnosis and effective counselling for the families.

WHAT SIGNS OR COMPLICATIONS OCCUR DURING FETAL LIFE?

Mitral valve accretions ('golf balls') are strongly associated with Down syndrome during fetal life (Thilaganathan et al. 1999). Postnatally, this condition causes no known concern and further echocardiography is not required. The higher incidence of increased nuchal thickness in Down syndrome is also independently a marker for CHD. Infants with Down syndrome are more likely to develop pleural and pericardial effusion in utero and immediately postnatally. The cause is not known.

HOW DOES CONGENITAL HEART DISEASE PRESENT IN THE NEONATAL PERIOD AND EARLY CHILDHOOD?

In the immediate postnatal period, the pulmonary vascular resistance in Down syndrome tends to remain high. This can cause marked cyanosis, even if there is no CHD present. In those with known large septal defects (such as ventricular or AVSD), the high pulmonary vascular resistance can lead to right-to-left shunting and profound cyanosis in the early postnatal period, often causing some diagnostic confusion. This will gradually resolve and give way to the more usual left-to-right shunt over ensuing weeks.

Children with CHD may present with murmurs, cyanosis, signs of heart failure, faltering growth or may be asymptomatic (Dennis et al. 2010). The current Down Syndrome Medical Interest Group (DSMIG) guidelines for UK and Ireland state that all children with Down syndrome must have an echocardiogram within the first month of life (DSMIG 2007). This is mainly because symptoms may not be immediately apparent and also that pulmonary hypertension may develop earlier in infants with Down syndrome. For those with suspected or proven CHD, a specialist cardiac opinion is required early to decide whether surgical correction or continuing review is required.

Medical management may be required before surgery. For those infants with heart failure and breathlessness due to a left-to-right shunt and a large septal defect, nutritional supplementation is often necessary. Nasogastric tube feeding is helpful to allow the administration of high-calorie feeds to encourage growth prior to surgery. This may be combined with diuretics such as furosemide and spironolactone or amiloride to encourage fluid loss. The drying effect allows the lungs to be less congested and the infant to feel more comfortable.

Addition of angiotensin-converting enzyme inhibitors has to be undertaken with caution since this group will often react by a precipitous fall in blood pressure, making careful observation and repeat renal function tests mandatory.

If children with Down syndrome have concomitant upper airway obstruction and left-to-right shunt through CHD, they may present much later than would the rest of the population. The relative hypoxaemia and hypercarbia will reduce pulmonary blood flow and may limit the symptoms of heart failure. It is important in these late presenters that a full assessment of their physiological status and pulmonary vascular resistance is made. Often, cardiac catheterization is required to determine the safety of forthcoming cardiac surgery. Those in whom the pulmonary vascular resistance is less than $7Um^2$, falling by >20% in nitric oxide, should undergo cardiac surgery (Andrews and Tulloh 2002).

Current best practice suggests that prompt surgical correction of cardiac defects is imperative to prevent the development of irreversible pulmonary vascular disease (Masuda et al. 2005). For those with AVSD or large VSD, routine surgical repair should take place in the first 3–6 months. For lesions without high pulmonary artery pressure, surgery may be offered later, with careful specialist monitoring in the interim.

Children with CHD may be particularly susceptible to respiratory infection. Advice to maximize preventative methods by uptake of routine childhood immunizations, careful hand-washing, avoidance of overcrowding, good hygiene at home and keeping siblings with infection away should be offered.

There is good evidence that Down syndrome brings an increased risk of respiratory syncytial virus (RSV; see Chapter 7). Prophylaxis is advised if there is pulmonary hypertension or unoperated, or only palliated, haemodynamically significant CHD before 2 years of age (Bloemers et al. 2007). Prophylaxis is currently with monoclonal antibody palivizumab given at hospital or community immunization clinics during the winter season.

How does congenital heart disease affect adults?
Despite screening in childhood, CHD may not be diagnosed until later life. A study in Holland found that 17% of people with Down syndrome living in residential homes with no cardiac history were found to have CHD on echocardiography (Vis et al. 2010) including mitral valve abnormalities, ASDs, AVSDs and PDA. Interestingly, all of these people were born before 1980 when childhood screening was not robust. The overall prevalence of CHD in the population studied was 33%.

Some units pursue a policy of screening by echocardiogram in early adult life, or prior to leaving paediatric services, as suggested in DSMIG UK (2007) guidelines. Others reserve screening for those who have not had an echocardiogram in childhood. In all cases, the possibility of previously undetected CHD, should be born in mind, and routine medical review should always include enquiry for possible symptoms and examination for signs of heart disease.

Those diagnosed with CHD in childhood, who have had percutaneous or surgical intervention, may develop further pathology and require further intervention in later life. For example, those with an AVSD often develop significant leaks of the atrioventricular valves.

Arrhythmia related to scarring from previous interventions can also be problematic, resulting in emergency admissions that require standard intervention.

Those newly diagnosed and those under long-term follow-up for adult congenital heart disease (ACHD) should have the same investigations and treatments as those without Down syndrome (although some may need to be under general anaesthetic). The risk of pulmonary hypertension remains raised in adulthood compared with the general population. Diagnostic cardiac catheterization prior to any intervention such as device closure of an ASD or surgical repair of an AVSD is more likely to be required to ensure it is safe to proceed. In older adults, a diagnostic coronary angiogram prior to surgery, which is usually not a requirement in children and young adults, may be needed because of the potential for significant coronary artery disease in later life.

The number of people with CHD in adulthood now exceeds the number of affected children and, with the growing and ageing population of those with ACHD, it is recommended that they are followed up within, or under, the umbrella of a specialist ACHD unit (Warnes et al. 2008, Baumgartner et al. 2010).

Sara, 45 years old, has Down syndrome. A heart lesion was suspected at a young age and after a diagnostic cardiac catheter procedure at age 7, her family was told that she had a hole in her heart, not requiring treatment, and she was not followed up.

By age 40, her exercise capacity had started to decline and she had to leave her job at McDonalds. She became more breathless on exertion, stopped looking after herself and had no energy, making it difficult for her elderly mother to care for her. She was admitted to hospital in heart and respiratory failure and required ventilation on intensive care. Subsequent assessment at a specialist ACHD unit found her to have an AVSD with a large VSD component and pulmonary hypertension as a result of Eisenmenger syndrome. Her breathing was affected by obesity-related hypoventilation similar to sleep apnoea.

With medical treatment, a more active lifestyle, a supervised diet and a move to sheltered accommodation, Sara lost a significant amount of weight with improvement in her exercise capacity. She is followed up at the ACHD pulmonary hypertension clinic. Sara's case highlights the importance of lifelong follow-up for everyone with Down syndrome.

Pulmonary arterial hypertension in children

Pulmonary arterial hypertension (PAH) can be characterized as an elevated pulmonary arterial pressure and is defined as a mean pulmonary arterial pressure greater than 25mmHg at rest or as a tricuspid regurgitation jet greater than 2.7m/s at echocardiography in the absence of right ventricular outflow tract obstruction (Tulloh 2005). Children with Down syndrome have a higher risk of developing PAH than the general population (Hawkins et al. 2011). This is for a variety of reasons, including the increased risk of CHD, structural lung disease and upper airway obstruction. Exposure to increased pulmonary blood flow due to left-to-right intracardiac shunting (Rowland and Nordstrom 1981)

Neonatal	Persistent pulmonary hypertension (idiopathic)
	Respiratory distress syndrome and subsequent chronic lung disease
	Infection, e.g. Streptococcus
	Structural disease, e.g. congenital diaphragmatic hernia
Cardiac	Left-to-right shunt, e.g. ASD, VSD, AVSD, PDA, AP window
	Obstructive lesions, e.g. TAPVC, MS, HLHS, HOCM, DCM
Acquired	Chronic hypoxia: Lymphangiectasia, high altitude
	Scoliosis
	Airway obstruction: tonsillar hypertrophy, tracheal stenosis
	Vasculitic: Connective tissue disease, rheumatoid arthritis, sickle cell
Idiopathic	Sporadic	20% genetic in origin
	Familial	60% genetic in origin

Fig. 8.1. Causes of pulmonary hypertension (Tulloh 2005); ASD, Atrial septal defect; VSD, Ventricular septal defect; AVSD, Atrioventricular septal defect; PDA, Persistent ductus arteriosus; AP, Aortopulmonary; TAPVC, Total anomalous pulmonary venous connection; MS, Mitral stenosis; HLHS, Hypoplastic left heart syndrome; HOCM, Hypertrophic obstructive cardiomyopathy; DCM, Dilated cardiomyopathy.

results in increased shear stress on pulmonary endothelial cells and may impair production of nitric oxide. The pathological changes are characterized by a process of vascular remodelling, eventually leading to the development of plexiform lesions and irreversible pulmonary vascular disease (Rabinovitch et al. 1984).

Amongst the numerous causes of PAH (Fig. 8.1), the presence of a left-to-right shunt and chronic upper airways obstruction (Hawkins et al. 2011) is frequently encountered in children with Down syndrome.

Obstructive sleep apnoea (OSA; de Miguel-Diez et al. 2003) is common in children with Down syndrome, affecting 30–50% compared with 3% of the general paediatric population (see Chapter 9). This may result from a number of factors, including hypotonic upper airway muscles, adeno-tonsillar hypertrophy, macroglossia, glossoptosis, flattened mid-face and narrowed nasopharynx. Down syndrome also brings an increased incidence of malacic airways, in particular laryngomalacia (Mitchell et al. 2003) and a tendency

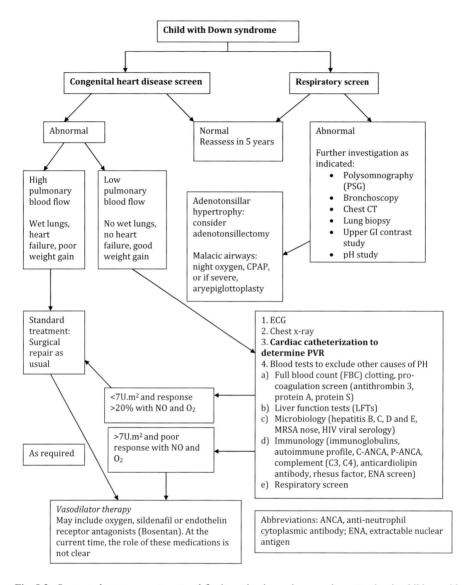

Fig. 8.2. Suggested management protocol for investigating pulmonary hypertension in children with Down syndrome.

towards gastro-oesophageal reflux, which may worsen airways disease (Martin et al. 2005). Upper airways obstruction with repeated episodes of systemic hypoxaemia is associated with the development of increased pulmonary vascular resistance and may contribute to the more rapid development of PAH in children with Down syndrome and left-to-right shunts, leading to irreversible pulmonary vascular disease.

The association of cardiac disease in Down syndrome with PAH has led to neonatal screening and early intervention for cardiac lesions in Down syndrome. It is clear that all those with large left-to-right shunts have the potential to develop pulmonary vascular disease but some do not demonstrate any symptoms due to the raised pulmonary vascular resistance, perhaps associated with upper airways obstruction (Kawai et al. 1995, DSMIG 2007). This is ameliorated, but not abolished by the screening programme and the advent of earlier corrective cardiac surgery at 3–6 months of age (Masuda et al. 2005). However, even with screening, a number will develop PAH and require investigation. Part of this assessment should be a rigorous search for other causes (especially respiratory). Despite recognition of the high prevalence for respiratory disorders in Down syndrome and their association with PAH, there is little published research. A review of 19 children with Down syndrome and PAH showed a wide range of causes (Hawkins et al. 2011). Some children required aggressive management of gastro-oesophageal reflux. Others required aryepiglottoplasty or continuous supplemental oxygen. As a result, a systematic management protocol that includes appropriate investigation and management of the role of airway and respiratory disorders has been suggested (Fig. 8.2). Attention to this subject might allow us to intervene at an early stage and modify the expected outcome.

How is pulmonary hypertension treated in children?

Currently, there is limited research regarding pulmonary hypertension in Down syndrome, and little advice on how it should be managed. It is well recognized that there may be cardiac and respiratory disease with pulmonary hypertension in children with Down syndrome, but there is little information in the literature on how these should be approached together. It is recommended that to ameliorate the symptoms of airways disease and to prevent the development of PAH, aggressive treatment of cardiac, gastro-oesophageal reflux and airways disease should be offered (DSMIG 2001).

Current best practice suggests that prompt surgical correction of cardiac defects is imperative to prevent the development of irreversible pulmonary vascular disease (Masuda et al. 2005). Respiratory disease should be treated aggressively using prophylactic antibiotics, inhaled corticosteroids where appropriate, alongside oxygen and physiotherapy (see Chapter 9). In those with evidence of night-time hypoxia from a sleep study, overnight oxygen therapy can be used. Adenotonsillectomy may be beneficial in those with significant airways obstruction and children with severe laryngo-tracheo-bronchomalacia may require treatment with home oxygen therapy, with or without continuous positive airways pressure, or even aryepiglottoplasty (Martin et al. 2005). Recent reports have suggested that the benefits of adenotonsillectomy in children with Down syndrome may be less clear (Eipe et al. 2009).

Notably, the high prevalence of asymptomatic obstructive airways disease in children with Down syndrome and the risks of developing irreversible PAH support routine sleep studies in children with Down syndrome, even those without symptomatic airway disease (Shott et al. 2006).

The diagnosis of PAH in children with Down syndrome is now important, since there are a number of disease-targeted therapies available, including sildenafil (phosphodiesterase type V inhibitor), riociguat (just licensed for pulmonary hypertension as a guanylate cyclase stimulator), endothelin receptor antagonists (such as bosentan and ambrisentan) and prostanoids—either intravenous epoprostenol or inhaled iloprost (Tulloh 2009). These therapies may be used preoperatively, postoperatively or palliatively. Currently, there are no national guidelines regarding the medical management of patients with PAH in Down syndrome. In practice, many of the methods in use in children without Down syndrome are employed. Ultimately, some may need to undergo transplantation, although referral rates remain low, in part due to concerns regarding postoperative complications and posttransplant malignancy secondary to immunosuppression (Leonard et al. 2000).

The relative contributions of cardiac and airways disease in children with Down syndrome and pulmonary hypertension have yet to be determined. We have also yet to establish the mechanism responsible for the fall in oxygen saturations seen in some of those with airways disease following the administration of nitric oxide. Crucially, further studies are required to facilitate the development of guidelines to establish which drugs are most appropriate for the management of PAH in this group of children.

Pulmonary arterial hypertension and Eisenmenger syndrome in adults with Down syndrome

Historically, children with Down syndrome may not have been offered surgical treatment options for cardiac lesions based on the presence of Down syndrome rather than technical feasibility or medical considerations. Thus, there is currently a large proportion of people with AVSDs and large VSDs who have developed Eisenmenger syndrome: PAH secondary to large left-to-right intracardiac shunts, with subsequent damage to the pulmonary vasculature, reversal of the direction of shunting from right to left and resultant chronic cyanosis. Whilst many will survive into the 4th and 5th decades of life, their life expectancy is reduced (Diller et al. 2006). In the future, with children with Down syndrome being offered the same initial treatments as children with typical development, the number of adults with Eisenmenger syndrome should fall.

There is also a high incidence of PAH in adults due to OSA. OSA may have been present in childhood, but other risk factors for OSA are more common in later life, particularly obesity and hypothyroidism. One American study screened 16 children with Down syndrome and a history of no or previously treated OSA and found 15 to have OSA (Trois et al. 2009). Twelve of these sixteen were obese and the severity of OSA was found to correlate with the degree of obesity.

The diagnosis of PAH and its underlying cause may be difficult in Down syndrome. Difficulty in understanding what is happening to them and fear of medical procedures can make investigation challenging. Often the development of Eisenmenger syndrome is obvious on transthoracic echocardiography (typically large septal defect with bidirectional or right-to-left shunting, right ventricular hypertrophy with flattening of the ventricular septum and dilated pulmonary arteries). This negates the need for diagnostic cardiac catheterization. In fact, catheterization may carry a greater risk in this group, as many require a general anaesthetic with the potential for respiratory/haemodynamic complications, the risk of thrombus formation and paradoxical embolus across the septal defect and problems with haemostasis.

Treatment options for PAH are similar to the paediatric population. Non-invasive ventilation, treatment of any underlying lung pathology and nocturnal oxygen should be used when appropriate. Oral pulmonary vasodilators are currently indicated in those who have significant symptoms of breathlessness. Phosphodiesterase V inhibitors (sildenafil or tadalafil) and/or endothelin receptor antagonists (bosentan and ambrisentan) are the mainstay of treatment. Oral treatments have been shown to improve symptoms and exercise capacity (Galiè et al. 2006, Raposo-Sonnenfeld et al. 2007, Duffels et al. 2009), and some early evidence suggests that treatment may improve survival (Dimopoulos et al. 2010). For those who deteriorate despite oral therapy, nebulized or intravenous prostanoids are an option but are less likely to be tolerated in those with Down syndrome (Galie et al. 2009).

Heart and lung transplantation in adults without Down syndrome who have Eisenmenger syndrome is very rare. Although some people with Down syndrome have received heart transplantation (Irving and Chaudhari 2011), the author is unaware of any who also had Eisenmenger syndrome.

As well as breathlessness, heart failure and reduced life expectancy it should be remembered that the chronic cyanosis of PAH and Eisenmenger syndrome affect many other systems affecting patient morbidity and mortality. Chronically low oxygen levels result in high haemoglobin levels in blood as a compensatory mechanism to increase oxygen-carrying capacity. This increase in blood viscosity can increase the risk of stroke and treatment for Eisenmenger syndrome used to include regular venesections to reduce the haemoglobin levels and packed cell volume. However, we now know that this results in iron deficiency and a relative anaemia that can exacerbate fatigue and shortness of breath. Practice has therefore changed and venesection should only be used if there are true symptoms of hyperviscosity syndrome (headaches, lassitude, visual or neurological symptoms) without dehydration.

WHAT NON-CONGENITAL CARDIOVASCULAR PROBLEMS OCCUR IN PEOPLE WITH DOWN SYNDROME?
Mean life expectancy in Down syndrome has changed dramatically over the last 50 years, from 12 years in the 1940s to a current mean of approximately 60 years. As for the general population, people with Down syndrome, with or without CHD, may develop cardiovascular problems as they age. However, despite premature ageing and the high prevalence of obesity, diabetes mellitus and dyslipidaemia, the prevalence of hypertension and coronary artery disease appears to be lower than the general population. In fact, a post-mortem study (Murdoch et al. 1977) proposed Down syndrome as an atheroma-free model and a review of mortality in Down syndrome found only 12 instances of coronary artery disease out of 150 deaths in adults with Down syndrome (Bittles et al. 2006). A lower incidence of hypertension and smoking in Down syndrome may contribute to the lower rate, but is unlikely to account for it fully. Increased cystathionine synthase activity may play a role. If coronary artery disease is diagnosed, standard management pathways should be followed including percutaneous coronary intervention.

The high prevalence of hypothyroidism in adults with Down syndrome affects myocardial function and systemic vascular resistance. This can result in a drop in cardiac output and an increase in diastolic blood pressure. Moreover, changes in the QT interval may predispose to ventricular arrhythmia (Vis et al. 2009). Conversely, hyperthyroidism causes increased cardiac output, sinus tachycardia or atrial fibrillation and increased systolic blood pressure (with an increase in pulse pressure). Either extreme can result in heart failure, palpitations or syncope (Klein and Danzi 2007). Hypothyroidism also has a strong association with hyperlipidaemia, which in combination with blood pressure changes could theoretically increase the risk of coronary artery disease. Treatment should be aimed at the underlying thyroid abnormality alongside the medical treatment of heart failure and arrhythmia. The high prevalence of thyroid dysfunction and potential for cardiac complications lend weight to the argument for routine screening of thyroid function in Down syndrome (see Chapter 11).

What general health issues need to be considered in people with Down syndrome who have cardiac disease?

Although CHD and pulmonary hypertension have historically been the main cardiac focus in Down syndrome, we are likely to see an increasing burden of other cardiovascular diseases as life expectancy increases. An emphasis on continuing cardiovascular prevention should therefore be present from early life with attention paid to weight, thyroid function, lipid disorders and regular exercise as well as screening for OSA and other causes of pulmonary hypertension. Investigations for undiagnosed CHD and pulmonary hypertension should be considered in any person with Down syndrome with symptoms of breathlessness or other cardiac symptoms.

Those affected by CHD will need to continue with sensible measures in the prevention of endocarditis: namely good dental hygiene with regular dental visits and the avoidance of tattoos and body piercing. The routine use of a large preventative dose of antibiotic prior to dental treatment is no longer recommended in some countries, but patients and carers can check the advice of their specialist cardiac centre (NICE Guidance UK 2008).

Unplanned pregnancy in Down syndrome can be a challenge, but unplanned pregnancy in the presence of significant cardiac abnormalities or pulmonary hypertension can also cause significant morbidity and mortality. Women should use a reliable form of contraception (usually hormonal) and if pregnancy is considered, those with cardiac problems should have an up-to-date review prior to stopping contraception to assess their cardiovascular risk in pregnancy. Despite some improvements in the care of pregnant women with pulmonary hypertension, it is still associated with significant maternal mortality (over 30%; Bedard et al. 2009) and termination of pregnancy is usually advised. For those with pulmonary hypertension and many congenital cardiac lesions, progesterone-only contraceptive should be used because of the higher risk of thrombosis with oestrogen-containing preparations. Intramuscular depot injections or a subdermal implant are often good choices, as they do not rely on women taking a pill on a regular basis (see Chapter 4).

The care of any person with Down syndrome and cardiovascular disease will need to be individualized. Some may tolerate regular medication, investigations and blood tests very well, whilst just attending a hospital may be a major hurdle for others. A multidisciplinary team including specialist cardiac centres, community services, family and carers should provide support. The importance of good communication between team members is often highlighted when admission to hospital is required for investigations and procedures. Careful preparation of the individual and family/carers prior to admission along with appropriate protocols and sufficient staffing will help inpatient management to run more smoothly.

Finally, despite all the advances in cardiovascular medicine and surgery, a significant number of individuals with Down syndrome will die from long-term complications of CHD and pulmonary hypertension before senescence (Bittles et al. 2006). Excellent palliative and end-of-life care will remain important services for all those with Down syndrome and should be a topic of continuing dialogue with carers, even if not required straightaway.

Key points
- 40–60% of children with Down syndrome will have a congenital heart anomaly.
- Congenital heart disease (CHD) is usually detectable during fetal life by a specialized fetal cardiologist.
- A normal echocardiogram does not rule out heart disease, but it should exclude the major conditions.
- Small holes, persistent arterial ducts and atrial septal defects may not be detected by examination or echocardiogram.
- The risk of pulmonary hypertension is greater in people with Down syndrome than in the general population.
- Pulmonary artery hypertension may be caused by the presence of CHD, with or without concurrent airways disease.
- Prompt surgical correction of cardiac defects can help prevent the development of irreversible pulmonary vascular disease.
- Failure to operate in a timely manner on significant lesions will lead to a shortened life expectancy and complications in middle adult life or earlier.
- All children should be offered the same management for heart disease, regardless of whether or not they have Down syndrome.
- Upper airways obstruction may be a significant contributing factor to the development of pulmonary hypertension.

REFERENCES

Andrews R, Tulloh R (2002) Pulmonary hypertension in pediatrics. *Curr Opin Pediatr* 14: 603–605.

Baraona F, Gurvitz M, Landzberg MJ, Opotowsky AR (2013) Hospitalizations and mortality in the United States for adults with Down syndrome and congenital heart disease. *Am J Cardiol* 111: 1046–1051. PubMed PMID: 23332593. doi: 10.1016/j.amjcard.2012.12.025.

Baumgartner H, Bonhoeffer P, De Groot NMS et al. (2010) ESC guidelines for the management of grown-up congenital heart disease (new version 2010). *Eur Heart J* 31: 2915. doi: 10.1093/eurheartj/ehq249.

Bedard E, Dimopoulos K, Gatzoulis MA (2009) Has there been any progress made on pregnancy outcomes among women with pulmonary arterial hypertension? *Eur Heart J* 30: 256. doi: 10.1093/eurheartj/ehn597.

Bittles AH, Bower C, Hussain R, Glasson EJ (2006) The four ages of Down syndrome. *Eur J Public Health* 17: 221. doi: 10.1093/eurpub/ckl103.

Bloemers BL, van Furth AM, Weijerman ME et al. (2007) Down syndrome: A novel risk factor for respiratory syncytial virus bronchiolitis—a prospective birth-cohort study. *Pediatrics* 120: e1076–e1081. doi: 10.1542/peds.2007-0788.

de Miguel-Diez J, Villa-Asensi J, Alvarez-Sala JL (2003) Prevalence of sleep-disordered breathing in children with Down syndrome: Polygraphic findings in 108 children. *Sleep* 26: 1006–1009.

Dennis J, Archer N, Ellis J, Marder L (2010) Recognising heart disease in children with Down syndrome. *Arch Dis Child Educ Pract Ed* 95: 98–104. PubMed PMID: 20688855. doi: 10.1136/adc.2007. 126672.

Diller GP, Dimopoulos K, Broberg CS et al. (2006) Presentation, survival prospects, and predictors of death in Eisenmenger syndrome: A combined retrospective and case-control study. *Eur Heart J* 27: 1737–1742. Epub 22 June 2006. doi: 10.1093/eurheartj/ehl116.

Dimopoulos K, Inuzuka R, Goletto S et al. (2010) Improved survival among patients with Eisenmenger syndrome receiving advanced therapy for pulmonary arterial hypertension. *Circulation* 121: 20. doi: 10.1161/CIRCULATIONAHA.109.883876.

Down Syndrome Medical Interest Group (DSMIG) (2001) Respiratory disorders with Down's syndrome: Overview with diagnostic and treatment options. http://www.dsmig.org.uk/ (accessed January 2014).

Down Syndrome Medical Interest Group (DSMIG) (2007) Basic medical surveillance essentials for people with Down's syndrome – cardiac disease: Congenital and acquired. http://www.dsmig.org.uk/ (accessed January 2014).

Duffels MG, Vis JC, van Loon RL et al. (2009) Effect of bosentan on exercise capacity and quality of life in adults with pulmonary arterial hypertension associated with congenital heart disease with and without Down syndrome. *Am J Cardiol* 103: 1309–1315. doi: 10.1016/j.amjcard.2009.01.021.

Eipe N, Lai L, Doherty D (2009) Severe pulmonary hypertension and adenotonsillectomy in a child with trisomy-21 and obstructive sleep apnoea. *Pediatr Anesth* 19: 541–553. doi: 10.1111/j.1460-9592.2009.02936.x.

Galie N, Beghetti M, Gatzoulis MA et al. (2006) Bosentan therapy in patients with Eisenmenger syndrome a multicenter, double-blind, randomized, placebo-controlled study. *Circulation* 114: 48. doi: 10.1161/CIRCULATIONAHA.106.630715.

Galie N, Hoeper MM, Humbert M et al. (2009) Guidelines for the diagnosis and treatment of pulmonary hypertension: The Task Force for the Diagnosis and Treatment of Pulmonary Hypertension of the European Society of Cardiology (ESC) and the European Respiratory Society (ERS), endorsed by the International Society of Heart and Lung Transplantation (ISHLT). *Eur Heart J* 30: 2493. doi: 10.1093/eurheartj/ehp297.

Greenwood RD, Nadas AS (1976) The clinical course of cardiac disease in Down's syndrome. *Pediatrics* 58: 893–897.

Hawkins A, Henderson J, Langton-Hewer S, Tulloh R (2011) Management of pulmonary hypertension in Down's syndrome. *Eur J Pediatr* 170: 915–921. doi: 10.1007/s00431-010-1378-1.

Irving CA, Chaudhari MP (2011) Cardiovascular abnormalities in Down's syndrome: Spectrum, management and survival over 22 years. *Arch Dis Child* 97: 326. doi: 10.1136/adc.2010.210534.

Kawai T, Wada Y, Enmoto T et al. (1995) Comparison of hemodynamic data before and after corrective surgery for Down's syndrome and ventricular septal defect. *Heart Vessels* 10: 154–157.

Klein I, Danzi S (2007) Thyroid disease and the heart. *Circulation* 116: 1725–1735. doi: 10.1161/CIRCULATIONAHA.106.678326.

Leonard H, Eastham K, Dark J (2000) Heart and heart lung transplantation in Down's syndrome. *BMJ* 320: 816–817.

Martin JE, Howarth KE, Khodaei I, Karkanevatos A, Clarke RW (2005) Aryepiglottoplasty for laryngomalacia: The Alder Hey experience. *J Laryngol Otol* 119: 958–960.

Masuda M, Kado H, Tanoue Y et al. (2005) Does Down syndrome affect the long-term results of complete atrioventricular septal defect when the defect is repaired during the first year of life? *Eur J Cardiothorac Surg* 27: 405–409. doi: 10.1016/j.ejcts.2004.11.027.

Mitchell RB, Call E, Kelly J (2003) Diagnosis and therapy for airway obstruction in children with Down syndrome. *Arch Otolaryngol Head Neck Surg* 129: 642–645. doi: 10.1001/archotol.129.6.642.

Murdoch JC, Rodger JC, Rao SS et al. (1977) Down's syndrome: An atheroma-free model? *BMJ* 2: 226.

NICE Clinical Guideline 64 (2008) Prophylaxis against infective endocarditis: Antimicrobial prophylaxis against infective endocarditis in adults and children undergoing interventional procedures. www.nice.org.uk/CG064.

Rabinovitch M, Keane JF, Norwood WI, Castaneda AR, Reid L (1984) Vascular structure in lung tissue obtained at biopsy correlated with pulmonary hemodynamic findings after repair of congenital heart defects. *Circulation* 69: 655–667. doi: 10.1161/01.CIR.69.4.655.

Raposo-Sonnenfeld I, Otero-González I, Blanco-Aparicio M et al. (2007) Treatment with sildenafil, bosentan or both in children and young people with idiopathic pulmonary hypertension and Eisenmenger's syndrome. *Rev Esp Cardiol* 60: 366–372.

Roizen NJ, Patterson D (2003) Down's syndrome. *Lancet* 361: 1281–1289. doi: 0.1016/S0140-6736 (03)12987-X.

Rowland TW, Nordstrom LG, Bean MS, Burkhardt H (1981) Chronic upper airway obstruction and pulmonary hypertension in Down's syndrome. *Am J Dis Child* 135: 1050–1052.

Sailani MR, Makrythanasis P, Valsesia A et al. (2013) The complex SNP and CNV genetic architecture of the increased risk of congenital heart defects in Down syndrome. *Genome Res* 23: 1410–1421. doi: 10.1101/gr.147991.112. Epub 19 June 2013. doi: 10.1101/gr.147991.112.

Shott SR, Amin R, Chini B, Heubi C, Hotze S, Akers R (2006) Obstructive sleep apnea: Should all children with Down syndrome be tested? *Arch Otolaryngol Head Neck Surg* 132: 432–436. doi: 10.1001/archotol.132.4.432.

Thilaganathan B, Olawaiye A, Sairam S, Harrington K (1999) Isolated foetal echogenic intracardiac foci or golf balls: Is karyotyping for Down's syndrome indicated? *Br J Obstet Gynaecol* 106: 1294–1297.

Trois MS, Capone GT, Lutz JA et al. (2009) Obstructive sleep apnea in adults with Down's syndrome. *J Clin Sleep Med* 5: 317.

Tulloh R (2005) Congenital heart disease in relation to pulmonary hypertension in paediatric practice. *Paediatr Respir Rev* 6: 174–180. doi: 10.1016/j.prrv.2005.06.010.

Tulloh R (2009) Etiology, diagnosis and pharmacologic treatment of pediatric pulmonary hypertension. *Pediatr Drugs* 11: 115–128. doi: 0.2165/00148581-200911020-00003.

Vis JC, de Bruin-Bon RH, Bouma BJ et al. (2010) Congenital heart defects are under-recognised in adult patients with Down syndrome. *Heart* 96: 1480. doi: 10.1136/hrt.2010.197509.

Vis JC, Duffels MG, Winter MM et al. (2009) Down syndrome: A cardiovascular perspective. *J Intellect Disabil Res* 53: 419. doi: 10.1111/j.1365-2788.2009.01158.x.

Warnes CA, Williams RG, Bashore TM et al. (2008) ACC/AHA 2008 guidelines for the management of adults with congenital heart disease: A report of the American College of Cardiology/American Heart Association Task Force on Practice Guidelines (writing committee to develop guidelines on the management of adult with congenital heart disease. *Circulation* 118: e714–e833. doi: 10.1161/CIRCULATIONAHA.108.190690.

Weijerman ME, van Furth AM, van der Mooren MD et al. (2010) Prevalence of congenital heart defects and persistent pulmonary hypertension of the neonate with Down syndrome. *Eur J Pediatr* 169: 1195–1199. PubMed PMID: 20411274. Pubmed Central PMCID: 2926442. doi: 10.1007/s00431-010-1200-0.

9
RESPIRATORY DISEASE

Hazel Evans, Katy Pike, Marian McGowan and Sally Shott

Introduction

Although children with Down syndrome are probably healthier today than they have ever been before and can look forward to a considerably increased life expectancy compared with previous generations, they continue to experience more illness than their peers with typical development. In particular, pre-school children often seem to go from one respiratory infection to another.

Respiratory illnesses are the predominant source of mortality in individuals with Down syndrome and the second most common cause of death during childhood (Bittles et al. 2007). In infants and young children, respiratory disease is the most likely reason for hospitalization (So et al. 2007) and also for intensive care admission (Hilton et al. 1999). While hospital data indicate that excess numbers of children with Down syndrome are admitted with lower respiratory infections, this number is overshadowed by the many episodes managed in the community.

Despite the prevalence of respiratory disease in children with Down syndrome, it is often under-recognized. Optimal care requires comprehensive monitoring for respiratory problems and aggressive treatment of reversible conditions including gastro-oesophageal reflux, recurrent pulmonary aspiration and poor immune function.

Why are people with Down syndrome prone to respiratory disease?

Structural anomalies of the respiratory tract, pulmonary vascular disease and immune dysfunction are all more common in Down syndrome. This confers increased vulnerability to lower respiratory disease, compounded by upper airway, cardiac and other problems frequently associated with Down syndrome (Box 9.1). Together these abnormalities predispose children with Down syndrome to airway obstruction and chronic or intermittent hypoxaemia (Fitzgerald et al. 2007).

Structure of airways

A number of the phenotypic features of Down syndrome narrow the upper airway (Shott 2006a). Significant phenotypic features include mid-face hypoplasia, mandibular hypoplasia, choanal stenosis, short palate, relative macroglossia, medially displaced tonsils and adenoids sitting in a contracted nasopharynx. These structural abnormalities may be exacerbated by functional abnormalities such as increased secretions, hypotonia and secondary effects of comorbid conditions, particularly tonsillar and adenoidal enlargement, gastro-oesophageal

---

Box 9.1 Contributors to respiratory disease

Congenital abnormalities of the respiratory tract
  • Pulmonary hypoplasia
  • Parenchymal lung disease
  • Subpleural cysts
  • Tracheobronchomalacia
Pulmonary vascular disease
Immune dysfunction
Comorbid conditions
  • Hypotonia
  • Relative obesity
  • Cardiac disease
  • GORD

---

reflux disease (GORD) and obesity. GORD, for example, can cause oedema of the posterior pharyngeal area, further decreasing the overall size of the airway.

Narrowing of the upper airway predisposes children with Down syndrome to obstructive sleep apnoea (OSA) and increases the severity of airway obstruction during episodes of infection. It also increases the difficulty and risk associated with anaesthesia and intubation. Laryngomalacia occurs in association with Down syndrome and is a common cause of upper airway obstruction, particularly in infancy (Mitchell et al. 2003).

Structural abnormalities of the upper airway may compound abnormalities of the lower airway structure. The most commonly associated lower airway abnormality is tracheobronchomalacia (Bertrand et al. 2003). Tracheomalacia is often attributable to extrinsic compression as a consequence of congenital heart disease (CHD) and usually presents in infancy with feeding difficulties, vomiting and biphasic stridor (Box 9.2). Bronchomalacia may be of similar aetiology but tends to present with recurrent chest infections or to be diagnosed following chest radiograph or bronchoscopy.

Subglottic stenosis is thought to be more common in Down syndrome but, as many children with Down syndrome are intubated for surgery, it may reflect acquired stenosis.

Box 9.2 Presenting features of tracheobronchomalacia

• Recurrent chest infections
• Stridor
• Monophonic wheeze or wheeze resistant to asthma therapy
• Cough
• Sudden collapse (caused by a vicious cycle of respiratory distress, increased intrathoracic pressure and airway compression)
• Failure to extubate or disproportionate ventilatory requirement relative to lung disease

---

The relatively high incidence of children with Down syndrome undergoing laryngotracheal reconstruction (Boseley et al. 2001) and tracheal dimensions, measured by MRI, suggests that children with Down syndrome do indeed have smaller airways (Shott 2000).

The likelihood of a tracheal bronchus in Down syndrome is up to 10 times higher than (estimated 2%) in the general population. The presence of a tracheal bronchus may predispose to atelectasis and infection in the right upper lobe, particularly in the first 2 years of life. In contrast, abnormal segmental bronchial branching, which is also often found in association with Down syndrome, is usually asymptomatic (Bertrand et al. 2003). Complete tracheal rings are also believed to occur with increased frequency. This condition may be symptomatic only during upper respiratory infections but can present with severe respiratory distress and laryngotracheal reconstruction may be required if airway growth is insufficient to relieve symptoms (Rutter et al. 2004).

Abnormal lung development and parenchymal lung disease

Down syndrome is associated with abnormal lung development, parenchymal abnormalities and pulmonary hypoplasia. Abnormalities of increased alveolar size, distended alveolar ducts and reduced alveolar number originate during early postnatal life suggesting that Down syndrome is characterized by inadequate alveolarization of the terminal lung units (Gonzalez et al. 1991).

Diffuse parenchymal lung disease in children with Down syndrome may be asymptomatic but more commonly presents as dyspnoea, wheezing, cough, crackles or hypoxia accompanied by persistent chest radiograph changes. Parenchymal abnormalities are a feature of pulmonary hypoplasia but also occur with interstitial lung diseases such as pulmonary lymphangiectasia or lymphoid interstitial pneumonitis. Importantly, parenchymal abnormalities may develop secondarily to chronic aspiration, cardiac or pulmonary vascular disease, infection or pulmonary haemorrhage.

The characteristic abnormalities of alveolar and connective tissues found in Down syndrome are believed to contribute to pulmonary cyst formation (Biko et al. 2008). Although rarely seen in the general population, they occur in 20–36% of children with Down syndrome (Gonzalez et al. 1991) and more commonly in those with coexistent CHD (Biko et al. 2008). Subpleural cysts are generally numerous, small (1–4mm diameter) and may communicate with more proximal air spaces (Gonzalez et al. 1991). CT imaging is needed to detect subpleural cysts since they are difficult to detect on plain chest films (Biko et al. 2008). Generally, individuals with subpleural cysts suffer no obvious impairment, although it is possible that subpleural cysts might increase the risk of pneumothorax during mechanical ventilation.

Pulmonary vascular disease

Persistent pulmonary hypertension (PHT) of the newborn occurs disproportionately commonly in infants with Down syndrome (Weijerman et al. 2010). Likely mechanisms for this include structural vascular abnormalities and genetic polymorphisms influencing regulators of pulmonary vascular resistance. The risk of pulmonary oedema, pulmonary haemorrhage, and Eisenmenger syndrome is also increased. PHT may occur as a consequence of chronic lung disease or OSA whilst pulmonary hypoplasia may be a further risk factor since development of the capillary bed in the lungs parallels that of the alveolar surface area. Pulmonary haemorrhage may be asymptomatic, present acutely with haemoptysis and respiratory failure, or present subacutely with iron deficiency, chronic dyspnoea or diffuse interstitial disease. Pulmonary haemorrhage in Down syndrome may be secondary to CHD (Aceti et al. 2012). Recurrent pneumonia, pulmonary aspiration, congenital lung malformations or autoimmune phenomena, such as capillaritis, also predispose to pulmonary haemorrhage. Children with Down syndrome appear to have particularly fragile pulmonary capillaries placing them at risk of developing pulmonary oedema.

Immune dysfunction
Immune dysfunction affecting both humoral and cellular immunity predisposes to respiratory infection (see Chapter 7). In recurrent infection, decreased salivary IgA and IgG may be important (Chaushu et al. 2003). Respiratory immune defence is functionally impaired by increased mucus secretion and by reduced respiratory cilia beat frequency, a likely consequence of recurrent respiratory infection (Piatti et al. 2001).

Gastro-oesophageal reflux disease
GORD is dealt with in detail in Chapter 13. It can precipitate significant respiratory morbidity and cause chronic cough, stridor, wheezing, recurrent pneumonia or apnoea. In the face of significant symptoms treatment with prokinetics, proton-pump inhibitors or fundoplication may be necessary.

How do respiratory disorders affect people with Down syndrome?
UPPER RESPIRATORY TRACT
Nasal Congestion
Parents often report that their child seems to go straight from one 'cold' to the next and certainly the picture of the chronically catarrhal child with an almost permanently running nose is a common sight in children with Down syndrome. Although often dismissed by doctors as a minor problem, these symptoms can result in much misery for the children and may be socially inhibiting as the sight of a constantly dripping nose may not endear a child to others.

Stridor
Infants with Down syndrome often present with stridor. This may be due to structural anomalies such as laryngomalacia, tracheomalacia and tracheal anomalies as described above, or may occur following intubation for respiratory illness or surgery. Any of these conditions, or generally smaller upper airways combined with hypotonia may predispose to stridor occurring in the context of upper airway infection.

Sleep-related upper airway obstruction
Many children with Down syndrome are reported to snore loudly, breathe deeply or have long respiratory pauses during sleep. They may sleep in unusual positions such as sitting

up, with neck extended or flopped forward in order to optimize their airways. Sleep-disordered breathing is a significant cause of morbidity in this population (Mitchell et al. 2003, Vernail et al. 2004, Shott 2006a).

Studies report a 50–100% incidence of OSA syndrome in individuals with Down syndrome with almost 60% having abnormal sleep studies by age 3.5–4 years (Shott et al. 2006b). Evidence shows that these numbers increase with age (Marcus et al. 1991, Levanon et al. 1999, Dyken et al. 2003). Fitzgerald et al. (2007) showed a 97% incidence of OSA in children with Down syndrome who snored, aged 0.2–19 years (4.9 years mean age).

Sleep-disturbed breathing has been shown to affect cognitive abilities, behaviour, growth rate and the more serious consequences of pulmonary hypertension and cor pulmonale (Southall et al. 1987, Bonnet 1989, Marcus et al. 1991, Breslin et al. 2014). Because of the high incidence of underlying congenital cardiac anomalies, there is a higher risk for children with Down syndrome to develop these more severe complications (Jacobs et al. 1996; Levine and Simpser 1982).

LOWER RESPIRATORY TRACT
The combined effects of immune and airway defects place children with Down syndrome at increased risk of respiratory infections (Davidson 2008). Admissions for respiratory illnesses other than asthma occur more commonly, last longer and are more costly when compared with individuals without Down syndrome (Hilton et al. 1999).

Lower respiratory tract infections occur more commonly in children with Down syndrome than in those without (Weir et al. 2007). The most common cause for admission to hospital, to intensive care and the primary indication for ventilatory support in children with Down syndrome is pneumonia. A comparison of rates of lower respiratory tract infection in individuals with Down syndrome and their healthy siblings suggests that reduced levels of IgG2, total lymphocytes, T-lymphocytes, invariant natural killer cells and regulatory T-cells might contribute to the higher susceptibility to lower respiratory tract infections associated with Down syndrome (Broers et al. 2012). Airway abnormalities and aspiration due to disordered swallowing (Frazier and Friedman 1996) and GORD (Weir et al. 2007) also contribute to the elevated risk.

Down syndrome has been identified as an independent risk factor for severe respiratory syncytial virus (RSV) bronchiolitis (Bloemers et al. 2007). This may be as a consequence of immune dysfunction or increased airway responsiveness. Hospitalization with RSV bronchiolitis is more common and, in contrast to children without Down syndrome, may occur beyond the first 2 years of life (Megged and Schlesinger 2010). Hospitalization may be prolonged in those with both Down syndrome and CHD (Hilton et al. 1999). Since children with Down syndrome appear particularly vulnerable to RSV bronchiolitis, it has been suggested that passive immunoprophylaxis should be considered for all children with Down syndrome (Fitzgerald 2009).

Wheeze
Recurrent wheeze is very common among children with Down syndrome, occurring in up to 36% (Bloemers et al. 2010). Treatment with antiasthmatic medication, however, is usually

unsuccessful (McDowell and Craven 2011) and important factors other than asthma such as hypotonia, reduced elastic recoil of lung tissue, chronic aspiration or tracheomalacia may account for recurrent wheeze (Bloemers et al. 2010). Many studies have reported decreased asthma prevalence in children with Down syndrome (Weijerman et al. 2011) and traditional risk factors for asthma including atopy (Weijerman et al. 2011) and previous RSV infection (Bloemers et al. 2010) are not associated with wheezing in Down syndrome. It appears likely that mechanisms separate to those responsible for asthma underlie wheeze in children with Down syndrome.

OXYGEN DEPENDENCY

Children with Down syndrome may need oxygen therapy to relieve symptoms and effects of hypoxemia due to pulmonary hypertension, interstitial lung disease or OSA. Individual management for the causes of hypoxemia should be addressed. For children with OSA, adenotonsillectomy should be considered as well as non-invasive ventilation. In those who do not tolerate facemask ventilation, oxygen can be used to correct hypoxemia. Long-term oxygen therapy for pulmonary hypertension may relieve symptoms (D'Alto and Mahadevan 2012). Following respiratory infection requiring hospitalization, children with Down syndrome often remain oxygen dependent for several weeks.

LIFE-THREATENING EVENTS

The pattern of comorbidities associated with Down syndrome increases the risk of apparent life-threatening events. During such an event of respiratory origin, children present with apnoea and cyanosis. Causes of apnoea in children with Down syndrome include GORD, viral lower respiratory tract infection (particularly bronchiolitis) and airway abnormality.

How should possible respiratory disease be investigated?

Investigation into possible underlying causes or factors contributing to respiratory problems in the child with Down syndrome requires a structured multidisciplinary approach (Box 9.3) involving clinicians from a number of different disciplines (Watts and Vyas 2013).

Given the frequency with which cardiac and upper airway problems cause lower airway symptoms, referral to cardiology and ear, nose and throat specialists should be made early. Upper gastrointestinal imaging is important to identify GORD and to exclude compression

---

Box 9.3 Steps for investigating of respiratory symptoms

1. Review cardiac status
2. Assess for upper airway obstruction
3. Check immune status
4. Upper GI contrast series
5. 24-hour pH probe
6. Flexible bronchoscopy
7. Repeat steps 1 and 2

---

of the trachea by vascular structures. Other useful investigations include a 24-hour pH probe, flexible bronchoscopy and oximetry. It is also important to consider an underlying immunodeficiency in any child presenting with recurrent pneumonia or other serious bacterial infection, so screening tests of immune function including serum immunoglobulins, IgG subclasses, standard vaccines responses and T- and B-cell subsets may be indicated.

How is sleep-disordered breathing assessed? Should we screen for it?
Although there is increasing awareness of sleep-related breathing disorders amongst the public and clinicians, the availability of diagnostic services is limited. Unpublished data (Hadjikoumi et al.—personal communication 2013) suggest not only a lack of parental awareness of the problem (although this is probably changing in the light of increased publicity) but also that paediatricians do not routinely enquire about potential symptoms during clinic appointments. Unfortunately, several studies have shown that parental reporting is unreliable with low correlation between parental reports regarding their child's sleep patterns and polysomnogram or sleep study results (Shott et al. 2006b).

The concern, therefore, is that the problem remains underdiagnosed and may be subject to the phenomenon of 'diagnostic overshadowing' with symptoms such as behavioural difficulties or somnolence being attributed to Down syndrome rather than to the underlying sleep disorder. Because of this, there have been suggestions that all children with Down syndrome should be screened for the presence of upper airway obstruction in sleep.

The Royal College of Paediatrics and Child Health (2009) Working Party on Sleep Physiology and Respiratory Control Disorders in Childhood recommended screening with pulse oximetry for all young children with Down syndrome. However, such a programme presents significant logistical challenges and unpublished data presented at a meeting of the UK and Ireland Down Syndrome Medical Interest Group in 2012 suggested that, 3 years later, only a handful of units in the UK had set up such screening programmes. A further difficulty is the emerging evidence that oximetry is not an adequate tool for screening as it carries a high false-negative rate.

A sleep study or polysomnogram continues to be the criterion standard test from which to evaluate sleep-disordered breathing and sleep apnoea. The most recent American Academy of Pediatrics (2001) guidelines for health care for children with Down syndrome (Bull 2011) recommend a sleep study in all children with Down syndrome by age 4 years. The need is for a simple, easily administered, highly sensitive and economical screening tool. Research initiatives in the UK are now addressing this question.

More detailed assessment may be required in some cases to establish the site of the upper airway obstruction. Examination of the nose should be done to rule out nasal septal deviation, nasal obstruction from enlarged nasal turbinates as well as regrowth of adenoid tissue. Lateral neck radiographs are helpful to evaluate for adenoid regrowth. Regrowth of adenoids was seen in over 60% of children with Down syndrome who had persistent OSA after previous adenotonsillectomy (tonsils and adenoids [T&A]) (Donnelly et al. 2004).

Flexible endoscopy, under general anaesthetic, can be good for diagnosing obstruction from nasal septal deviation, adenoid regrowth and from enlarged lingual tonsils or base of tongue lesions. The position of the base of tongue and epiglottis can be assessed. Endoscopy may also help diagnose tracheomalacia or laryngomalacia, which may only be seen while the child is relaxed and asleep.

Flexible endoscopy does have some limitations. The general anaesthesia level that is required for airway instrumentation may exacerbate airway collapse and give false-positive findings. As only one airway level can be viewed at a time, primary and secondary sites of obstruction cannot be established.

Cine MRI is another way to evaluate the airway. This is a high-resolution, dynamic examination of the airway where 128 MRI images of the airway are taken over 2 minutes. The images are obtained with snoring or oxygen desaturations. This study is done with sedation but less than that needed for airway instrumentation and is especially useful in those with complex airways. It provides both static and dynamic images for evaluation of site(s) of obstruction and allows assessment of multiple levels of airway at the same time, so one can more easily identify primary and secondary levels of obstruction. Studies have shown that the cine MRI has high success in identifying sites of residual obstruction in children with Down syndrome who continue to have OSA after T&A (Donnelly et al. 2004).

How do we treat respiratory problems?

Treatment of respiratory problems may also require a structured multidisciplinary approach (Box 9.4). Management aims are to reduce lung damage and minimize hypoxemia. Most commonly, this involves identification and treatment of reversible causes of airway obstruction and parenchymal disease, the specific treatment in each case reflecting the underlying condition.

Box 9.4 Treatment of respiratory symptoms

- Treat cardiac disease aggressively
- Treat GORD aggressively
- Treat upper airway disease aggressively
- Treat lower airway disease
- Consider physiotherapy during relapse
- Consider supplementary oxygen
- Non-invasive ventilation rarely needed

A 6-month-old girl with Down syndrome and previously repaired VSD was admitted with severe respiratory distress (Fig. 9.1).

Following stabilization, she was investigated as follows:

1. Cardiac echo—stable cardiodynamics
2. pH probe—significant reflux with a reflux index 13%
3. Bronchoscopy and bronchoalveolar lavage—haemosiderin-laden macrophages

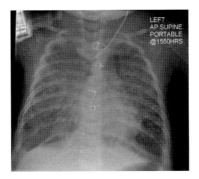

Fig. 9.1. Upon admission with respiratory distress the lungs were hyperinflated with bilateral air space shadowing showing more confluent perihilar distribution. There was a small right-sided pleural effusion and a suggestion of septal lines particularly on the right, raising the possibility of interstitial lung disease.

The differential diagnosis included inflammatory, infectious and fibrosing disease as well as pulmonary venous congestion. She was commenced on lansoprazole for GORD and, given that pulmonary fibrosis might be an indication for long-term steroids, an open lung biopsy was performed. The biopsy revealed

1. *parenchymal changes consistent with Down syndrome (poor alveolar development, subpleural cysts and fibrosis),*
2. *changes consistent with CHD (muscularization of the intra-acinar arteries mild haemosiderosis),*
3. *mild venous changes consistent with venous obstruction,*
4. *prominent lymphangiectasia.*

In view of these findings, a medium-chain triglyceride-based milk was started to reduce infiltration of the lymphatics. During outpatient follow-up, blood was sent for full blood count and immunoglobulin screen, and an overnight pulse oximetry study was conducted to assess oxygen requirement and azithromycin prophylaxis started for the winter months. One year after her initial presentation, the girl's chest was clear and she was able to discontinue home oxygen (Fig. 9.2).

If cardiac disease is present, this should be treated aggressively to minimize pulmonary oedema, PHT or airway compression. Similarly, GORD should be treated aggressively to minimize the possibility of aspiration pneumonia. Airway malacia is sometimes treated with oxygen, although ventilation or surgery to relieve compression or reconstruct the airway may be required. Lower airways disease may benefit from continuous prophylactic antibiotics. Useful once-daily prophylactic antibiotics include azithromycin, co-trimoxazole, amoxicillin with clavulanic acid or cefixime. RSV prophylaxis is indicated at least in children with CHD and vaccination should be considered for all children with Down syndrome.

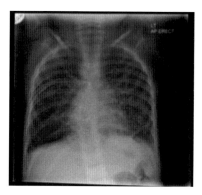

Fig. 9.2. Chest X-ray at outpatient review. Multiple nodules and septal lines throughout the lungs. The lungs appear to be of increased volume, with flattening of the diaphragms. The left heart border is a little indistinct suggesting there may be some inflammatory shadowing.

Cardiovascular or respiratory disease qualifies many children for polysaccharide pneumococcal vaccine (PPV), and it has been recommended that both PPV and influenza vaccination be considered (Down Syndrome Medical Interest Group 2013). The treatment of acute lower respiratory infections is standard according to the pathogens most likely to be present and local resistance patterns (Grant et al. 2009). Bacterial lower respiratory tract infections require broad-spectrum cover with high-dose penicillins. Staphylococcal infection should be considered in complicated cases. Physiotherapy may be a useful adjunct in those children who will tolerate this, particularly children with bronchomalacia. Children who recover from respiratory infection slowly may require supplemental oxygen for a prolonged period of time, which can then be gradually weaned in the community.

The increased vulnerability of children with Down syndrome to pulmonary oedema may need to be considered if planning a trip to altitude or even a commercial airflight.

Managing Nasal Congestion
There are few evidence-based management suggestions for this problem. However, in clinical settings, many practitioners have found one or a combination of the following approaches helpful:

• Teaching even young children to blow their noses is a surprisingly overlooked manoeuvre, which yields dividends. Encouraging nose blowing at bedtime may help to allay sleep disturbance arising from a blocked nose.
• A simple salt-water nasal spray can be bought from pharmacies and helps promote clearance of the nasal cavity when followed by vigorous nose blowing. Even children who are too young to do this can benefit as the use of the spray often produces a vigorous sneeze.
• Mechanical decongestors are also available from pharmacies and are used to suck out accumulated thick secretions from the nasal cavity. This can be particularly helpful on

waking as it enables secretions that have accumulated during the night to be cleared. While parents initially undertake the manoeuvre, many children become adept at doing it themselves.

- Non-sedating antihistamines have sometimes been thought to be helpful.
- Although there is no published evidence to support this measure, some parents report upper airway symptom improvement after cow's milk and other dairy products are excluded from their child's diet. Doctors may avoid this approach that families find difficult to implement. If parents are keen on a few weeks' trial, there are no reasons to discourage them. If the child seems to benefit and parents wish to continue, a paediatric dietician should advise on continuing the exclusion diet and essential nutrients.

The following vignette illustrates the fact there is no single 'cure' for nasal congestion.

Tom and Sally, both aged 2, attended a group for children with Down syndrome and their mothers had become good friends. Both bemoaned the fact that their children had constantly 'snotty' noses and that their doctors seemed to have little advice to offer. Sally's mother read an article which suggested a dairy-free diet. Both mothers spoke to their paediatrician about this but were informed that there was no evidence that dairy products caused the problem. Nevertheless, the two mothers agreed that they would try excluding all dairy products for 2 months. After 6 weeks, Tom's blocked/runny nose was much better and his mother felt that he was functioning better and was more alert. In contrast, Sally's symptoms failed to improve. She had always been a fussy eater and was very distressed at not being allowed some of her favourite foods. Her mother decided there was no point in continuing the diet. Sally did however start using a decongestor, with some benefit.

Management of sleep-disordered breathing

Adenotonsillectomy

Removal of the tonsils and adenoids (T&A) is the most common first-line surgical treatment for OSA. Because of the higher rate of respiratory complications after T&A in children with Down syndrome, overnight observation in hospital after this surgery is recommended (Bower and Richmond 1995). As with all surgery, the anaesthetist needs to be made especially aware of the higher incidence of cranio-vertebral instability in Down syndrome (see Chapter 15) and to avoid neck hyperextension.

Although T&A is the most common initial surgical intervention, studies have shown that residual airway obstruction after this surgery is possible and further interventions may be needed, both surgical and medical (Shott and Donnelly 2004, Shott et al. 2006b, Merrell and Shott 2007). This has recently also been shown to be more common, than previously believed, in children with typical development with OSA. Mitchell (2007) showed a 10–20% incidence of persistent sleep apnoea in a group of 79 'typical' children after T&A, defining 'success' as a postoperative apnoea/hypopnea index (AHI) of less than 5. Tauman et al. (2006) using a much more strict definition of surgical cure, requiring a postoperative AHI of 1 or less, showed persistent OSA after T&A in 75% of their test population of 'typical' children. A large, multicentred study, evaluating over 570 'typical' children, showed that only 27% had an AHI of 1 or less after T&A, with 73% continuing to have OSA (Bhattacharjee et al. 2010). Risk factors identified included obesity, older age at operation, underlying asthma in non-obese children and more severe AHI preoperatively.

The outcome is unfortunately worse for children with Down syndrome. In the paper by Shott et al. (2006b) if all components of the sleep study are evaluated, including AHI less than 1, hypoxemia, hypercarbia and the arousal index, there was only a 5% success rate seen in a group of children with Down syndrome. On the other hand, if an AHI of 5 or less is acceptable (i.e. including mild OSA in the 'success' group), 50–70% of the children in this study continued to have OSA after T&A.

TREATMENT OPTIONS IF OBSTRUCTIVE SLEEP APNOEA PERSISTS AFTER ADENOTONSILLECTOMY

If there is oedema of the nasal turbinates and only mild residual OSA, nasal steroid sprays may be a useful treatment to treat the obstruction (Brouillette et al. 2001). If the child is overweight, weight loss is helpful. In very young children, especially if less than 1 year old, oxygen supplementation may be considered with a repeat polysomnogram in 6 months to reassess the OSA. Positive pressure ventilation with continuous or biphasic positive airway pressure is another option. For this to be successful, it must be worn at least 5 hours per night. This is frequently difficult to achieve in children. At Cincinnati Children's Hospital, a higher compliance rate was found if the children undergo mask desensitization with several days of hospital admission and close follow-up in the Sleep Disorders Clinic.

Palate expanders have been shown to be helpful, especially in children with high-arched palates (Villa et al. 2007). Chronic rhinitis and sinusitis should be addressed aggressively to minimize obstructive associated effects from the nasal congestion and obstruction. Oedema of the posterior oropharynx can cause further narrowing of the airway and treatment for chronic rhinitis, postnasal drainage and GORD may improve this.

Surgical options include procedures that address adenoid regrowth, lingual tonsil hypertrophy, macroglossia and glossoptosis. Cine MRI studies show that the base of the tongue is one of the most common sites for residual obstruction despite previous T&A (Donnelly et al. 2004). Surgical procedures to treat this include lingual tonsillectomy, midline posterior glossectomy and genioglossus suspension procedures. Airway obstruction causing OSA in children with Down syndrome is also more likely to be multilevel and several surgeries may be needed. Success rates, however, are currently in the 60% range and therefore continuous positive airway pressure is often tried prior to considering surgical intervention (Wooten and Shott 2010). Tracheostomy may also need to be considered where there is severe sleep apnoea with associated pulmonary hypertension, severe hypoxaemia and/or cardiac complications. Postoperative sleep studies should be done following surgical intervention to ensure adequate treatment.

Part of the challenge of managing children with Down syndrome, some of whom may be seeing different specialists, is keeping an overview of the whole picture and understanding how reported symptoms may provide a clue to problems in other systems, as is illustrated in the following vignette.

Ahmed displayed poor weight gain during the first year and was 'posseting' several times a day. His paediatrician diagnosed reflux and empirically prescribed anti-reflux medication. The vomiting reduced markedly and his weight tracked upwards across centile lines. By the time he was 2, however, Ahmed had become very averse to taking medication. Getting him to do so regularly turned into a pitched battle, especially when his father was not at home, and regularly reduced his mother to tears. As Ahmed was so much better and giving medication was so difficult, his parents stopped it. Over the next few months, there was occasional vomiting but the family felt this was not a problem. He became unsettled at night, regularly waking and crying. The parents mentioned this to the paediatrician at his routine appointment but omitted to tell him that they had stopped the medication. The paediatrician suspected that Ahmed might be restless because of upper airway obstruction. He was admitted for a sleep study, which was normal, although the nurses noted that the child woke several times and appeared to be in discomfort. Over the same period, Ahmed had been seen numerous times by his GP with symptoms of chest infections and had received several courses of antibiotics. The same pattern continued over the next year until he was eventually admitted with pneumonia. The doctors then ascertained that Ahmed had not been receiving his reflux medication. He underwent a pH study that confirmed severe continuing reflux. Omeprazole was restarted. The nighttime waking settled quickly and he had no courses of antibiotics over the following winter. The clinical psychologist set up a programme to help with getting him to accept medication.

Key points
- Children with Down syndrome have significant respiratory morbidity, which accounts for a large number of hospitalizations.
- Risk factors include CHD, congenital abnormalities of the airways and parenchyma, pulmonary vascular disease and immune dysfunction.
- Important contributory comorbidities include OSA, pulmonary aspiration, GORD, hypotonia and obesity.
- Common presentations are nasal congestion, sleep-disordered breathing, respiratory infections and recurrent wheeze. It is important to recognize multifactorial contributors, particularly those amenable to therapy.
- Respiratory symptoms should be treated early and aggressively to avoid progression to more serious illness.
- Additional immunizations, including RSV prophylaxis, PPV and influenza vaccine should be considered.

REFERENCES

Aceti A, Sciutti R, Bracci PR, Bertelli L, Melchionda F, Cazzato S (2012) Idiopathic pulmonary haemosiderosis in a child with Down's syndrome: Case report and review of the literature. *Sarcoidosis Vasc Diffuse Lung Dis* 29: 58–61.
American Academy of Pediatrics (2001) Health supervision for children with Down syndrome. *Pediatrics* 107: 442–449.

Bertrand P, Navarro H, Caussade S, Holmgren N, Sanchez I (2003) Airway anomalies in children with Down syndrome: Endoscopic findings. *Pediatr Pulmonol* 36: 137–141. doi.org/10.1002/ppul.10332.

Bhattacharjee R, Kheirandish-Gozal L, Spruyt K, et al. (2010) Adenotonsillectomy outcomes in treatment of obstructive sleep apnea in children: A multicenter retrospective study. *Am J Respir Crit Care Med* 2010, 182: 676–683.

Biko DM, Schwartz M, Anupindi SA, Altes TA (2008) Subpleural lung cysts in Down syndrome: Prevalence and association with coexisting diagnoses. *Pediatr Radiol* 38: 280–284.

Bittles AH, Bower C, Hussain R, Glasson EJ (2007) The four ages of Down syndrome. *Eur J Public Health* 17: 221–225.

Bloemers BL, van Furth AM, Weijerman ME et al. (2007) Down syndrome: A novel risk factor for respiratory syncytial virus bronchiolitis—a prospective birth-cohort study. *Pediatrics* 120: e1076–e1081.

Bloemers BL, van Furth AM, Weijerman ME et al. (2010) High incidence of recurrent wheeze in children with Down syndrome with and without previous respiratory syncytial virus lower respiratory tract infection. *Pediatr Infect Dis J* 29: 39–42.

Bonnet MH (1989) The effect of sleep fragmentation on sleep and performance in younger and older subjects. *Neurobiol Aging* 10: 21–25. doi.org/10.1016/s0197-4580(89)80006-5.

Boseley ME, Link DT, Shott SR, Fitton CM, Myer CM, Cotton RT (2001) Laryngotracheoplasty for subglottic stenosis in Down syndrome children: The Cincinnati experience. *Int J Pediatr Otorhinolaryngol* 57: 11–15. doi.org/10.1016/s0165-5876(00)00426-2.

Bower CM, Richmond D (1995) Tonsillectomy and adenoidectomy in patients with Down syndrome. *Int J Pediatr Otorhinolaryngol* 33: 141–148. doi.org/10.1016/0165-5876(95)01207-r.

Breslin J, Spanò G, Bootzin R, Anand P, Nadel L, Edgin J (2014) Obstructive sleep apnea syndrome and cognition in Down syndrome. *Dev Med Child Neurol* Jan 29. doi: 10.1111/dmcn.12376 [Epub ahead of print].

Broers CJ, Gemke RJ, Weijerman ME, Kuik DJ, van Hoogstraten IM, van Furth AM (2012) Frequency of lower respiratory tract infections in relation to adaptive immunity in children with Down syndrome compared to their healthy siblings. *Acta Paediatr* 101: 862–867. doi.org/10.1111/j.1651-2227.2012.02696.x.

Brouillette RT, Manoukian JJ, Ducharme FM et al. (2001) Efficacy of fluticasone nasal spray for pediatric obstructive sleep apnea. *J Pediatr* 138: 838–844. doi.org/10.1067/mpd.2001.114474.

Bull MJ (2011) Health supervision for children with Down syndrome. *Pediatrics* 128: 393–406.

Chaushu S, Yefe Nof E, Becker A, Shapira J, Chaushu G (2003) Parotid salivary immunoglobulins, recurrent respiratory tract infections and gingival health in institutionalized and non-institutionalized subjects with Down's syndrome. *J Intellect Disabil Res* 47: 101–107. doi.org/10.1046/j.1365-2788.2003.00446.x.

D'Alto M, Mahadevan VS (2012) Pulmonary arterial hypertension associated with congenital heart disease. *Eur Respir Rev* 21: 328–337. doi.org/10.1183/09059180.00004712.

Davidson MA (2008) Primary care for children and adolescents with Down syndrome. *Pediatr Clin North Am* 55: 1099–1111. doi.org/10.1016/j.pcl.2008.07.001.

Donnelly LF, Shott SR, LaRose CR, Amin RS (2004) Causes of persistent obstructive sleep apnea despite previous tonsillectomy and adenoidectomy in children with trisomy 21 as depicted on MR cine studies. *Am J Roentgenol* 183: 175–181. doi.org/10.2214/ajr.183.1.1830175.

Down Syndrome Medical Interest Group (2013) Schedule for health checks [online]. http://www.dsmig.org.uk/publications/pchrhealthchk.html (accessed 26 October 2013).

Down Syndrome Medical Interest Group (2013) Key points-Down syndrome: Immunisation [online]. http://www.dsmig.org.uk/library/keypoints-immunisations.html (accessed 26 October 2013).

Dyken ME, Lin-Dyken DC, Poulton S, Zimmerman MB, Sedars E (2003) Prospective polysomnographic analysis of obstructive sleep apnea in Down syndrome. *Arch Pediatr Adolesc Med* 157: 655–660. doi.org/10.1001/archpedi.157.7.655.

Fitzgerald DA (2009) Preventing RSV bronchiolitis in vulnerable infants: The role of palivizumab. *Paediatr Respir Rev* 10: 143–147. doi: 10.1016/j.prrv.2009.06.002.

Fitzgerald DA, Paul A, Richmond C (2007) Severity of obstructive apnoea in children with Down syndrome who snore. *Arch Dis Child* 92: 423–425. doi: 10.1136/adc.2006.111591.

Frazier JB, Friedman B (1996) Swallow function in children with Down syndrome: A retrospective study. *Dev Med Child Neurol* 38: 695–703. doi.org/10.1111/j.1469-8749.1996.tb12139.x.

Gonzalez OR, Gomez IG, Recalde AL, Landing BH (1991) Postnatal development of the cystic lung lesion of Down syndrome: Suggestion that the cause is reduced formation of peripheral air spaces. *Pediatr Pathol* 11: 623–633. doi.org/10.3109/15513819109064794.

Grant GB, Campbell H, Dowell SF et al. (2009) Recommendations for treatment of childhood non-severe pneumonia. *Lancet Infect Dis* 9: 185–196. doi: 10.1016/S1473-3099(09)70044-1.

Hilton JM, Fitzgerald DA, Cooper DM (1999) Respiratory morbidity of hospitalized children with trisomy 21. *J Paediatr Child Health* 35: 383–386. doi.org/10.1046/j.1440-1754.1999.00386.x.

Jacobs IN, Gray RF, Todd NW (1996) Upper airway obstruction in children with Down syndrome. *Arch Ororlaryngol Head Neck Surg* 122: 945–950. doi.org/10.1001/archotol.1996.01890210025007.

Levanon A, Tatasiuk A, Tal A (1999) Sleep characteristics in children with Down syndrome. *J Pediatr* 134: 755–760. doi.org/10.1016/s0022-3476(99)70293-3.

Marcus CL, Keens TG, Bautista DB, von Pechmann WS, Davidson Ward SL (1991) Obstructive sleep apnea in children with Down syndrome. *Pediatrics* 88: 132–139. doi.org/10.1007/978-1-60761-725-9_22.

McDowell KM, Craven DI (2011) Pulmonary complications of Down syndrome during childhood. *J Pediatr* 158: 319–325. doi: 10.1016/j.jpeds.2010.07.023.

Megged O, Schlesinger Y (2010) Down syndrome and respiratory syncytial virus infection. *Pediatr Infect Dis J* 29: 672–673. doi: 10.1097/INF.0b013e3181d7ffa5.

Merrell JA, Shott SR (2007) OSAs in Down syndrome: T&A versus T&A plus lateral pharyngoplasty. *Int J Pediatr Otorhinolaryngol* 71: 1197–1203. doi.org/10.1016/j.ijporl.2007.04.009.

Mitchell RB (2007) Adenontonsillectomy for obstructive sleep apnea in children: Outcome evaluated by pre- and postoperative polysomnography. *Laryngoscope* 117: 1844–1854. doi.org/10.1097/mlg.0b013e318123ee56.

Mitchell RB, Call E, Kelly J (2003) Diagnosis and therapy for airway obstruction in children with Down syndrome. *Arch Otolaryngol Head Neck Surg* 129: 642–645. doi.org/10.1001/archotol.129.6.642.

Piatti G, Allegra L, Ambrosetti U, De Santi MM (2001) Nasal ciliary function and ultrastructure in Down syndrome. *Laryngoscope* 111: 1227–1230. doi.org/10.1097/00005537-200107000-00016.

Royal College of Paediatrics and Child Health (RCPCH) (2009) Working party on sleep physiology and respiratory control disorders in childhood. Standards for services for children with disorders of sleep physiology.

Rutter MJ, Willging JP, Cotton RT (2004) Nonoperative management of complete tracheal rings. *Arch Otolaryngol Head Neck Surg* 130: 450–452. doi: 10.1001/archotol.130.4.450.

Shott SR (2000) Down syndrome: Analysis of airway size and a guide for appropriate intubation. *Laryngoscope* 110: 585–592. doi: 10.1097/00005537-200004000-00010.

Shott SR (2006a) Down syndrome: Common otolaryngologic manifestations. *Am J Med Genet C Semin Med Genet* 142C: 131–140. doi: 10.1002/ajmg.c.30095.

Shott SR, Amin R, Chini B, Heubi C, Hotze S, Akers R (2006b) Obstructive sleep apnea: Should all children with Down syndrome be tested? *Arch Otolaryngol Head Neck Surg* 132: 432–436. doi: 10.1001/archotol.132.4.432.

Shott SR, Donnelly LF (2004) Cine magnetic resonance imaging: evaluation of persistent airway obstruction after tonsil and adenoidectomy in children with Down syndrome. *Laryngoscope* 114: 1724–1729. doi.org/10.1097/00005537-200410000-00009.

So SA, Urbano RC, Hodapp RM (2007) Hospitalizations of infants and young children with Down syndrome: Evidence from inpatient person-records from a statewide administrative database. *J Intellect Disabil Res* 51: 1030–1038. doi: 10.1111/j.1365-2788.2007.01013.x.

Southall DP, Stebbens VA, Mirza R, Lang MH, Croft CB, Shinebourne EA (1987) Upper airway obstruction with hypoxaemia and sleep disruption in Down syndrome. *Dev Med Child Neurol* 29: 734–742. doi.org/10.1111/j.1469-8749.1987.tb08818.x.

Tauman R, Gulliver TE, Krishna J et al. (2006) Persistence of obstructive sleep apnea syndrome in children after adenotonsillectomy. *J Pediatr* 149: 803–808. doi.org/10.1016/j.jpeds.2006.08.067.

Vernail F, Gardiner Q, Mondain M (2004) ENT and speech disorders in children with Down's syndrome: An overview of pathophysiology, clinical features, treatments, and current management. *Clin Pediatr* 43: 783–791. doi.org/10.1177/000992280404300902.

Villa MP, Malagola C, Pagani J et al. (2007) Rapid maxillary expansion in children with obstructive sleep apnea syndrome: 12-month follow-up. *Sleep Med* 8: 128–134. doi.org/10.1016/j.sleep.2006.06.009.

Watts R, Vyas H (2013) An overview of respiratory problems in children with Down's syndrome. *Arch Dis Child* 98: 812–817. doi.org/10.1136/archdischild-2013-304611.

Weijerman ME, Brand PL, van Furth MA, Broers CJ, Gemke RJ (2011) Recurrent wheeze in children with Down syndrome: Is it asthma? *Acta Paediatr* 100: e194–e197. doi.org/10.1111/j.1651-2227.2011. 02367.x.

Weijerman ME, van Furth AM, van der Mooren MD et al. (2010) Prevalence of congenital heart defects and persistent pulmonary hypertension of the neonate with Down syndrome. *Eur J Pediatr* 169: 1195–1199. doi: 10.1007/s00431-010-1200-0.

Weir K, McMahon S, Barry L, Ware R, Masters IB, Chang AB (2007) Oropharyngeal aspiration and pneumonia in children. *Pediatr Pulmonol* 42: 1024–1031. doi: 10.1002/ppul.20687.

Wooten C, Shott SR (2010) Evolving therapies to treat retroglossal and base of tongue obstruction in pediatric obstructive sleep apnea. *Arch Otolaryngol Head Neck Surg* 136: 983–987. doi.org/10.1001/archoto. 2010.178.

10
GROWTH

Jennifer Dennis and Liz Marder

Introduction

Growth in Down syndrome from late intrauterine life through to adulthood differs in many ways from the rest of the population. Much of this variation is biologically determined. Environmental factors can play a part, and a range of both major and minor pathologies may further compromise growth.

Short stature is a recognized characteristic as is a tendency to overweight. For the majority, the cause of growth retardation is not known. Average height at most ages is around the 2nd centile for the general population. Associated medical problems may jeopardize growth and include congenital heart disease (Torfs and Christianson 1998, Dennis et al. 2010), sleep-related upper airway obstruction (Stebbens et al. 1991), coeliac disease (Jansson and Johansson 1995, George et al. 1996), nutritional inadequacy due to feeding problems (Spender et al. 1996) and thyroid hormone deficiency (Sharav et al. 1988, Karlsson et al. 1998). Bearing this in mind, regular health surveillance, as suggested by the UK Down Syndrome Medical Interest Group (DSMIG) schedule of health checks for the personal child health record (PCHR) insert (Charleton et al. 2010, DSMIG 2012a) or the American Academy of Pediatrics (Bull 2011), is essential for the early identification of problems that may lead to poor growth or excessive weight gain.

Are there special growth charts for children with Down syndrome?

United Kingdom/Republic of Ireland growth charts for healthy children with Down syndrome from birth to 18 years are available (Styles et al. 2002) and recently revised (DSMIG 2011b) (Fig 10.1). They are also included in the special Down syndrome insert for the parent-held PCHR (DSMIG 2011a). These reference values are essential for assessing linear growth. However, as many older children and adults with Down syndrome are overweight, the reference values for weight should not be used as a standard to be achieved! A Down syndrome body mass index (BMI) conversion chart is included on the UK charts to aid the assessment of those who may be overweight. A fact sheet that gives detailed information on how to use these charts is available (DSMIG 2012b). Growth reference charts are also available for populations in Sicily (Piro et al. 1990), Holland (Cremers et al. 1996), Sweden (Myrelid et al. 2002), USA (Cronk et al. 1988, Rosenbloom et al. 2010) and Egypt (Meguid et al. 2004).

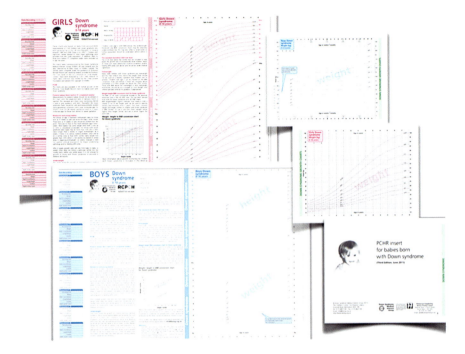

Fig. 10.1. UK Down syndrome growth charts (DSMIG 2011) (with thanks to Harlow Printing plc. for permission to reproduce.).

Does intrauterine growth of infants with Down syndrome differ from that of other infants?

In Down syndrome, preterm birth is common and mean birthweight is lower than in the general population. This has generally been attributed to deficient intrauterine growth (Smith and McKeown 1954, Cronk and Anneren 1992). However, studies of first-trimester growth restriction and aneuploidy (Bahado-Singh et al. 1997, Schemmer et al. 1997) have shown normal first trimester growth. We have known for a long time that the modal gestational age at birth is 38 weeks (Smith and McKeown 1954, Clementi et al. 1990), and it has recently been shown by Boghossian et al. (2012) and Morris et al. (2013) that prior to 38 weeks weight distribution is similar to other infants (Figs. 10.2a and 10.2b). At 38 weeks, males are only 107g lighter and females 51g lighter than their unaffected peers.

From 38 weeks' gestation, weight gain slows and by 40 weeks the shortfall compared with typical infants is considerable. It appears that any intrauterine growth restriction is usually confined to the last weeks of pregnancy and is likely to reflect an earlier onset of postmaturity. It is possible that this is an early manifestation of premature biological ageing, but there is no hard evidence to support this view.

It is clear from the above that Down syndrome-specific birthweight charts are not needed up to 38 weeks' gestation and until this age, within the UK, it is appropriate to use the UK neonatal and infant close monitoring growth charts (NICM) (RCPCH 2009). There

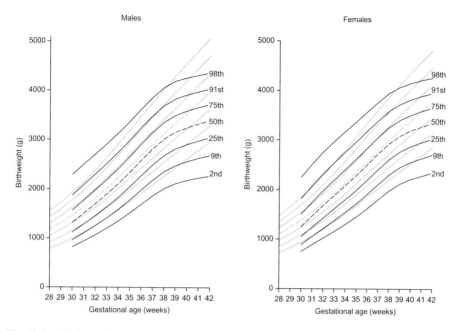

Fig. 10.2a. Birthweight centiles by gestation: Down syndrome (black lines) compared with UK 1990 growth reference charts (UK90) (grey lines).

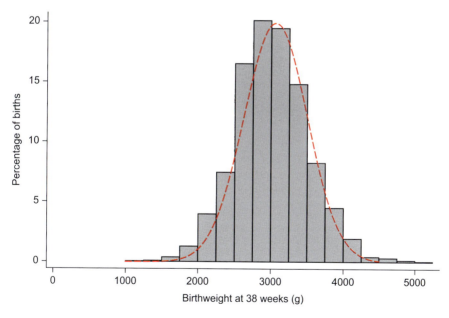

Fig. 10.2b. Birthweight in infants with Down syndrome at 38 weeks (grey) compared to birthweight in unaffected infants at 38 weeks (red line). From Morris et al. (2013).

are no appropriate birthweight reference charts for those born between 38 and 42 weeks but the birthweight centile distributions at these ages are presented in Fig 10.2b Morris et al. (personal communication 2013).

Do infants with Down syndrome gain weight in the first weeks of life in the same way as other infants and is breastfeeding advisable?
Analysis of data from the UK National Down Syndrome Cytogenetic Register (www.wolfson .qmul.ac.uk/ndscr) shows that for 800 boys with Down syndrome born at 40 weeks the mean birthweight was 3252g and for 810 girls 3195g (Morris et al. personal communication, 2013). Those born before 37 completed weeks' gestation can, once they have reached their expected date of delivery, be plotted on the charts taking into account the degree of prematurity. As with all preterm infants, this correction for preterm birth should be made until the end of the first year (corrected age) for infants born after 32 weeks and up to two corrected age years for those born at less than 32 weeks' gestation.

The UK Down syndrome growth charts charts (Styles et al. 2002) were produced using data from healthy infants born at or after 37 completed weeks' gestation. It is essential that these charts rather than the regular UK WHO charts are used when assessing an infant's growth; otherwise, undue anxiety about supposed faltering growth will arise.

Amelia had uncomplicated Down syndrome and was a flourishing little girl during her first year of life. However, her health visitor was extremely concerned because her weight was consistently on the lowest centile on the national weight charts. She thought that nutritional intake might be inadequate or that there might be some deficiency in parenting skills. Her mother pointed out to the health visitor that Amelia's height and weight were entirely consistent one with the other and that she appeared to be growing at an acceptable rate, though on the lowest centile. The health visitor remained unconvinced. At around age 1, all measurements were replotted on the Down syndrome-specific charts that had recently become available. This showed that measurements for height, weight and head circumference were proportionate and that all fell on the 50th centile for a child with Down syndrome.

Parental perspective. The concrete demonstration using the Down syndrome charts that became available during this child's first year of life confirmed that the mother's interpretation was entirely correct and empowered her to continue to have confidence in her own mothering skills and opinions.

Health professionals' perspective. This demonstrated a lack of liaison between the specialist Down syndrome team and the local primary health care team and the importance of ensuring that Down syndrome-specific growth charts are readily available both to parents and to health care professionals.

As with the 2009 UK WHO charts (RCPCH 2009), no centile lines are printed for the first 2 weeks. This is because, like all infants, weight loss after birth is common and the pattern of weight gain thereafter is very individual. In Down syndrome, early weight loss may be more than 10% and it may take longer than 2 weeks to regain birthweight. However, this is an area where there is a dearth of adequate information. Epidemiologically, sound information about growth patterns of infants with Down syndrome in the early weeks of life is urgently needed. There is general consensus, however, that by 4 weeks, if there is no serious medical problem, most will be on a centile close to their birth centile. By contrast, early weight loss greater than 10% that is not quickly recovered or undue delay in regaining birthweight (more than 4 weeks) indicates a need for careful clinical evaluation for feeding difficulties or major underlying pathology (see Chapter 4 for information on feeding and feeding difficulties).

What about the growth of children with Down syndrome who have additional medical problems?

Medical problems affecting growth, such as significant congenital heart disease, should ideally be detected very early in life but an infant whose early growth is not following an acceptable pattern should be carefully assessed for possible underlying medical problems that may have been missed. Faltering growth secondary to feeding problems may continue and may remain undiagnosed in the face of coexistent medical problems (diagnostic overshadowing).

Chloe had multiple small ventricular septal defects and her weight fell progressively from the lower centile lines (Fig. 10.3a). This was attributed to the fact that she had both Down syndrome and a cardiac defect despite the fact that the defects were not thought to be of haemodynamic significance. At age 13 months, she was admitted for a period of hospital observation where it was found that she had major problems with oral motor coordination to the extent that her mother had been terrified to feed her anything other than a very limited diet. Hence, her very poor growth proved to be nutritionally determined. Following careful and intensive work with her family to enable them to feed her with confidence, her measurements gradually reached an acceptable level (Fig. 10.3b).

Chloe's mother had mild intellectual disability. Chloe was her sixth child. Her older children had all fed easily. She was fearful in general and overwhelmed by this new baby who had a syndrome she had never heard of and also a heart problem. She did her best for the child but did not communicate readily and had never expressed to health care professionals any anxiety about feeding Chloe.

***Parental perspective.** Chloe's mother responded well to hands on help and was very reassured to find herself able to look after this infant more adequately.*

***Health care professional perspective.** This is an example of diagnostic overshadowing that can occur when a child's poor growth is attributed not only to the fact they have Down syndrome but that they also have a cardiac defect. It illustrates a need to be open-minded and for a practical hands on approach when looking after disadvantaged mothers and families.*

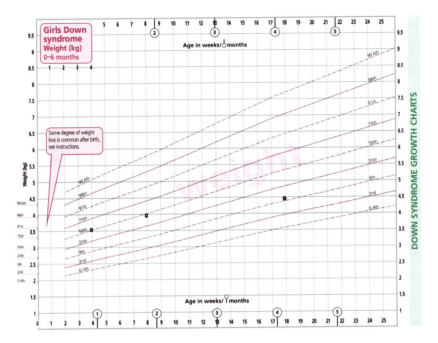

Fig. 10.3a. Chloe's growth chart 0–6 months.

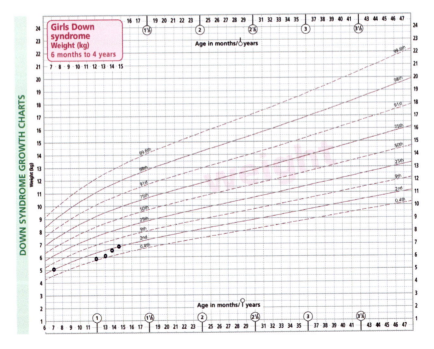

Fig. 10.3b. Chloe's growth chart from 6 months.

As with other children, it is not unusual for growth to proceed in a pattern of spurts and plateaux but in Down syndrome these tend to be more prolonged and this must be taken into account when reviewing growth. After age of 4 weeks, infants may not follow a particular centile line but usually track within one centile space. As the UK charts were constructed from data obtained in healthy children with Down syndrome, those with additional medical needs, including commonly those with congenital heart problems, are likely to be on the lower centiles. Some with additional problems may be very underweight but the inclusion of a −4 standard deviation line on the charts enables professionals to gain an idea of whether those children are growing at a reasonable rate and whether they are showing signs of 'catch up' growth. Some, however, will already be experiencing excessive weight gain.

Is overweight common in adolescents with Down syndrome?
As adolescence approaches, the weight distribution of the whole population becomes increasingly skewed in the direction of overweight. The data collected by Styles et al. showed that 30% of those aged 10 or more had a BMI greater than the 91st centile and 20% greater than the 98th centile for the general population (Styles et al. 2002). Whilst environmental factors in the form of excess calorie intake and deficient exercise undoubtedly contribute to this tendency to overweight, biological factors also play a part.

A recent epidemiological study on Down syndrome from the Netherlands (van Gameren-Oosterom et al. 2012) showed 'alarmingly high prevalence rates of overweight and obesity' during childhood and adolescence. This exceeded that in the general population and was found not only in healthy youngsters but also in those with heart disease and other medical conditions. Anecdotally, however, within the UK there is an impression that the prevalence of overweight is less than previously thought, possibly because parents are well informed with regard to management. However, we urgently need a contemporary epidemiological study to investigate possible secular change.

How do adolescents with Down syndrome grow during puberty?
The way the growth curves are generated means that they do not show an adolescent growth spurt. This does however occur in young people with Down syndrome but is less marked and often occurs earlier than in the general population. Final height may be achieved earlier (Arnell et al. 1996, Kimura et al. 2003) and may be even more limited if early onset of puberty occurs. (See Chapter 4 for information on other aspects of puberty).

Why are adults with Down syndrome shorter than other people? Why do they tend to be overweight and can anything be done about this?
By age 18, the mean height for males (158cm) and females (146cm) is around the 0.4th centile for the general population. The cause of short stature is not understood. Growth hormone levels are normal. There is, however, a selective deficiency of insulin-like growth factor and Castells et al. (1996) suggest that hypothalamic rather than pituitary function may be at fault.

For some individuals, problems with weight control tend to persist throughout life. This is graphically represented by the charts and can be extreme and life threatening. There are powerful biological variables as well as environmental factors that underpin this tendency to obesity.

Short stature means that calorie requirements for individuals with Down syndrome are less than those of their adult peers and dietary control can be very difficult to achieve. It is likely that those with Down syndrome have a reduced resting metabolic rate (Luke et al. 1996). Luke suggests that this acts as 'an inherent metabolic risk factor for expending less total energy, hence placing those with Down syndrome at risk for developing obesity'. Furthermore, although there are some fine athletes and dancers with Down syndrome, for many sustained exercise is problematic and disinclination arises on account of fundamental physiological factors. There is extensive literature on this subject, which is comprehensively reviewed by Mendonca et al. (2010). This concludes that reduced exercise capacity and motor performance are limited by fundamental biochemical and cardiorespiratory responses and poor motor coordination (Eberhard et al. 1991, Mendonca et al. 2010). Appropriate management strategies designed to combat excessive weight gain in this population are excellently covered in the Down Syndrome Nutrition Handbook (Medlen 2006).

Is there a place for growth hormone treatment for those with Down syndrome?
The use of growth hormone for those with Down syndrome is still being evaluated. There is no evidence that it should be prescribed except in the unusual situation of concurrent primary growth hormone deficiency (Anneren et al. 2000). Investigations over many years by Anneren and his group in Sweden (Anneren et al. 1999) show that short-term treatment in infancy and childhood accelerates growth during the course of treatment but there is no effect on final height. Following this short-term treatment in childhood, adolescents showed an increased head growth standard deviation score and there may be some small improvement in fine motor skills and in some areas of cognitive function but motor tone remains unchanged (Myrelid et al. 2010).

Key points on growth
- Down syndrome-specific growth charts should be used to assess growth in a child with Down syndrome. Short stature is a recognized feature of Down syndrome.
- Children identified as being particularly short or underweight on the Down syndrome chart should be thoroughly investigated for underlying causes.
- People with Down syndrome are commonly overweight but it is not an inevitable part of the syndrome and should be assessed and managed as for the general population.
- Weight for height should be assessed using standard BMI charts or the Down syndrome BMI conversion included on the UK Downs syndrome growth charts..
- The use of growth hormone remains investigational and is not currently recommended.

REFERENCES

Anneren G, Tuvemo T, Carlsson-Skwirut C et al. (1999) Growth hormone treatment in young children with Down's syndrome: Effects on growth and psychomotor development. *Arch Dis Child* 80: 334–338.
Anneren G, Tuvemo T, Gustafsson J (2000) Growth hormone therapy in young children with Down syndrome and a clinical comparison of Down and Prader-Willi syndrome. *Growth Horm IGF Res* 10: S87–S91.

Arnell H, Gustafsson J, Ivarsson SA, Annerén G (1996) Growth and pubertal development in Down syndrome. *Acta Paediatr* 85: 1102–1106.

Bahado-Singh RO, Lynch L, Deren O et al. (1997) First-trimester growth restriction and fetal aneuploidy: The effect of type of aneuploidy and gestational age. *Am J Obstetr Gynecol* 176: 976–980.

Boghossian NS, Horbar JD, Murray JC, Carpenter JH (2012) Anthropometric charts for infants with trisomies 21, 18, or 13 born between 22 weeks gestation and term: The VON charts. *Am J Med Genet A* 158A: 322–332.

Bull MJ (2011) Health supervision for children with Down syndrome. *Pediatrics* 128: 393–340.

Castells S, Beaulieu I, Torrado C, Wisniewski KE, Zarny S, Gelato MC (1996) Hypothalamic versus pituitary dysfunction in Down's syndrome as cause of growth retardation. *J Intellect Disabil Res* 40 (Pt 6): 509–517.

Charleton PM, Dennis J, Marder E (2010) Medical management of children with Down syndrome. *Paediatr Child Health* 20: 331–337.

Clementi M, Calzolari E, Turolla L, Volpato S, Tenconi R (1990) Neonatal growth patterns in a population of consecutively born Down syndrome children. *Am J Med Genet* Suppl 7: 71–74.

Cremers MJ, van der Tweel I, Boersma B, Wit JM, Zonderland M (1996) Growth curves of Dutch children with Down's syndrome. *J Intellect Disabil Res* 40: 412–420.

Cronk C, Crocker AC, Pueschel SM et al. (1988) Growth charts for children with Down syndrome: 1 month to 18 years of age. *Pediatrics* 81: 102–110.

Cronk CE, Anneren G (1992) Growth. In: Pueschel SM, Pueschel JK, editors. *Biomedical Concerns in Persons with Down's Syndrome*, 19–37. Baltimore, MD: Paul H. Brookes Publishing Co.

Dennis J, Archer N, Ellis J, Marder L (2010) Recognising heart disease in children with Down's syndrome. *Arch Dis Child Educ Pract Ed* 95: 98–104.

DSMIG (2011a) Down Syndrome Medical Interest Group. Personal child health record insert for babies with Down syndrome. Available from Harlow Printing www.healthforallchildren.com.

DSMIG (2011b) Down Syndrome Medical Interest Group. Growth charts for children with Down syndrome. Available from Harlow Printing www.healthforallchildren.com.

DSMIG (2012a) Down Syndrome Medical Interest Group Guidelines for Essential Medical Surveillance - Growth. http://www.dsmig.org.uk/publications/index.html (accessed 1 January 2015).

DSMIG (2012b) RCPCH/DSMIG Growth chart fact sheet. http://www.dsmig.org.uk/pdf/ChartFactSheetA4 4pp.pdf (accessed 1 January 2015).

Eberhard Y, Eterradossi J, Therminarias A (1991) Biochemical changes and catecholamine responses in Down's syndrome adolescents in relation to incremental maximal exercise. *J Ment Defic Res* 35: 140–146.

George EK, Mearin ML, Bouquet J et al. (1996) High frequency of celiac disease in Down syndrome. *J Pediatr* 128: 555–557.

Greenwood RD, Nadas AS (1976) The clinical course of cardiac disease in Down's syndrome. *Pediatrics* 58: 893–897.

Jansson U, Johansson C (1995) Down syndrome and celiac disease. *J Pediatr Gastroenterol Nutr* 21: 443–445.

Karlsson B, Gustafsson J, Hedov G, Ivarsson SA, Annerén G (1998) Thyroid dysfunction in Down's syndrome: Relation to age and thyroid autoimmunity. *Arch Dis Child* 79: 242–245.

Kimura J, Tachibana K, Imaizumi K, Kurosawa K, Kuroki Y (2003) Longitudinal growth and height velocity of Japanese children with Downs syndrome. *Acta Paediatr* 92: 1039–1042.

Luke A, Sutton M, Schoeller DA, Roizen NJ (1996) Nutrient intake and obesity in pre-pubescent children with Down syndrome. *J Am Diet Assoc* 96: 1262–1267.

Medlen J (2006) *The Down Syndrome Nutrition Handbook: A Guide to Promoting Healthy Lifestyles.* Portland, OR: Phronesis Publishing.

Mendonca GV, Pereira FD, Fernhall B (2010) Reduced exercise capacity in persons with Down syndrome: Cause, effect, and management. *Therapeut Clin Risk Manag* 6: 601–610.

Meguid NA, El-Kotoury AI, Abdel-Salam GM, El-Ruby MO, Afifi HH (2004) Growth charts of Egyptian children with Down syndrome (0–36 months). *East Mediterr Health J* 10: 106–115.

Morris JK, Cole T, Dennis J (2013) Birthweight and gestation for babies with Down syndrome in England and Wales: An epidemiological study with implications for clinical practice. Personal communication.

Myrelid A, Bergman S, Elfvik Strömberg M et al. (2010) Late effects of early growth hormone treatment in Down syndrome. *Acta Paediatr* 99: 763–769.

Myrelid A, Gustafsson J, Ollars B, Annerén G (2002) Growth charts for Down's syndrome from birth to 18 years of age. *Arch Dis Child* 87: 97–103.

Piro E, Pennino C, Cammarata M et al. (1990) Growth charts of Down syndrome in Sicily: Evaluation of 382 children 0–14 years of age. *Am J Med Genet* Suppl 7: 66–70.

Rosenbloom ST, McGregor TL, Chen Q, An AQ, Hsu S, Dupont WD (2010) Specialized pediatric growth charts for electronic health record systems: The example of Down syndrome. *AMIA Annu Symp Proc* 687–691.

RCPCH (2009) UK-WHO Growth Charts. http://www.rcpch.ac.uk/child-health/research-projects/uk-who-growth-charts/uk-who-growth-charts (accessed 1 January 2015).

Schemmer G, Wapner RJ, Johnson A, Schemmer M, Norton HJ, Anderson WE (1997) First-trimester growth patterns of aneuploid fetuses. *Prenat Diagn* 17: 155–159.

Sharav T, Collins RM Jr, Baab PJ (1988) Growth studies in infants and children with Down's syndrome and elevated levels of thyrotropin. *Am J Dis Child* 142: 1302–1306.

Smith A, McKeown T (1955) Prenatel growth of mongoloid defectives. *Arch Dis Child*. Jun; 30 (151): 257–259.

Spender Q, Stein A, Dennis J, Reilly S, Percy E, Cave D (1996) An exploration of feeding difficulties in children with Down syndrome. *Dev Med Child Neurol* 38: 681–694.

Stebbens VA, Dennis J, Samuels MP, Croft CB, Southall DP (1991) Sleep related upper airway obstruction in a cohort with Down's syndrome. *Arch Dis Child* 66: 1333–1338.

Styles ME, Cole TJ, Dennis J, Preece MA (2002) New cross sectional stature, weight, and head circumference references for Down's syndrome in the UK and Republic of Ireland. *Arch Dis Child* 87: 104–108.

Torfs CP, Christianson RE (1998) Anomalies in Down syndrome individuals in a large population-based registry. *Am J Med Genet* 77: 431–438.

van Gameren-Oosterom HB, van Dommelen P, Schönbeck Y, Oudesluys-Murphy AM, van Wouwe JP, Buitendijk SE (2012) Prevalence of overweight in Dutch children with Down syndrome. *Pediatrics* 130: e1520. doi: 10.1542/peds.2012-0886.

11
ENDOCRINE DISORDERS

11a. Thyroid Disorders

Malcolm Donaldson and Kath Leyland

Introduction—what are the problems which can affect the thyroid gland in Down syndrome?

The thyroid gland in Down syndrome is known to be vulnerable to acquired disease related to autoimmune mechanisms. Although the reason for this predisposition is not understood, the diagnosis and management of disorders such as Hashimoto thyroiditis and Graves disease is reasonably standard.

More controversial in terms of diagnosis and management is thyroid dysfunction in Down syndrome during the first year of life. The literature commonly refers to congenital hypothyroidism occurring frequently in Down syndrome. However, typical thyroid dysgenesis has not been reliably reported, while thyroid dyshormonogenesis would not be expected to occur more commonly in Down syndrome, given that the various defects are inherited in autosomal recessive fashion.

What is established is that levels of thyroid-stimulating hormone (TSH) from the pituitary gland may be raised in Down syndrome during the neonatal period, while levels of thyroid hormones tend to be at the lower end of the normal range. At present, there is no strong evidence to indicate that such mild derangement of thyroid function ought to be managed with thyroxine replacement but this remains an area of interest and uncertainty.

The purpose of this chapter is to discuss the challenges posed by altered thyroid function in infancy and then to focus on diagnosis and management of both underactivity and overactivity of the thyroid thereafter. As well as referring to the relevant published literature in these areas, the chapter draws on the authors' experience in Scotland, including the Newborn Screening Programme, and particularly concerning the school-based capillary TSH screening programme for hypothyroidism.

What are the important definitions and reference ranges for thyroid dysfunction in Down syndrome?

Table 11a.1 gives reference ranges for TSH, free thyroxine (fT4), total T4, free triiodothyronine (fT3) and total T3 in relation to age, along with the principal thyroid autoantibodies: antithyroid peroxidase (TPO) and anti-TSH receptor. It should be noted that normal TSH levels are higher during the first week of life when there is a postnatal TSH surge. T4 is now usually measured as fT4 to avoid problems with conditions such as thyroid-binding globulin deficiency and medications interfering with thyroid hormone binding. Assessment of antibody status is important in people with Down syndrome, given their vulnerability to autoimmune attack. Thyroid autoantibodies against TPO, thyroglobulin (Tg) and thyroid microsomal tissue are often, but not always, present in Hashimoto disease. TSH receptor antibodies (TRAB), which are measured in terms of inhibition of binding of labelled TSH or monoclonal antibody, are found in Graves disease, usually together with TPO antibodies. Measurements of thyroid microsomal and Tg antibodies are outdated, so only TPO and TRAB are shown in Table 11a.1.

Definitions in thyroid disease are important since simple terms may mean different things to different people. Hypothyroidism is a state in which function of the hypothalamo–pituitary–thyroid axis is jeopardized, resulting either in compensated hypothyroidism when the axis is still able to maintain levels of thyroid hormones within the reference range or decompensated hypothyroidism when thyroid hormone levels are below the reference range. The site of dysfunction in the axis is classified as primary (thyroid), secondary (pituitary) and tertiary (hypothalamic). The term 'hyperthyrotropinemia' is purely descriptive and has no precise definition. It is usually applied to situations where thyroid hormones are normal but TSH is mildly elevated (e.g. 6–10mU/L). Hyperthyroidism, almost invariably primary in nature, is when thyroid hormones are elevated above and TSH is suppressed below their respective reference ranges. The term 'incipient hyperthyroidism' can be used when fT4 and/or T3 are either at or slightly above the upper limit of normal, and TSH is suppressed.

Should we search for elevation of thyroid-stimulating hormone in Down syndrome at birth and during infancy? If we do discover elevated thyroid-stimulating hormone with or without low fT4, how should this be managed?

Only a small percentage of newborn infants with Down syndrome are detected as having elevated capillary TSH on newborn screening. In Scotland from 1979 to 2013, only 28 of 899 referrals by the Newborn Screening laboratory were for infants with Down syndrome—an estimated 1% of the population with Down syndrome during the 34-year period. Classic congenital hypothyroidism due to thyroid dysgenesis is not common in Down syndrome—only 1 of the 28 infants referred has had true hypothyroidism

TABLE 11a.1
Normative values for thyroid hormones and autoantibodies

	Free T4 (pmol/L)	Total T4 (nmol/L)	Free T3 (pmol/L)	Total T3 (pmol/L)	TSH (mU/L)	TPO-ab (IU/mL)	TSHR-ab (u/L)
Neonatal period	8.5–30.5	80–160	4.5–10	1.5–3.4	1.3–16	<50	<10
1–12 mo	9–25	80–160	4.6–7.6	1.5–3.4	0.9–7.7		
Childhood and adolescence	10–23	80–160	4–7.5	1.6–3.0	0.6–5.5		
>18 y		80–140		0.9–2.8			

T4, thyroxine; T3, tri-iodo-thyronine; TPO-ab, thyroid peroxidase antibody; TSH, thyroid-stimulating hormone; TSHR-ab, thyroid stimulating receptor antibody.

138

confirmed. This infant has a heterozygous *PAX8* mutation, inherited from the mother, causing hypoplasia *in situ* which could be coincidental to the trisomy 21 (Hermanns et al. 2014). Moreover, work from France on 13 fetuses with Down syndrome showed normal glands on gross examination, although follicular size was reduced (Luton et al. 2012).

By contrast, mild TSH elevation is common in Down syndrome during infancy and there is evidence that this begins *in utero*. Thus, the French study of Luton et al. showed TSH elevation and low fT4 in 6 of the 13 fetuses examined. The authors noted that this thyroid dysfunction did not result in thyroid enlargement (goitre), which suggests a mild decrease in responsiveness to TSH in fetuses with Down syndrome.

In keeping with this prenatal finding, a recent study from Israel involving 428 individuals with Down syndrome aged 6 months to 64 years confirmed a significant shift of the TSH distribution curve to higher values compared with the general population (Meyerovitch et al. 2012). Work from the Netherlands has shown that the distribution curve for capillary T4 in 284 newborn infants with Down syndrome was shifted significantly downwards (van Trotsenburg et al. 2003, 2006). These data suggest that the thyroid hormone/TSH circuit may be 'set' at a higher level in Down syndrome compared with the general population.

Given the tendency for higher thyroid-stimulating hormone values during infancy in Down syndrome, what should be done concerning treatment?
The Dutch group (van Trotsenburg et al. 2005, 2006) went on to randomize 196 infants with Down syndrome to treatment either with thyroxine or placebo between birth and two years. Assessment at the age of two years showed less mental developmental delay in the treated group but this difference did not reach significance. The group also found an improvement in growth, the treated subjects being longer and slimmer, a change which did reach significance. A recently published follow up report of this study cohort, mean age now 10.7 years, has shown no apparent benefit of early L-T4 treatment on either motor or mental development (Marchal et al. 2014). However, the improvement in linear growth in the treated group compared with controls has been maintained.

Faced with this information, how should the clinician caring for a newborn infant with Down syndrome proceed?
At present, there is no hard evidence to justify routine treatment of infants with Down syndrome with thyroxine when thyroid function is normal nor is there a clear case for rescreening newborn infants with Down syndrome at 15 and 30 days to detect subtle postnatal thyroid dysfunction as carried out by some centres for at-risk infants (e.g. infants <33 weeks' gestation). However, some centres do currently elect to rescreen their infants with Down syndrome (Vigone et al. 2014).

At present, therefore, we do not recommend retesting thyroid function in infancy provided that newborn screening at 4–6 days is negative and there are no features to suggest hypothyroidism. This approach may change if further long-term follow-up studies were to show a significant cognitive benefit in children who were treated with thyroxine during infancy.

How should infants with Down syndrome be managed when raised venous thyroid-stimulating hormone values and/or low fT4 values are detected during infancy?

This might occur, for example, following referral by the newborn screening laboratory because of capillary TSH elevation, or when a direct parental request has led to testing, or when there is clinical suspicion of hypothyroidism. Raised venous TSH may indicate thyroid dysgenesis, and ultrasound and/or radioisotope imaging should be considered.

In keeping with the Congenital Hypothyroidism Consensus Guidelines published recently by Léger et al. (2014), we recommend treating all infants with fT4 <10pmol/L with thyroxine, keeping infants with venous TSH values of 6–10mU/L and normal fT4 levels under observation, discussing thyroxine treatment for TSH values of 10–20mU/L and recommending treatment with values higher than this. The starting dose of thyroxine should be 25µg daily, titrating fT4 and TSH values against dosage to achieve fT4 10–23pmol/L and TSH 0.5–3mU/L. All infants receiving thyroxine treatment in these borderline situations should be retested off treatment to reassess the thyroid axis and confirm that the disturbance in thyroid function was transient in nature, which it is in 70% of cases (Claret et al. 2013). The age of stopping thyroxine and retesting should be from 2 years onwards, after the period of most rapid brain growth and maturation. There is an argument for deferring retesting until 3 years in order to protect the brain and because logistically, imaging and venepuncture may be easier in older children.

Key points—thyroid function during the first year of life
- Classic congenital hypothyroidism does not commonly occur.
- There is a shift towards the upper limit of normal for TSH and the lower limit for fT4.
- Frank elevation of TSH in the newborn period can occur, but only 1% of infants will test positive on newborn screening.
- If venous TSH elevation is found, we suggest managing according to the consensus guidelines of the European Society for Paediatric Endocrinology (Leger et al. 2014).
- At present, there is no clear evidence to justify giving thyroxine treatment to infants with Down syndrome if they have normal thyroid function.

How do we detect and manage thyroid underactivity (including mild thyroid-stimulating hormone elevation) between the end of the first year of life up to young adulthood?

PREVALENCE

Beyond infancy, hypothyroidism due to Hashimoto disease becomes increasingly common with an estimated prevalence of not less than 5.7% in children and adolescents in Scotland (McGowan et al. 2011). This figure is lower than in adults, Prasher reporting decompensated hypothyroidism (low T4, increased TSH) in 13 out of 160 (8.1%) cases while 19 (11.9%) were described as having increased TSH with normal T4, although this figure may include some individuals with marginal TSH elevation (Prasher 1994).

Not only is the prevalence of hypothyroidism in people with Down syndrome of all ages high, but clinical diagnosis is difficult (see Fig. 11a.1). This is because symptoms of hypothyroidism including slow growth, cold intolerance, constipation, dry skin and hair and tiredness are relatively common in the population of people with Down syndrome.

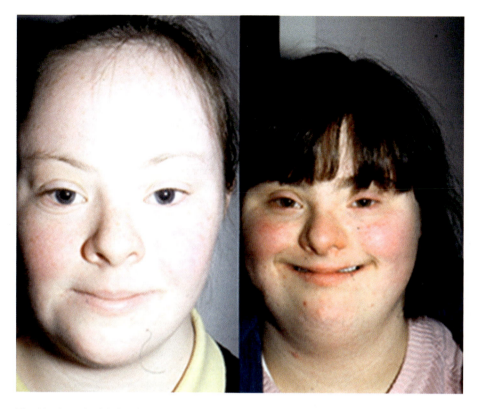

Fig. 11a.1. Both girls in this picture have Down syndrome and were referred with capillary thyroid-stimulating hormone (TSH) elevation on school-based screening. One would think that the girl on the left may well have decompensated hypothyroidism while the one on the right looks euthyroid. In fact the girl on the left, aged 14.5 years, has compensated hypothyroidism with capillary TSH of 14mU/l, venous TSH 14.5mU/l and free thyroxine (fT4) 13.1pmol/l, thyroid peroxidase (TPO) antibodies >1000IU/ml; while the girl on the right, aged 11.8 years, has decompensated hypothyroidism with capillary TSH 55mU/l, venous TSH 79mU/l and fT4 8.7pmol/l!

Who should be screened for hypothyroidism in Down syndrome and at what age?
Given the increasing prevalence of hypothyroidism with age in Down syndrome, a screening programme should be in place throughout life, as recommended by the Down Syndrome Medical Interest Group (DSMIG 2001). Elevated TSH and decreased fT4 as well as thyroid autoantibodies can be detected by venepuncture performed either once every 1 or 2 years. An alternative method is to measure capillary TSH using modified filter strips via the newborn screening laboratory (see Fig. 11a.1). In 1996, a system of school-based capillary blood spot screening was developed in the West of Scotland. This was in response to per-ceived difficulty in achieving consistent universal screening with venepuncture, which entails hospital attendance and sometimes a degree of restraint with which staff felt uncom-fortable. This approach has been found to be both feasible and effective (Noble et al. 2000)

and the most recent review of the Scottish programme found the method to have been adopted virtually nationwide (McGowan et al. 2011). This review has also confirmed that screening needs to be annual when the capillary TSH method is used. 56 of 132 children referred from 1997 to 2009 had tested negative during the previous year. Currently, the capillary TSH cut-off for referral by the Newborn Screening Laboratory is set at ≥4mU/L of whole blood.

By contrast, measurement of thyroid autoantibodies appears to be of limited value in screening for hypothyroidism. In the study of McGowan et al. (2011), TPO antibodies were detected in all age groups, including 8 of 22 participants younger than 8 years, which is in contrast to previous reports (Karlsson et al. 1998). However, although TPO antibody status correlated with TSH elevation, antibodies were negative in 23 of 67 patients referred with TSH elevation.

What are the clinical features of hypothyroidism in Down syndrome and how does it present?

The characteristics of hypothyroidism in children and adolescents with Down syndrome are mainly as for the general paediatric population but with some important differences. The sex distribution is equal, in contrast to the female preponderance found in the general population (Popova et al. 2008, McGowan et al. 2011). Also, goitre does not occur commonly, which makes clinical screening even more difficult. Although the median age at presentation is around 9 years, hypothyroidism may occur at a young age and be severe.

Profound hypothyroidism due to Hashimoto disease in a pre-school child

A boy with trisomy 21 who was attending the cardiac clinic with a small secundum atrial septal defect was found on review aged 3.6 years to be markedly lethargic with dry skin and constipation. On examination, he was pale with dry skin, thyroid not palpable. Using UK 1990 reference data for standard deviation score (SDS) and the revised UK 2011 growth charts for Down syndrome (Freeman et al. 1995, McGowan et al. 2011), height at 90cm was −2.59 SDS and 50th centile, and weight at 14kg was −1.16 SDS and 50th centile. Echocardiogram showed a pericardial effusion from which 98ml of fluid were aspirated. Thyroid function tests showed fT4 <6pmol/L, TSH >1100mU/L and TPO antibodies 961IU/mL. Treatment with thyroxine 12.5mcg daily for 2 weeks, 25mcg daily for 2 weeks and then 37.5mcg daily greatly improved his energy levels and constipation but he proved more difficult to manage due to poor sleeping pattern and more temper tantrums than before. In retrospect, his parents thought that he had been cold intolerant since the age of 2 years and increasingly lethargic over the previous 12 months.

TREATMENT

Based on the experience in Scotland with capillary TSH screening and the known tendency for TSH in Down syndrome to fluctuate, the following algorithm has been developed (see Table 11a.2).

142

TABLE 11a.2
Algorithm for the management of children and adolescents with Down syndrome referred with TSH elevation on capillary screening based on data from the screening programme for Down syndrome in Scotland 1997–2009 (McGowan et al. 2011)

TSH ≥ 6mU/L and **either** fT4 <9pmol/L, **or** child has symptoms or both	Start L-T4 treatment without delay
TSH ≥ 21mU/L	Start L-T4 treatment irrespective of clinical and fT4 status
TSH 6–<11mU/L, fT4 9–23pmol/L, and child is symptom free	Immediate treatment not indicated; continue annual screening **but** advise family to attend earlier if symptoms suggestive of hypothyroidism (e.g. tiredness and cold intolerance)
TSH 11–20.9mU/L, fT4 within the reference range, child is symptom free	**Recommend** thyroxine treatment since therapy is likely to be required eventually. **Advise** family of the alternative, that is surveillance, with early recourse to venous testing if the child develops symptoms

TSH, thyroid-stimulating hormone; fT4, free thyroxine.
Note: TSH and fT4 values refer to *venous* and not *capillary* blood.

In terms of thyroxine dosage, we recommend starting with 25µg daily and gradually increasing the dose according to clinical features and thyroid function tests (see above). It is important for the family to realize that in Hashimoto disease, which is the most common cause of TSH elevation in Down syndrome, thyroid function may fluctuate in severity. Thus, although the tendency is towards the development of true permanent hypothyroidism, the condition may remain stable or even improve. The family should therefore be made aware of symptoms of overtreatment with thyroxine (sweating, poor sleep, thirst, diarrhoea) as well as symptoms of under treatment (cold intolerance, constipation, lethargy). Once treatment has started, it is prudent to recheck thyroid function every 6 months until the child is stable, but thereafter annual TSH screening to confirm TSH suppression/compliance should suffice.

Key points—hypothyroidism after the first year of life
- The prevalence of autoimmune (Hashimoto) thyroiditis increases with age in Down syndrome, affecting about 5–6% of the paediatric population.
- Clinical diagnosis is difficult because of an overlap in features shared between hypothyroidism and Down syndrome itself (e.g. constipation, dry skin and hair).
- Screening for hypothyroidism is essential in Down syndrome and should be put in place for life.
- Capillary TSH testing using the filter strip papers, designed for newborn screening, is a practical method and can be easily implemented within the community.
- Children with mild venous TSH elevation (<10mU/L) and normal fT4 levels can be observed rather than treated immediately, provided that they appear symptom free.

Is overactivity of the thyroid gland (hyperthyroidism) more common in people with Down syndrome, and how should we diagnose and manage this problem?

PREVALENCE

The incidence of hyperthyroidism in Down syndrome is increased; a study of older participants (mean age 16y 9mo) gave an estimate of 6.5 per 1000 (Goday-Arno et al. 2009). As with all children, this incidence is much less than for hypothyroidism. In the Glasgow clinic, 84 children and adolescents with Down syndrome with thyroid problems were seen between 1989 and 2012 of whom only 7 (5 females and 2 males) had hyperthyroidism.

WHAT ARE THE CLINICAL FEATURES OF THYROTOXICOSIS IN DOWN SYNDROME?

The classic features of thyrotoxicosis occur in Down syndrome as described by Goday-Arno and colleagues. This group studied 12 individuals (5 males), mean age 16.8 years, who had Graves disease (mean TRAB very high 128.1U/L) in whom the most common symptoms were heat intolerance, irritability and weight loss with diffuse goitre in all and exophthalmos in two. All patients had diffuse goitre at physical examination and two patients presented with exophthalmos.

Experience in Glasgow in the paediatric age group suggests that the clinical course in Graves disease may be atypical, with fluctuating thyroid, as illustrated by the following case studies. Presentation was biphasic in one girl with Hashimoto thyroiditis and this was relatively easy to manage:

Hashimoto disease causing mild TSH elevation followed by incipient hyperthyroidism followed by barely compensated symptomatic, hypothyroidism in an adolescent female

A girl underwent school-based hypothyroid screening at 14 years and was referred with a capillary TSH value of 17mIU/L. On examination at age 14.3 years, she was clinically euthyroid. Height at 144.6cm was −2.47 SDS (50–75th centiles for Down syndrome) and weight at 63.3kg was +1.31 SDS (75th–91st centiles for Down syndrome), (mid-parental height −0.2 SDS). Venous thyroid function tests showed fT4 11.3pmol/L and TSH 7.8mU/L. Thyroid microsomal antibodies were positive with a titre of 1/6400. The family were advised that thyroxine treatment was not needed at this time and arrangements were made to recheck thyroid function in a year, or sooner if symptoms developed. At 15.3 years, fT4 was high at 29.9pmol/L, T3 borderline high at 2.8nmol/L and TSH suppressed at 0.04mU/L. Two weeks later, thyroid function was similar—fT4 29.2pmol/L and TSH <0.03mU/L, TPO antibodies were raised at 82.0IU/mL, but serum thyroid receptor antibody showed <10% inhibition of TSH binding. No treatment was started but the girl was kept under close observation. Three months later, she developed fatigue, somnolence and cold intolerance. Thyroid function now showed fT4 9.9pmol/L, TSH 20.6mU/L, T3 2nmol/L and haemoglobin 12.9g/dL. Following thyroxine treatment, building to a final dose of 100mcg daily, there was a self-limiting period of hair loss. The tiredness gradually improved so that after 5 months of treatment energy levels had become normal.

144

Three of seven children, all with positive TSH receptor antibodies, have pursued a markedly fluctuating course between hypo- and hyperthyroidism that has proved difficult to manage. One of these developed unsightly exophthalmos aged 13 years, at which point she was euthyroid on a small thyroxine replacement dose having become permanently hypothyroid. Management was particularly difficult in another girl:

Fluctuating thyroid status in a girl with positive TPO and TSH receptor antibodies
A girl presented at 7.3 years with palpitations and TSH suppression (<0.03mU/L) but normal fT4 (13.9pmol/L). She was untreated initially but after 1 month developed decompensated hypothyroidism with fT4 7.3pmol/L and TSH 33.5mU/L. TPO antibodies were elevated at 525IU/mL and TSH receptor antibodies very elevated at 108U/L. She was treated with thyroxine for 5 months but after 6 months became borderline hyperthyroid (fT4 29pmol/L; TSH <0.03mU/L) and treatment was stopped. Subsequently, 18 months after initial presentation, at age 8.8 years, she developed manifest hyperthyroidism (fT4 42.6pmol/L; TSH <0.03mU/L) and was treated with carbimazole. During the next 3.5 years, her biochemical status fluctuated between mild hyperthyroidism and compensated hypothyroidism, and her carbimazole dose was titrated accordingly. At 12.4 years, 5 years after presentation, she became frankly hypothyroid with raised TSH (12.7mU/L) and fT4 just within the normal range (10.8pmol/L) and has required permanent thyroxine replacement, developing type 1 diabetes at 18 years.

Comment: *In retrospect, a block and replace regime (see below) would have been more appropriate in this child.*

TREATMENT

Incipient hyperthyroidism with negative TSH receptor antibodies is probably best left untreated. If TSH receptor antibodies are positive and significant hyperthyroidism occurs, our limited experience suggests that the so-called 'block and replace' regime is best, at least for the first 2 or 3 years. The block and replace regime consists of giving an antithyroid drug such as carbimazole in the dose of 0.75mg/kg/day, continuing this until the fT4 has fallen to around 15pmol/L. Then, instead of reducing the carbimazole dose according to thyroid function—the dose titration method—the carbimazole is maintained in its current dose to 'block' production by the gland, and treatment with thyroxine is introduced to replace the deficit, usually in the dose of 50–75µg daily, adjusting this to keep the fT4, T3 or fT3 and TSH normal.

Block and replace treatment works well when the family is compliant with medications, but such management is specialized and we recommend that it should either be supervised by a paediatric endocrinologist, or as a shared care package between paediatric endocrinologist and general paediatric/community paediatric colleague.

After 2–3 years of block and replace treatment, thyroxine can be withdrawn to examine thyroid status. If the child's thyroid function tests show hypothyroidism a few weeks after stopping thyroxine, this is a sign that the condition has become less severe, may have remitted or may have evolved into hypothyroidism. If so, carbimazole can be reduced or stopped accordingly and thyroxine replacement reintroduced, if necessary.

Key points—hyperthyroidism in Down syndrome
- Hyperthyroidism is less common in Down syndrome than hypothyroidism, but still occurs more commonly than in the general population.
- Hashimoto thyroiditis may include a hyperthyroid phase, sometimes causing incipient hyperthyroidism which can be simply observed. More severe cases may need treatment with antithyroid drugs such as carbimazole.
- Graves disease, in which TSH receptor antibodies are found, can pursue a prolonged and fluctuating course in Down syndrome. In such cases, combined treatment with carbimazole and thyroxine (so-called block and replace therapy) may be preferable to carbimazole alone.

How should adults with Down syndrome be managed in terms of being monitored and treated for an underactive thyroid gland?
Screening for hypothyroidism should continue throughout life. Given that underactivity of the thyroid gland becomes more common with increasing age, it is particularly important to ensure that people with Down syndrome do not miss being screened once they have left school, and annual blood tests are recommended. Hypothyroidism is an important diagnosis to consider in those presenting with symptoms of depression or decline in cognitive function.

Acknowledgements
We thank Dr Jane McNeilly from the Department of Biochemistry at the Royal Hospital for Sick Children in Glasgow for her help with Table 1, and Professor Paul van Trotsenburg for his helpful comments regarding the thyroid management of Down syndrome during infancy.

REFERENCES

Claret C, Goday A, Benaiges D et al. (2013) Subclinical hypothyroidism in the first years of life in patients with Down syndrome. *Pediatr Res* 73: 674–678.

Down Syndrome Medical Interest Group (DSMIG) (2001) Basic medical surveillance essentials for people with Down syndrome – thyroid disorder. http://www.dsmig.org.uk/library/articles/guideline-thyroid-6.pdf (accessed 1 January 2015)

Goday-Arno A, Cerda-Esteva M, Flores-Le-Roux JA, Chillaron-Jordan JJ, CorretgerJM, Cano-PérezJF (2009) Hyperthyroidism in a population with Down syndrome (DS). *Clin Endocrinol* (Oxford) 71: 110–114. doi: 10.1111/j.1365-2265.2008.03419.x. Epub 12 September 2008.

Hermanns P, Shepherd S, Mansor M et al. (2014) A new mutation in the promoter region of the *PAX8* gene causes congenital hypothyroidism in a girl with Down's syndrome. *Thyroid* 24: 939–44. doi: 10.1089/thy.2013.0248.

Karlsson B, Gustafsson J, Hedov G, Ivarsson SA, Annerén G (1998) Thyroid dysfunction in Down's syndrome: Relation to age and thyroid autoimmunity. *Arch Dis Child* 79: 242–245.

Léger J, Olivieri A, Donaldson M et al. (2014). European Society for Paediatric Endocrinology consensus guidelines on screening, diagnosis and management of congenital hypothyroidism. *J Clin Endocrinol Metab.* 99: 363–84. doi: 10.1210/jc.2013–1891.

Luton D, Azria E, Polak M et al. (2012) Thyroid function in fetuses with Down syndrome. *Horm Res Paediatr* 78: 88–93.

Marchal JP, Maurice-Stam H, Ikelaar NA, Klouwer FCC, Verhorstert KWJ, Witteveen ME, et al. (2014) The effect of early thyroxine treatment on development and growth at the age of 10.7 years: Follow-up of a randomized placebo-controlled trial in children with Down syndrome. *JCEM* doi.org/10.1210/jc.2014-2849.

McGowan S, Jones J, Brown A et al. (2011) Capillary TSH screening programme for Down syndrome in Scotland 1997–2009. *Arch Dis Child* 96: 1113–1117. doi: 10.1136/archdischild-2011-300124.

Meyerovitch J, Antebi F, Greenberg-Dotan S, Bar-Tal O, Hochberg Z (2012) Hyperthyrotropinaemia in untreated subjects with Down's syndrome aged 6 months to 64 years: A comparative analysis. *Arch Dis Child* 97: 595–598. doi: 10.1136/archdischild-2011-300806.

Noble SE, Leyland K, Findlay CA et al. (2000) School based screening for hypothyroidism in Down's syndrome by dried blood spot TSH measurement. *Arch Dis Child* 82: 27–31.

Popova G, Paterson WF, Brown A, Donaldson MDC (2008) Hashimoto's thyroiditis in Down's syndrome: Clinical presentation and evolution. *Horm Res* 70: 278–284.

Prasher VP (1994) Prevalence of thyroid dysfunction and autoimmunity in adults with Down syndrome. *Down Syndr Res Pract* 2: 67–70.

van Trotsenburg AS, Vulsma T, van Santen HM, Cheung W, de Vijlder JJ (2003) Lower neonatal screening thyroxine concentrations in Down syndrome newborns. *J Clin Endocrinol Metab* 88: 1512–1515.

van Trotsenburg AS, Kempers MJ, Endert E, Tijssen JG, de Vijlder JJ, Vulsma T (2006) Trisomy 21 causes persistent congenital hypothyroidism presumably of thyroidal origin. *Thyroid* 16: 671–680.

van Trotsenburg ASP, Vulsma T, van Rozenburg-Marres SLR et al. (2005) The effect of thyroxine treatment started in the neonatal period on development and growth of two-year-old Down syndrome children: A randomized clinical trial. *J Clin Endocrinol Metab* 90: 3304–3311. Epub 8 March 2005.

Vigone MC, Caiulo S, Di Frenna M et al. (2014) Evolution of thyroid function in preterm infants detected with congenital hypothyroidism. *J Pediatr* 164: 1296–1302. doi: 10.1016/j.jpeds.2013.12.048.

11b Diabetes in Children with Down Syndrome

Hilary Hoey and Pat Charleton

Introduction

Diabetes mellitus is a group of metabolic disorders characterized by chronic hyperglycaemia resulting from defects in insulin secretion, insulin action or both. The two main groups are known as type 1 (insulin-dependent) diabetes and type 2, previously known as maturity onset diabetes.

What proportion of people with Down syndrome will develop diabetes?

People with Down syndrome are more likely to have diabetes mellitus than the general population. Dutch researchers have reported a threefold increase in the prevalence of type 1 and type 2 diabetes (Burch and Milunsky 1969; Van Goor et al. 1997).

A National Danish Study showed that the prevalence of Down syndrome in people with type 1 diabetes (T1DM) was 4.2 times higher compared with the background population, or 1 in 60 children with Down syndrome compared with 1 in 250 in the general population (Bergholdt et al. 2006).

It tends to present at a younger age, with a bimodal age distribution peaking under 2 years of age and again around 12 years (compared to a Gaussian distribution normally). In the general population, very few children develop T1DM before 1 year of age, whereas this has been reported in up to 15% of children with Down syndrome. Twenty-two percent of these children developed T1DM before 2 years of age compared with only 7% of children in the general population (Shield et al. 1999; Rohrer et al. 2010).

Type 2 diabetes, associated with insulin resistance, being overweight and obesity, is the most common type of diabetes in adults with Down syndrome, as in the general population. Rates are increasing in children and adolescents. Though there are no good statistics available, it is generally accepted that young people with Down syndrome are at greater risk of insulin resistance than the general population if they are overweight or obese (Fonseca et al. 2005; Bergholdt et al. 2006).

Why does type 1 diabetes develop in Down syndrome?

As in the general population, over 90% of diabetes in children with Down syndrome is T1DM. The precise aetiology is unknown; however, there are a number of contributory factors including immune, genetic and environmental influences.

148

There is evidence to suggest that humerol and cell-mediated autoimmune ß-cell damage leads ultimately to T1DM, one of the autoimmune conditions over-represented in Down syndrome. These conditions commonly occur together, especially autoimmune thyroid disease (in up to one-third of people with T1DM) and coeliac disease (in up to one-fifth) (Villiano et al. 2009). This is further discussed in Chapter 7.

Early presentation of T1DM may be explained by a particularly aggressive autoimmune phenotype, destroying islet cells more rapidly, or it may be that the islet cell population is reduced or particularly susceptible to cell-mediated destruction. Islet autoimmunity in children with Down syndrome is increased with circulating autoantibodies found in similar frequencies to other children with T1DM. In Down syndrome, there have also been reports of a higher frequency of subclinical islet autoimmunity and antibodies persisting for longer after the presentation of diabetes. The frequency of T1DM HLA genotypes is reduced in Down syndrome compared to age-matched controls suggesting other factors, including some possible genes on chromosome 21, may increase the penetrance of T1DM in this condition (Gillespie et al. 2006; Rohrer et al. 2010; Aitken et al. 2013).

Although autoimmunity in T1DM has become an established concept, the initiating event is unknown. Environmental agents, especially viruses, have been proposed. These combine with genetic factors early in life to cause T1DM.

Is type 2 diabetes an autoimmune condition?
No. **Type 2 diabetes** is generally associated with being overweight/obesity, a positive family history, the absence of immune and HLA markers of T1DM and is generally treatable without insulin (Craig et al. 2009; Rosenbloom et al. 2009). The management of type 2 diabetes in Down syndrome is as for the general population.

How does diabetes present in Down syndrome?
Clinical presentation in people with Down syndrome is similar to that in the general population (Craig et al. 2009), although it may be more acute and present at a younger age. There is a greater incidence of diabetes in children under 2 years of age and they are more likely to present with diabetic ketoacidosis (DKA), largely due to the slower recognition of symptoms. Presentation in older children may be delayed due to diagnostic over shadowing, because symptoms such as weight gain, general malaise and skin infections are common in Down syndrome and may therefore be over looked.

How is diabetes diagnosed?
Most children with T1DM, whether they have Down syndrome or not, present with symptoms and raised blood glucose levels, glycosuria and ketonuria (American Diabetes Association 2013). Diabetes should be considered in any child presenting with impaired consciousness and/or acidosis, tachypnoea, abdominal pain or secondary enuresis. Any child with suspected diabetes should be referred to the local paediatric diabetes centre on the same day.

Are there any differences in the management of people with Down syndrome and diabetes, compared with the general population?

There are few reports of the clinical management and outcome of diabetes in Down syndrome. The principles of diabetes care are the same as for all people with T1DM—obtaining optimal blood sugar levels, absence of hypoglycaemic episodes, normal growth and psychosocial development, in addition to providing support for the young person and family in developing strategies to cope with a life and diabetes (Silverstein et al. 2005; Hoey 2009).

Are there any differences in acute management of diabetic ketoacidosis?

Approximately 25% of young children present with DKA. No difference has been observed in the presentation or severity of DKA in those with Down syndrome, and management should follow the same protocols as for other children. DKA and associated dehydration is a medical emergency for all children and must be treated urgently in hospital according to local DKA management guidelines. Children who are not ketotic can usually be managed with oral fluids and subcutaneous insulin, often at home with close expert supervision and instruction on insulin injections and diet from the paediatric diabetes team.

What are the principles of long-term management in people with Down syndrome and type 1 diabetes?

The principal diabetes management tools are the same for all children including those with Down syndrome. These include insulin, a healthy, balanced diet, home glucose monitoring, together with psychological support and a life style including regular exercise (Anderson et al. 2009; Smart et al. 2009). Specialized paediatric care is required for all children with diabetes to provide the appropriate medical, social, economic and emotional support. Structured self-management education is the keystone of successful diabetes care (Swift 2009) and diabetic educators should teach people with Down syndrome and their carers so that their diabetes is managed as effectively as with anyone else. All carers, at home, school or college should understand a personalized management plan and be empowered to adjust food and insulin based upon blood glucose data generated. They should know probable signs of hypoglycaemia in the person they are responsible for, as this can vary between individuals and people with Down syndrome may be less good at recognizing or communicating to others about hypoglycemic events.

What are the particular issues in very young children with Down syndrome and type 1 diabetes?

The increased prevalence of young children under 2 years with Down syndrome and diabetes is important as treatment of this group can be difficult mainly due to their variable eating and feeding patterns, which make adjusting insulin doses challenging. It is hypothesized that insulin pumps may have a particular role in future for these children.

Poppy, an 18-month-old girl with Down syndrome presented semi-conscious with DKA after a short vomiting illness. She required active resuscitation in the intensive care unit. After the initial crisis, her parents felt overwhelmed as to how they would manage, especially as she was strong willed and a fussy eater. By discharge, they had built up trust in the diabetes team, felt confident with basic management but were angry with their community team for not warning them that this could happen.

Over the next 2 years, her parents became highly knowledgeable about diabetes management, her insulin requirements were low and she had no hospital admissions, but she gained weight as her parents encouraged frequent snacks to avoid hypoglycaemia. She also developed an aversion to fingerprick blood tests, though she did not mind insulin injections. She was well integrated into her local nursery with a clear personal passport which she carried in her bag. This detailed her normal insulin regimen, how she tended to behave when hypo, exactly what to do if it occurred and who to contact if there were concerns.

How does insulin treatment of older children with Down syndrome and type 1 diabetes compare with usual protocols for type 1 diabetes?

All modern intensive treatment options including multiple injections, analogue insulins and infusion pumps (Scaramuzza et al. 2009; Swift 2009; American Diabetes Association 2013) should be considered for people with Down syndrome. There is a trend towards simpler insulin treatment regimens, with fewer injections per day and lower doses, in this group compared to others with T1DM. Interestingly, it was also noted that their glycaemic control is better despite the simpler regimen and their learning disabilities. It is suggested that a simpler lifestyle and acceptance of routine may explain this (Anwar et al. 1998; Rohrer et al. 2010).

Encouraging general independence in teenage years can be more difficult. In this group, the diabetes may play a larger role in prolonging reliance on parents than the intellectual disability. Children with Down syndrome are usually older than typically developing children when they take over management of their diabetes. For some, independent management is never possible. The importance of appropriate respite, clear communication with community health teams and careful transition to adult services cannot be overstated. Supporting, educating and motivating the child, family and all carers is the cornerstone of good control and this is the main purpose of the diabetic clinic.

What are the complications of childhood diabetes?

These can be divided into the early complications (hyperglycaemic ketoacidosis, hypoglycaemia, psychological problems, skin lesions, e.g. moniliasis) and late complications associated with microvascular disease (retinopathy, nephropathy, neuropathy) and macrovascular disease (ischaemic heart disease, peripheral vascular disease). Microvascular complications may develop in puberty or early adulthood whereas macrovascular complications affect older adults (Gale EA 2005, White NH et al. 2010).

Are early complications more common in Down syndrome?

No. Intercurrent illness, hyperglycaemia and hypoglycaemia are common to everyone with diabetes including those with Down syndrome. It is important that everyone, including parents, family, carers and school personnel, is trained to recognize and manage these conditions, as people with Down syndrome may not be able to interpret correctly or clearly inform others when they develop symptoms.

What psychological difficulties should families expect?

The diagnosis of diabetes is usually a shock for a family and associated with grief and sadness. Parents of children with Down syndrome may have coped with and anticipated other medical issues but are rarely prepared for diabetes (Hillege et al. 2013). Panic feelings may occur concerning their ability to cope with the vast amount of things to be learned. There may be uncertainty of how their child's learning disabilities might complicate management and how diabetes might limit their potential. With good support, most families soon become competent and confident. Diagnosis of diabetes may also be a shock to the child who may be unable to express his or her feelings and may react negatively to changes in routine. Simple explanations and demonstrations at the right level for the child's understanding will help ensure he or she accepts a new routine and learns to self-care to the level of his or her ability. Simple social stories and booklets appropriate for age and cognitive ability will help.

How do late complications differ in people with Down syndrome?

Children and teenagers who have had diabetes for several years may display asymptomatic features of incipient or established microvascular complications, including excessive urinary albumin excretion, cardiovascular indices of autonomic neuropathy, sensory nerve damage, retinopathy, cheiroarthropathy and reduced hyperaemic responses to skin vasculature. All have been noted in people with Down syndrome, but are not significantly different to the general population and might be expected to become more common as life expectancy increases. There is a suggestion that older people with Down syndrome and diabetes have a lower prevalence of diabetic retinopathy (Fulcher et al. 1998) but more research on this and the impact of late complications is needed.

Should diabetes be routinely screened for in Down syndrome?

Screening for diabetes in Down syndrome is not recommended. A high index of suspicion and low threshold for checking blood glucose is recommended due to the increased prevalence, especially in young children and those with other autoimmune conditions, for example, thyroid and coeliac disease. Screening for type 2 diabetes in adults with Down syndrome should be considered, particularly for those who are overweight. Those with the syndrome may be less able to recognize or describe symptoms, and it may be useful to add glycated haemoglobin (HbA1c) to the annual thyroid function tests. Screening should be carried out for autoimmune hypothyroidism which occurs more commonly in people with Down syndrome who have diabetes (Villiano et al. 2009).

Molly was diagnosed with juvenile chronic arthritis at 9 years of age. By the age of 14, her hands, shoulders and knees were affected. She became overweight and was troubled by frequent skin infections following her menarche. She then developed secondary enuresis. The presence of glycosuria led to a diagnosis of T1DM. This was managed at home and she responded remarkably well on twice daily insulin injections and developed a weekly food and snack diary. She learned to give her own insulin injections when her dexterity, sometimes limited by stiff hand joints, permitted and tolerated fingerprick tests. Glycaemic control was good, her skin infections slowly improved and though very dependent on her parents, diabetes did not stop her enjoying favoured activities. At the age of 17, asymptomatic autoimmune hypothyroidism was detected on her annual TSH screen. The addition of thyroxine has not affected her overweight BMI but she feels more active and manages to give her own insulin injections more often.

Key points
- There is an increased prevalence of diabetes in people with Down syndrome.
- Diabetes presents at a younger age in Down syndrome than in the general population.
- Management aims, treatment options and outcomes are no different than those for other people with T1DM.
- Insulin regimens in people with Down syndrome tend to be simpler and metabolic control better, perhaps because they have simpler lifestyles, accept routine and adherence is better as they are more reliant on adult carers.
- T1DM is one of the autoimmune conditions over-represented in Down syndrome.
- It commonly occurs with autoimmune thyroid disease and coeliac disease, so routine screening for these conditions should be performed.
- As in the general population, the prevalence of type 2 diabetes in people with Down syndrome is expected to increase, as the prevalence of obesity increases.

REFERENCES

Aitken RJ, Mehers KL, Williams AJ et al. (2013) Early-onset, coexisting autoimmunity and decreased HLA-mediated susceptibility are the characteristics of diabetes in Down syndrome. *Diabetes Care* 36: 1181–1185. doi: 10.2337/dc12-1712.

American Diabetes Association (2013) Clinical practice recommendations. *Diabetes Care* 36: S11–S15.

Anderson BJ, Holmbeck G, Iannotti R et al. (2009) Dyadic measures of the parent-child relationship during the transition to adolescence and glycemic control in children with type 1 diabetes. *Families, Systems & Health* 27: 141–152. doi: 10.1037/a0015759.

Anwar AJ, Walker JD, Frier BM (1998) Type 1 diabetes mellitus and Down's syndrome: Prevalence, management and diabetic complications. *Diabetic Medicine* 15: 160–163.

Bergholdt R, Eising S, Nerup J, Pociot F (2006) Increased prevalence of Down's syndrome in individuals with type 1 diabetes in Denmark: A nationwide population-based study. *Diabetologia* 49: 1179–1182.

Burch PR, Milunsky A (1969) Early-onset diabetes mellitus in the general and Down's syndrome populations. Genetics, aetiology and pathogenesis. *Lancet* 1: 554–558.

Craig ME, Hattersley A, Donaghue KC (2009) Definition, epidemiology and classification of diabetes in children and adolescents. *Pediatric Diabetes* 10: 3–12. doi: 10.1111/j.1399-5448.2009.00568.x.

Fonseca CT, Amaral DM, Ribeiro MG, Beserra IC, Guimaraes MM (2005) Insulin resistance in adolescents with Down syndrome: A cross-sectional study. *BMC Endocrine Disorders* 5: 6.

Fulcher T, Griffin M, Crowley S, Firth R, Acheson R, O'Meara N (1998) Diabetic retinopathy in Down's syndrome. *British Journal of Ophthalmology* 82: 407–409.

Gale EA (2005) Type 1 diabetes in the young: The harvest of sorrow goes on. *Diabetologia* 48: 1435–1438.

Gillespie KM, Dix RJ, Williams AJ et al. (2006) Islet autoimmunity in children with Down's syndrome. *Diabetes* 55: 3185–3188.

Hillege S, Gallagher S, Evans J (2013) The challenges for families managing an adolescent with an intel-lectual disability and type 1 diabetes. *Australian Journal of Advanced Nursing* 30: 26–32.

Hoey H (2009) Psychosocial factors are associated with metabolic control in adolescents: Research from the Hvidoere Study Group on Childhood Diabetes. *Pediatric Diabetes* 10: 9–14. doi: 10.1111/j.1399 -5448.2009.00609.x.

Rohrer TR, Hennes P, Thon A et al. (2010) DPV initiative Down's syndrome in diabetic patients aged <20 years: An analysis of metabolic status, glycaemic control and autoimmunity in comparison with type 1 diabetes. *Diabetolgia* 53: 1070–1075. doi: 10.1007/s00125-010-1686-z.

Rosenbloom AL, Silverstein JH, Amemiya S, Zeitler P, Klingensmith GJ (2009) Type 2 diabetes in children and adolescents. *Pediatric Diabetes* 10: 17–32. doi: 10.1111/j.1399-5448.2009.00584.x.

Scaramuzza AE, Giani E, Riboni S et al. (2009) Insulin pump therapy for type 1 diabetes treatment in a girl with Down's syndrome. *Diabetes Research and Clinical Practice* 85: 16–18. doi: 10.1016/j.diabres. 2009.06.008.

Shield JP, Wadsworth EJ, Hassold TJ, Judis LA, Jacobs PA (1999) Is disomic homozygosity at the APECED locus the cause of increased autoimmunity in Down's syndrome? *Archives of Disease in Childhood* 81: 147–150.

Silverstein J, Klingensmith G, Copeland K et al. (2005) Care of children and adolescents with type 1 diabetes. *Diabetes Care* 28: 186–212.

Smart C, Aslander-van Vliet E, Waldron S (2009) Nutritional management in children and adolescents with diabetes. *Pediatric Diabetes* 10: 100–117. doi: 10.1111/j.1399-5448.2009.00572.x.

Swift PG (2009) Diabetes education in children and adolescents. *Pediatric Diabetes* 10: 51–57. doi: 10.1111/j.1399-5448.2009.00570.x.

Van Goor JC, Massa GG, Hirasing R (1997) Increased incidence and prevalence of diabetes mellitus in Down's syndrome. *Archives of Disease in Childhood* 77: 186.

Villiano MJ, Huber AK, Greenberg DA, Golden BK, Concepcion E, Tomer Y (2009) Autoimmune thyriditis and diabetes: Dissecting the joint genetic susceptibility in a large cohort of multiplex families. *Journal of Clinical Endocrinology & Metabolism* 94: 1458–1466. doi: 10.1210/jc.2008-2193.

White NH, Sun W, Cleary PA et al. (2010) DCCT-EDIC Research Group. Effect of prior intensive therapy in type 1 diabetes on 10-year progression of retinopathy in the DCCT/EDIC: Comparison of adults and adolescents. *Diabetes* 59: 1244–1253. doi: 10.2337/db09-1216.

12
HAEMATOLOGICAL DISORDERS

Beki James and Shiela Puri

Introduction

Down syndrome is associated with a wide variety of haematological changes, some of which can be first apparent *in utero*. The haematological manifestations range from asymptomatic variations in the full blood count to an increased incidence of acute myeloid and lympho-blastic leukaemia. There has been considerable research in this field over the last decade, which has greatly extended our understanding. This chapter will review haematological disorders associated with Down syndrome at three key stages: as neonates, during childhood and in adulthood.

What are the haematological abnormalities commonly seen in the neonatal period?

Neonates with Down syndrome have a distinct haematological profile. It is vital that this is recognized when interpreting a full blood count result to make an appropriate clinical decision in the neonatal period. Two recent studies have set out to characterize the haema-tological profile of neonates with Down syndrome (Henry et al. 2007; B James, personal communication, 2013). The latter study, 'Children with Down Syndrome Study' (CDSS; www.cdss.org.uk), is a prospective birth cohort set within the UK. Down syndrome-specific reference ranges for the neonatal period from the CDSS are provided in Table 12.1.

Red blood cell changes

Polycythaemia has been reported in up to 33–54% of neonates with Down syndrome during the first week of life (Henry et al. 2007, James 2013). Both the haemoglobin and haema-tocrit fall over time and polycythaemia is rare by the fourth week of life. Treatment is only necessary for symptomatic polycythaemia. An increased haematocrit does not appear to be associated with increased erythropoietin levels or concurrent cardiac disease. Recent data suggest that the nucleated red blood cell counts tend to be increased and to persist. The red blood cell count is similar to that of the general population, although an increased mean cell volume persists throughout the first year of life.

Platelet changes

Thrombocytopenia associated with an increased mean platelet volume is commonly observed (Henry et al. 2007, James 2011). As larger platelets are typically more active in terms of their haemostatic function, the thrombocytopenia is usually asymptomatic and resolves spontaneously (Kivivuori et al. 1996).

TABLE 12.1
Reference ranges for neonates with Down syndrome

Parameter	0–7 d Range (95% centile)	8–14 d Range (95% centile)	15–21 d Range (95% centile)	22–28 d Range (95% centile)
Red blood cell parameters				
Red cell count ($\times 10^{12}$ cells/l)	4.3–6.6	3.1–6.2	3.3–4.8	3.7–6.7
Haemoglobin (g/dl)	16.8–25.3	9.5–19.6	11.6–17.6	13.2–23.2
Mean cell haemoglobin (pg)	33.8–41.3	28.6–39.5	31.7–39.6	32.9–39.5
Haematocrit (%)	0.51–0.76	0.3–0.69	0.36–0.58	0.4–0.71
Mean cell volume (fl)	102.1–128.5	84.6–127.1	97.3–127.2	95.1–123.5
Nucleated RBC ($\times 10^9$ cells/l)	0–20.3	0	0–0.2	0–0.2
White blood cell parameters				
White cell count ($\times 10^9$ cells/l)	6.1–24.2	8.1–10.7	4.3–12.3	5.7–22.0
Neutrophils ($\times 10^9$ cells/l)	1.9–16.0	2.2–4.8	1.2–6.0	1.6–11.1
Lymphocytes ($\times 10^9$ cells/l)	1.5–7.5	3.4–4.9	1.5–5.5	1.2–7.4
Basophils ($\times 10^9$ cells/l)	0–0.6	0.08–0.19	0–0.11	0.02–0.38
Eosinophils ($\times 10^9$ cells/l)	0–0.4	0.01–0.31	0.09–0.2	0.01–0.5
Monocytes ($\times 10^9$ cells/l)	0.3–2.0	0.6–2.7	0.1–1.1	0.5–2.1
Platelet parameters				
Platelet count ($\times 10^9$ cells/l)	35–255	102–463	167–451	61–333
Mean platelet volume (fl)	10.4–13.9	10.2–12.6	10.5–12.9	10.9–14.3

White blood cell changes

Neutrophilia with a relative lymphopenia has been observed in up to 80% of neonates with Down syndrome (Henry et al. 2007, James 2011).

Blood cell morphology

Blasts are common findings in blood films from neonates with Down syndrome with *and* without a transient myeloproliferative disorder (TMD). Interpretation of neonatal blood films can be difficult, and advice should be sought from an experienced paediatric haematologist if there are any concerns.

Transient myeloproliferative disorder

TMD (also referred to as transient abnormal myelopoiesis or transient leukaemia) is linked uniquely to trisomy 21 and manifests in the fetal or neonatal period. It is associated with a pathognomonic mutation of *GATA1*, producing a short form of GATA1 (GATA1s) (Kanezaki et al. 2010). It is encoded on the X chromosome and has a phosphorylated double zinc finger structure. Both zinc fingers help GATA1 bind DNA and interact with other proteins. Mutation of GATA1 is acquired *in utero*, probably in the third trimester. The mutation becomes undetectable as the TMD resolves, but may recur with the development of acute megakaryoblastic leukaemia (AMkL) (Shimada et al. 2004, Xu et al. 2006, Kanegane et al. 2007).

The most complete data on the incidence of transient myeloid disorder comes from a retrospective analysis of Guthrie cards of 590 children with Down syndrome. This found a GATA1 mutation in 3.8%—a much lower incidence of TMD than previously reported, although Hispanic children with Down syndrome were noted to have an increased incidence of 7.6% compared with 2.9% of non-Hispanic children (Pine et al. 2007).

What is the clinical course of transient myeloproliferative disorder?
Typically the child is asymptomatic, with no clinical stigmata, and the disorder resolves spontaneously within 3 months (Zipursky et al. 1997). The disorder can progress in a small but significant proportion of children, with uncontrolled proliferation of mega-karyoblasts and fibrosis involving liver, heart, marrow, pancreas and skin. The spleen, lungs and kidneys may also be affected. The central nervous system seems to be spared in TMD.

There is usually a moderate leukocytosis, with white cell counts often in the range of $20–40 \times 10^9$/L. Higher white cell counts of $>100 \times 10^9$/L are associated with severe disease and a poorer prognosis. Coagulopathy is reported in less than 10% of children with TMD, and may indicate disseminated intravascular coagulopathy, which is a poor prognostic factor (Klusmann et al. 2008).

Hepatomegaly is common and usually regresses spontaneously. Development of hepatorenal syndrome, hepatic failure or respiratory failure secondary to diaphragmatic elevation due to massive hepatomegaly is associated with a poor outcome. TMD is thought to arise from the fetal hepatic haemopoietic system rather than bone marrow haematopoiesis.

Splenomegaly only occurs in the presence of portal hypertension rather than due to infiltration or fibrosis. There may be asymptomatic pancreatic involvement with blast infiltration and fibrosis. Ascites and hydrops fetalis are associated with a poor five-year survival if present at the initial presentation (Gamis 2011; Klusmann et al. 2008). Hydrops is usually a result of anaemia, cardiac leukemic infiltration and fibrosis. The outcome is worse if it is associated with congenital heart disease.

TMD can also manifest as a vesiculo-pustular rash, often involving the face and easily mistaken for erythema toxicarum. Biopsy results of the skin lesions demonstrate leukae-mic infiltration with blasts. The rash typically resolves spontaneously as the blast count falls.

How is transient myeloproliferative disorder diagnosed?
Given the association of GATA1s and TMD, it may well be that assessment of GATA1 status will form part of future diagnostic criteria for TMD; however, currently the following diagnostic criteria are used (Gamis et al. 2011):

Less than 3 months of age at presentation with any non-erythroid blasts in the peripheral blood and any one of the following:

- Verification of blasts with a second sample of peripheral blood
- >5% non-erythroid bone marrow blasts
- Hepatomegaly or splenomegaly
- Lymphadenopathy (this is uncommon)
- Cardiac or pleural effusions

If TMD is suspected, then further management should be discussed with a paediatric haematologist. Most children are asymptomatic, but if a child is unwell with life-threatening symptoms then urgent intervention should be initiated with cytotoxic chemotherapy. A single course of intravenous cytarabine can induce long-lasting remission.

In a child who remains clinically well, it is appropriate to repeat the full blood count and blood film once or twice weekly until the blasts have cleared, and the blood film and count have normalized.

In our centre, children are initially seen every 3 months in the paediatric haematology clinic for clinical review, full blood count and blood film. After the age of 2 years, they are seen every 6 months until they have passed their fifth birthday due to an increased associated risk of developing childhood leukaemia—over and above the increased risk for all children with Down syndrome. It is not possible at present to predict with confidence which children with the disorder are likely to develop subsequent leukaemia. Acute myeloid leukaemia (AML) has been reported in 17–23%, with a median age of diagnosis in the second year of life and about 1–2% have subsequently developed acute lymphoblastic leukaemia (ALL), a two-fold increase compared with all children with Down syndrome (Klusmann et al. 2008, Gamis et al. 2011).

What are the haematological abnormalities commonly seen in childhood?
Benign haematological findings
Red blood cell parameters
The haematocrit and mean cell volume are increased in children with Down syndrome (James 2011). The life span of red blood cells, folate and vitamin B12 levels are similar to the general population (David et al. 1996). The persistence of an increased mean cell volume has important clinical implications. A child with Down syndrome and iron deficiency might have a mean red cell volume which appeared normal when compared with standard reference charts. The iron deficiency might be missed and remain untreated with adverse health consequences. This concern has recently been substantiated by a study of 114 children with Down syndrome, which set out to determine the prevalence of iron deficiency in this population (Dixon et al. 2010). It found that 13 out of 15 children who were diagnosed with iron-deficiency anaemia would have been missed if red blood cell indices alone had been used as a means of screening as a result of the elevated mean red cell volume in this group.

White blood cell parameters
Lower absolute neutrophil, lymphocyte, granulocyte and monocyte counts have been reported in children with Down syndrome (James 2011). However, specific subpopulations appear to be increased. For example, there is a 1.5-fold increase in $CD14^{dim}$ $CD16^+$

monocytes which are pro-inflammatory. It may be that these play a role in the many chronic inflammatory conditions associated with Down syndrome. The T- and B-lymphocyte expansion normally seen in children in the first few years of life is not seen in Down syndrome. In particular, there is a lower percentage of naïve T-cell CD4 and CD8 counts (see Chapter 7, Immune Disorders).

Platelet parameters
The platelet count rises throughout the neonatal period and is similar to the general population thereafter (Kivivuori et al. 1996, James 2011).

Acute leukaemia
The first reported case of leukaemia in an infant with Down syndrome was in 1930. Since then, large epidemiological studies have consistently reported that children with Down syndrome have a 20-fold increased risk of both ALL and AML compared with the general population. Although ALL is by far the more common leukaemia in the general population, both ALL and AML occur with roughly equal incidence in Down syndrome.

How does acute myeloid leukaemia differ in children with Down syndrome?
AML is characterized by a rapidly multiplying clone of immature white blood cells called myeloblasts derived from the myeloid lineage. Children with Down syndrome have a 500-fold increased risk of specifically developing AMkL compared with the general population (Zipursky et al. 1992, Khan et al. 2011).

ML-DS occurs at a much younger age, with 95% presenting by the age of 4 compared with only 35% of AML in the general population. Similarly, the median age at diagnosis in children with Down syndrome has been reported to be 1.8 years compared with 7.5 years in the general population.

The prognosis of ML-DS in children with Down syndrome is good, with reported event-free survival ranging between 80% and 100% compared with 35–45% in the general population. This is related to favourable response to chemotherapy as the blasts are very chemosensitive. There is a low incidence of CNS leukaemia in children with Down syndrome.

What is the pathogenesis of acute myeloid leukaemia in Down syndrome?
TMD is considered to be a precursor to ML-DS only in children with Down syndrome. Both GATA1s mutations, as described earlier in the chapter, and the presence of trisomy 21 are a prerequisite for the development of both TMD and ML-DS (Wechsler et al. 2002). GATA1s is uniformly found in all children with Down syndrome who have TMD and ML-DS, but not in children with Down syndrome who have either ALL or ALL in remission, or children who do not have Down syndrome but have AMkL.

It is still not clear what triggers the resolution of TMD or the subsequent occurrence of ML-DS. Up to 20% of children with Down syndrome will develop ML-DS after the clinical resolution of TMD.

Cytogenetic analysis typically shows absence of favourable chromosomal translocations such as *t*(8;21), *t*(15;17), inv 16, *t*(1;22), although unbalanced translocations, particularly +8, del 6q, +11, +21 appear to be increased (James et al. 2008). Recent genome-wide DNA studies involving specimens from different stages of the disease have been undertaken to explore the sequential epigenetic changes defining the biological phenotype of ML-DS in Down syndrome (Malinge et al. 2013). They demonstrated that this process probably occurs in two distinct epigenetic waves. The first wave is directly linked to chromosome 21, resulting in genome-wide hypomethylation. They postulate that hypomethylation occurs, as in trisomy 21 there is an overexpression of cystathionine β-synthetase leading to lower S-adenosylmethionine levels. The developmental disorder associated with Down syndrome is considered to be related specifically to the hypomethylation process. The second wave of aberrant DNA methylation results in hypermethylation at a definite set of target genes, specific to haematological development and cell cycle regulation, and including cell death in TMD. The mechanisms through which these epigenetic changes become established are yet to be identified. This process is believed to contribute to the distinct biological features of ML-DS associated with trisomy 21, particularly the higher sensitivity to cytarabine and other chemotherapeutic agents.

Sporadic acute myeloid leukaemia
Myeloid leukaemia in children 4 years or older with Down syndrome often lacks a GATA1 mutation, and the cytogenetic changes and risk of relapse are similar to AML in the general population with an event-free survival of only 33%. Analysis of AML subtypes by several groups has suggested that acute erythrocytic leukaemia may be specifically increased in children with Down syndrome (Lange et al. 1998, James et al. 2008), whilst other studies have shown a spread of subtypes (Agarwal et al. 2005; Abella et al. 2008). However the clinical management of AML in children with Down Syndrome is the same across the age range, even though the leukemogenesis process is different in the younger child.

What is the management of acute myeloid leukaemia in Down syndrome?
Children with a suspected diagnosis of AML should be referred urgently to a paediatric haematology specialist and wherever possible should be offered opportunities to participate in the current trials.

In 2013, the UK recommendations are for four courses of chemotherapy. In view of the sensitivity of the blasts, the excellent outcome and low relapse rate, a lower anthracycline dose is required, which should in turn reduce cardiotoxicity. Typically, anthracycline-containing regimens are given for the first two courses and high-dose cytarabine alone for the last two courses.

Acute lymphoblastic leukaemia
ALL occurs with a 24-fold increased risk in children with Down syndrome and presents as a more heterogeneous disease ML-DS. In absolute terms, ALL is at least as common as AML in children with Down syndrome (James et al. 2008).

What is the pathogenesis of acute lymphoblastic leukaemia in Down syndrome?
Precursor B-cell ALL is the predominant form, with T-cell ALL being extremely rare in Down syndrome though represents 15% of the total ALL in the general population (James

et al. 2008, Maloney et al. 2010). High hyperdiploidy is typically underrepresented, and chromosomal translocations associated with adverse outcomes such as 11q23/MLL, *t*(9;22), *t*(1;19) are often absent (James et al. 2008, Maloney et al. 2010). An activating mutation of *JAK2* localized has been demonstrated in 18% of children with Down syndrome compared with 10% of children in the general population. The mutations involve the highly conserved arginine residue and induce independent growth of Ba/F3 cells (Bercovich et al. 2008).

JAK 2 mutations have also been described by Kearney et al. (2009) in 28% of children with Down syndrome. A high proportion of children with Down syndrome and ALL have been found to have mutations involving *CRLF2* gene which has been associated with activation of JAK2 mutations. It has been postulated that children with Down syndrome ALL and JAK2 mutations represent a subset of children in which JAK2-STAT pathway activation is linked to the pathogenesis of ALL.

What is the clinical presentation of acute lymphoblastic leukaemia in Down syndrome?

The age of presentation of ALL in children with Down syndrome is similar to that of the general population, although it is rare in children with Down syndrome to present in before one year of age. This is in contrast to 2–6% of children within the general population (Bassal et al. 2005, James et al. 2008). The presenting features are similar to ALL in children without Down syndrome (Maloney 2011). The most common signs and symptoms arise from pancytopenia with anaemia and infection. Bone pain is also common. Presentation with a mediastinal mass or overt central nervous system disease is rare.

What is the management of acute lymphoblastic leukaemia in Down syndrome?

Again, a child with a suspected diagnosis of ALL should be referred urgently to a paediatric haematology specialist and wherever possible should be offered opportunities to participate in the current trials. Children with Down syndrome and ALL were previously reported to have a less favourable overall survival. However, in recent studies with improved supportive guidelines and therapeutic modifications to reduce toxicity, the overall survival of children with ALL and Down syndrome is improving and is approaching that of the general population. Most studies have found that children with Down syndrome are more susceptible to treatment toxicities, particularly infections and mucositis (Maloney 2011). A higher percentage of children with Down syndrome develop steroid-induced hyperglycaemia. In addition, they experience increased risks of anthracycline cardiotoxicity. This may be due to the localization of superoxide dismutase and carbonyl reductase 1 genes on chromosome 21, resulting in altered anthracycline metabolism, increased production of oxygen radicals and apoptosis.

How does the management of acute lymphoblastic leukaemia in Down syndrome differ?

In view of the excess morbidity and mortality in children with Down syndrome the following treatment modifications have been recommended:
- Anthracyclines are omitted in induction unless there is a poor response on the day 15 bone marrow.

- Males should receive the same duration of maintenance as females and not have an extra year of therapy.
- A broad-spectrum antibiotic such as a fluoroquinolone should be given as a primary prophylaxis.
- There should be a low threshold for diagnosing neutropenic sepsis, which may present with non-specific symptoms rather than a classic pyrexia, and early administration of broad-spectrum intravenous antibiotics according to the local protocol.
- Intensive care should be involved early if there are any features of septic shock.

Adults

WHAT ARE THE HAEMATOLOGICAL FINDINGS SEEN IN ADULTS WITH DOWN SYNDROME?

There is a lack of literature and evidence of haematological findings in adults with Down syndrome. Some of the changes described in children appear to persist into adulthood, but these changes should be investigated as there are no validated normative references ranges available for adults with Down syndrome.

A study from Ireland describes its findings in nine adults with Down syndrome over a 7-year period. Two adults were diagnosed with a myelodyplastic syndrome presenting at age 33 and 50 years. The 33-year-old adult required treatment for neutropenia, whilst the 50-year-old was asymptomatic. In the remaining seven adults, macrocytosis, a raised haematocrit and leucopoenia were observed. They recommend exclusion of associated conditions such as sleep apnoea, antiepileptic medication, hypothyroidism, B12 and folate deficiency and suggest that intensive follow-up of the haematological abnormalities is not warranted (McLean et al. 2009).

Key points

- Non-specific haematological abnormalities, particularly polycythaemia, red cell macro-cytosis and thrombocytopenia, are commonly seen in the neonatal period.
- All neonates should have a full blood count and blood film assessment. The results should be correlated clinically and referenced to the published haematological reference ranges specific to neonates with Down syndrome.
- Transient myeloproliferative disorder (TMD) may be seen in up to 10% of neonates. Most are asymptomatic and 20% may develop acute leukaemia in childhood. A paediatric haematologist should interpret the blood film.
- In childhood there is a 20-30-fold increased risk of developing acute leukaemias.
- Myeloid leukemia of Down syndrome has a good prognosis with an event-free survival of 80–100%. It is uniquely associated with prior TMD and a GATA1 mutation.
- Sporadic acute myeloid leukaemia can occur, but has a less favourable outcome.
- Acute lymphoblastic leukemia with a modified regime and intensive supportive therapy has a similar prognosis to the general population.
- Treatment-related toxicity is more common in ALL and should be modified accordingly.
- Leukaemias have been rarely reported in adults, but non- specific haematological abnormalities are commonly seen.

REFERENCES

Bassal M, La MK, Whitlock JA et al. (2005) Lymphoblast biology and outcome among children with Down syndrome and ALL treated on CCG-1952. *Pediatr Blood Cancer* 44: 21–28.

Bercovich D, Ganmore I, Scott LM et al. (2008) Mutations of JAK2 in acute lymphoblastic leukaemias associated with Down's syndrome. *Lancet* 372: 1484–1492.

David O, Fiorucci CC, Tosi MT et al. (1996) Hematological studies in children with Down syndrome. *Pediatr Hematol Oncol* 13: 271–275.

Dixon NE, Crissman BG, Smith PB, Zimmerman SA, Worley G, Kishnani PS (2010) Prevalence of iron deficiency in children with Down syndrome. *J Pediatr* 157: 967.e1–971.e1. doi: 10.1016/j.jpeds.2010.06. 011. Epub 21 July 2010.

Forestier E, Izraeli S, Beverloo B et al. (2008) Cytogenetic features of acute lymphoblastic and myeloid leukemias in pediatric patients with Down syndrome: An iBFM-SG study. *Blood* 111: 1575–1583.

Gamis AS, Alonzo TA, Gerbing RB et al. (2011) Natural history of transient myeloproliferative disorder clinically diagnosed in Down syndrome neonates: A report from the Children's Oncology Group Study A2971. *Blood* 118: 6752–6759.

Henry E, Walker D, Wiedmeier SE, Christensen RD (2007) Hematological abnormalities during the first week of life among neonates with Down syndrome: Data from a multihospital healthcare system. *Am J Med Genet A* 143: 42–50.

James R (2011) A study of the neonatal haematology of children with Down syndrome. http://etheses .whiterose.ac.uk/id/eprint/4063.

James R, Lightfoot T, Simpson J et al. (2008) Acute leukemia in children with Down's syndrome: The importance of population based study. *Hematol J* 93: 1262–1263.

Kanegane H, Watanabe S, Nomura K, Xu G, Ito E, Miyawaki T (2007) Distinct clones are associated with the development of transient myeloproliferative disorder and acute megakaryocytic leukemia in a patient with Down syndrome. *Int J Hematol* 86: 250–252.

Kanezaki R, Toki T, Terui K et al. (2010) Down syndrome and GATA1 mutations in transient abnormal myeloproliferative disorder: Mutation classes correlate with progression to myeloid leukemia. *Blood* 116: 4631–4638. doi: 10.1182/blood-2010-05-282426. Epub 20 August 2010.

Kearney L, Gonzalez De Castro D, Yeung J et al. (2009) Specific JAK2 mutation (JAK2R683) and multiple gene deletions in Down syndrome acute lymphoblastic leukemia. *Blood* 113: 646–648. doi: 10.1182/ blood-2008-08-170928. Epub 16 October 2008.

Khan I, Malinge S, Crispino J (2011) Myeloid leukemia in Down syndrome. *Crit Rev Oncog* 16: 25–36.

Kivivuori SM, Rajantie J, Siimes MA (1996) Peripheral blood cell counts in infants with Down's syndrome. *Clin Genet* 49: 15–19. doi: 10.1111/j.1399-0004.1996.tb04318.x.

Klusmann J-H, Creutzig U, Zimmermann M et al. (2008) Treatment and prognostic impact of transient leukemia in neonates with Down syndrome. *Blood* 111: 2991–2998.

Lange BJ, Kobrinsky N, Barnard DR et al. (1998) Distinctive demography, biology, and outcome of acute myeloid leukemia and myelodysplastic syndrome in children with Down syndrome: Children's Cancer Group Studies 2861 and 2891. *Blood* 91: 608–615.

Malinge S, Chlon T, Doré LC et al. (2013) Development of acute megakaryoblastic leukemia associated with sequential epigenetic changes. *Blood* 122: e33–e43. doi: 10.1182/blood-2013-05-503011.

Maloney K (2011) Acute lymphoblastic leukaemia in children with Down syndrome: An updated review. *Br J Haematol* 155: 420–425.

Maloney KW, Carroll WL, Carroll AJ et al. (2010) Down syndrome childhood acute lymphoblastic leukemia has a unique spectrum of sentinel cytogenetic lesions that influences treatment outcome: A report from the Children's Oncology Group. *Blood* 116: 1045–1050.

McLean S, McHale C, Enright H (2009) Hematological abnormalities in adult patients with Down's syndrome. *Irish J Med Sci* 178: 35–38.

Pine SR, Guo Q, Yin C, Jayabose S, Druschel CM, Sandoval C (2007) Incidence and clinical implications of GATA1 mutations in newborns with Down syndrome. *Blood* 110: 2128–2131.

Shimada A, Xu G, Toki T, Kimura H, Hayashi Y, Ito E (2004) Fetal origin of the GATA1 mutation in identical twins with transient myeloproliferative disorder and acute megakaryoblastic leukemia accompanying Down syndrome. *Blood* 103: 366.

Wechsler J, Greene M, McDevitt MA et al. (2002) Acquired mutations in GATA1 in the megakaryoblastic leukemia of Down syndrome. *Nat Genet* 32: 148–152.

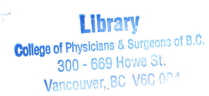

Xu G, Kato K, Toki T, Takahashi Y, Terui K, Ito E (2006) Development of acute megakaryoblastic leukemia from a minor clone in a Down syndrome patient with clinically overt transient myeloproliferative disorder. *J Pediatr Haematol/Oncol* 28: 696–698.

Zipursky A, Brown E, Christensen H, Sutherland R, Doyle J (1997) Leukemia and/or myeloproliferative syndrome in neonates with Down syndrome. *Semin Perinatol* 21: 97–101.

Zipursky A, Poon A, Doyle J (1992) Leukemia in Down syndrome: A review. *Pediatr Hematol Oncol* 9: 139–149.

13
GASTROINTESTINAL DISORDERS

Patricia D Jackson, Peter Gillett and Sarah Almond

This chapter will consider the gastrointestinal conditions which frequently occur, or are specific to children with Down syndrome.

What types of gastrointestinal tract disorders occur in Down syndrome?
We shall consider the following disorders: structural anomalies, disorders of nutrient absorption for healthy growth, infections, motility dysfunction and disorders of the large bowel.

What are the common gastrointestinal symptoms in childhood?
Gastrointestinal conditions account for at least 19% of hospital admissions (Van Trotsenberg et al. 2006). Children with Down syndrome have the same range of symptoms as other children. Interpretation of symptoms takes care, attention and time. Consideration should be given to the person's ability level, method of communication and advice sought from parents and carers. The practitioner needs to be aware of the danger of *diagnostic overshadowing*, the presumption that complaints are 'part of the syndrome' and not worthy of further investigation (Minnes and Steiner 2009).

What types of structural anomalies are commonly seen in the child with Down syndrome?
OESOPHAGEAL ATRESIA
Underlying Biology/Genetics
Between 0.5% and 1% of children with Down syndrome will have oesophageal atresia (Bianca et al. 2002). A failure of complete separation of the respiratory primordia from the foregut of the developing embryo is thought to be the cause, but the developmental mechanisms underpinning this remain uncertain (Ioannides and Copp 2009). Oesophageal atresia is characterized by a blind-ending upper oesophageal pouch, separated from the distal oesophagus by a variable distance, although in most instances the 'gap' is less than three vertebral bodies.

The following subtypes have been described:

- Eighty-five percent have a distal tracheoesophageal fistula (TOF) connecting the lower oesophageal pouch with the trachea.
- Six percent have 'pure' oesophageal atresia with no fistula.

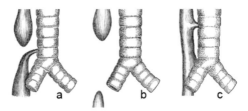

Fig. 13.1. Common anatomical types of oesophageal atresia. (a) Oesophageal atresia with distal tracheoesophageal fistula (86%). (b) Isolated oesophageal atresia without tracheoesophageal fistula (7%). (c) H-type tracheoesophageal fistula (4%).

© 2007 Spitz; Licensee BioMed Central Ltd.

- The remainder have a proximal TOF of an 'H-type' (see Fig. 13.1—Spitz 2007).

Pure oesophageal atresia is much more frequent in Down syndrome, accounting for 50% of cases. The majority of the rest have oesophageal atresia with a distal TOF (Beasley et al. 1997).

How Does Oesophageal Atresia Present in Children with Down Syndrome?
Antenatally oesophageal atresia occurs with polyhydramnios in association with a small fetal stomach. and in the neonatal period with a history of choking and aspiration on attempted feeding A later presentation occurs with episodes of respiratory distress during feeding due to an H-type TOF.

Approach to Management
Besides aiding diagnosis, the passage of a nasogastric tube enables continuous suction of the upper oesophageal pouch to prevent aspiration of secretions. A radiograph will show the position of the tube and outlines the upper oesophagus. Absence of distal bowel gas indicates either pure oesophageal atresia or a proximal TOF; a gas-filled distal bowel indicates the presence of a distal TOF (Spitz 2007).

Ventilation of infants with oesophageal atresia is contraindicated as air will be forced across a distal TOF inflating the bowel and splinting the diaphragm. Prior to surgery, a thorough examination for associated anomalies is recommended, with an echocardiogram to delineate cardiac anatomy (Spitz 2007).

In pure oesophageal atresia, the most common form in children with Down syndrome, primary repair is rarely possible. Enteral feeding by gastrostomy supports the child's nutrition for a period of 2–3 months. Growth of the oesophagus during this period may permit delayed primary oesophageal anastomosis, or oesophageal replacement using the stomach, colon or jejunum to 'bridge the gap' (Gupta and Sharma 2008). For those with oesophageal atresia and distal TOF, a primary repair of the oesophagus to establish continuity is usually achieved.

Outcome

Children with oesophageal atresia in association with Down syndrome have increased complication and mortality rates (Beasley et al. 1997). Contributory factors are the increased incidence of both cardiac defects with pure oesophageal atresia, and a technically more challenging operation, associated with preoperative hospitalization and gastrostomy feeding (Lopez et al. 2006, Gupta and Sharma 2008).

Early complications following oesophageal atresia repair include anastomotic leak, stricture and recurrent fistula. Most leaks settle with conservative management, but strictures require dilatation under anaesthetic and recurrent fistulae are unlikely to resolve without further surgery. In the long term, children often have symptoms of dysphagia and gastro-oesophageal reflux, as a consequence of oesophageal dysmotility (Spitz 2007).

DUODENAL ATRESIA

Duodenal atresia has an overall incidence of 1 in 10 000 live births rising to 247 in 10 000 live births with Down syndrome (Kallen et al. 1996, Best et al. 2012). It arises through failure of recanalization of the duodenum during early fetal life (Best et al. 2012). Choudhry et al. (2009) found 46% of 61 children with duodenal atresia presenting over a 10-year period to have Down syndrome, whereas a European epidemiological study found the association in only 16.6% of infants (Best et al. 2012). Frequent associations are malrotation of the gut, congenital heart disease and vertebral, anorectal, cardiac, tracheo-oesophageal, renal, limb (VACTERL) anomalies.

Duodenal obstruction is classified as either stenosis, or atresia of which there are three types:

1. Type I, duodenum in continuity with a mucosal web within the lumen
2. Type II, duodenal ends connected by a fibrous cord
3. Type III, complete separation of the duodenal ends

Any can be associated with an annular pancreas, which is thought to arise as a consequence of duodenal atresia, rather than being a cause of it (Kamisawa et al. 2001).

The most common anomaly is a type I atresia; 80% are distal to the insertion of the common bile duct on the medial aspect of the second part of the duodenum (Choudhry et al. 2009).

How Do Children Present?

Antenatal. A distended fetal stomach and duodenum at the 20 week anomaly scan, particularly in the presence of polyhydramnios, is highly suggestive, with a low false-positive rate (Choudhry et al. 2009). In view of the strong association with Down syndrome, a suspected diagnosis of duodenal atresia should prompt antenatal counselling for Down syndrome.

Postnatal. Vomiting is typically bilious (80% of obstructions being distal to the opening of the common bile duct) and/or profuse (due to complete obstruction of the duodenum). The minority with incomplete obstruction present after weeks or months with a history of less severe vomiting (Saha et al. 2012). This is more commonly seen in those children with a proximal membrane and associated non-bilious vomiting. An urgent upper gastrointestinal contrast study to exclude malrotation is mandated by episodes of bilious vomiting.

Differential diagnoses include jejunal and ileal atresia, incarcerated inguinal hernia and more distal obstructions such as a meconium plug, meconium ileus or imperforate anus. Abdominal distension is **not** generally a feature of duodenal atresia due to the proximal level of the obstruction.

Approach to Management

An abdominal radiograph should be undertaken in all neonates with bilious or persistent non-bilious vomiting and/or an antenatal history of polyhydramnios or dilated stomach. The double-bubble sign on radiograph is characteristic (Fig. 13.2). The presence of distal bowel gas raises the possibility of an alternative diagnosis but does not exclude a diagnosis of duodenal atresia, incomplete atresia or unusual variants. An upper gastrointestinal contrast study may be required to exclude malrotation and volvulus, or if uncertainty persists, urgent laparotomy is required (Gilbertson-Dahdal et al. 2009).

Preoperative assessment should include screening for congenital heart lesions, fluid resuscitation, nasogastric tube drainage of aspirates and correction of electrolyte balance. Surgery is generally performed during the first week of life to enable early enteral feeding.

Outcome of surgery

Outcomes following surgery for duodenal atresia are good, although complications are more common in children with associated anomalies (Choudhry et al. 2009). Early complications of anastomotic leak or stricture are infrequent. A prolonged postoperative ileus may necessitate parenteral nutrition. Both reflux and blind loop syndrome are associated with a very dilated proximal duodenum with poor peristalsis. These complications generally resolve over time but are amenable to further surgical intervention when necessary (Choudhry et al. 2009).

ANORECTAL MALFORMATIONS

Anorectal malformations (ARMs) affect 1:5000 live births in the general population. Two percent of children with ARM have Down syndrome and 95% of them have an imperforate anus *without* fistula. The rectum is blind-ending approximately 2cm above the perineal skin, and a well-developed sphincter complex is present. ARM is considered to be of multifactorial aetiology (Torres et al. 1998).

Other subtypes with fistula are more commonly seen in children without Down syndrome. The rectum fails to locate within the sphincter complex, resulting in an abnormally placed rectal fistula. In females, the fistula can open onto the perineum, vestibule or within the vagina. In males, it is either perineal or opens along the urethra (Levitt and Pena 2007).

How Do Children Present?

Presentation is in the neonatal period with failure to pass meconium or with an abnormal 'anus' noted on postnatal examination. Rectal examination is essential.

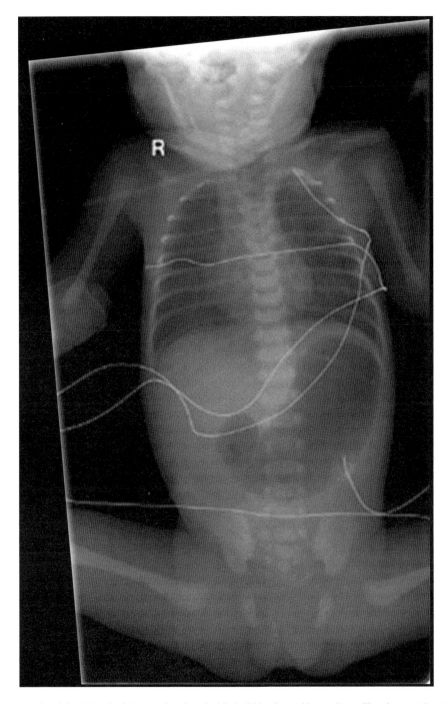

Fig. 13.2. Plain abdominal X-ray showing double bubble sign with gas in a dilated stomach and proximal duodenum.

When a fistula is present, the small calibre of the opening causes difficulty in passing stool. A very small number of infants can present later with constipation.

How Are Anorectal Malformations Managed?
Management of ARMs is surgical. Most children with Down syndrome will not have a perineal fistula/opening, so initial management involves formation of a colostomy to enable stooling, followed by definitive surgery at a few months of age.

Children with ARMs and perineal fistula can generally undergo surgery to reposition the anus within the first few days of life, with the aim of placing the rectum within the sphincter complex to enable normal stooling and continence. The most commonly performed procedure is posterior sagittal anorectoplasty. Closure of the colostomy is undertaken at a later stage (Levitt and Pena 2007).

Outcomes of surgery
The outcome is assessed by capacity for voluntary bowel opening, faecal continence and constipation. For the common imperforate anus without fistula seen in Down syndrome, 80% achieve voluntary bowel opening. Constipation and occasional soiling affect 46%. In contrast to other anomalies discussed in this chapter, the association with Down syndrome does not significantly worsen outcomes (Torres et al. 1998).

ABSORPTION AND MOTILITY
The essential function of the gastrointestinal system is to ensure intake and absorption of nutrients. Even in the absence of any structural anomaly this can be a significant problem for infants with Down syndrome, disadvantaged by poor early feeding. Subsequently, it is hard to establish good breast or bottle-feeding technique. Breast feeding has been shown to be less popular in mothers of children with Down syndrome, and mothers are often discouraged from persisting. The mechanism of feeding by breast or bottle can be affected by the infant's poor orofacial muscle control (see Chapter 18a), the shape of the palate and the sleepiness associated with a higher incidence of neonatal jaundice. Gastro-oesophageal reflux can lead the infant to associate feeding with pain. Loss of nutrients also occurs because of associated vomiting. All of these are compounded if the infant has a cardiac problem.

Dick had pyloric stenosis with classic symptoms. This was treated surgically at 6 weeks. However, following this procedure, weight gain was inadequate and he continued to fall further away from the lowest centiles on the charts. He was quite a distressed baby. He had watery green stools and was breastfeeding. He was the third child of a paediatric nurse who was convinced that he was sucking adequately. However, we decided to test weigh him and this revealed that he was getting less than 50mL of milk at every feed. Supplementation with bottle feeding rapidly brought him back to the expected centile.

Parental perspective. *Dick's mother, a very competent, paediatric nurse, initially felt guilty that she had failed to pinpoint the cause of her baby's distress and poor* *weight gain. She did however take comfort in the fact that it had raised awareness of the problem of underfeeding at the breast by babies with Down syndrome.*

Health professionals' perspective. *Another case of diagnostic overshadowing but fortunately one which did not persist for long before the true nature of the problem was revealed.*

Why is gastro-oesophageal reflux disorder more common?

Poor oro-muscular tone and coordination, laxity of the gastro-oesophageal junction and lower diaphragmatic and abdominal muscle tone increase the risk for gastro-oesophageal reflux (Frazier and Friedman 1996). This risk is prolonged because of the associated motor impairment. Gastro-oesophageal reflux disorder (GORD) may be implicated as a cause of conductive hearing loss, due to inflammation not only within the oesophagus, but also affecting the Eustachian tubes (see Chapter 5).

HOW DOES THIS PRESENT AND HOW TO TREAT?

Children will present in the first few months of life with poor feeding, vomiting after feeds and general irritability. Increased severity is indicated by blood in the vomit, and delay or decelerating weight gain and growth, as measured on the Down syndrome-specific growth charts. Good postfeeding posture is essential as well as early intervention with treatment for their reflux. Given the high incidence of GORD in Down syndrome, a low threshold to treat when we suspect the condition seems appropriate. The treatment approach is the same as for any child with GORD (Mancchini et al. 2011).

MOTILITY

Motility studies in children with Down syndrome who are well show no evidence of abnormality in gastric emptying and gut transit. The high incidence of constipation in otherwise healthy children on healthy diets suggests that abdominal muscle hypotonicity is a significant contributor, as is diminished physical activity related to developmental level and/or opportunities for exercise.

Research indicates that the motility of the bile duct is affected, encouraging accumulation of deposits and gall stone development. There is conflicting evidence as to whether these are more likely to be symptomatic in children with Down syndrome. It is not felt useful to screen for gall stones, but to await the presentation of symptoms (Boechat et al. 2007).

Constipation

Significant constipation is a problem, despite the lack of any obvious underlying gut abnormality. It is so common that there is a case for starting more active bowel management at an early stage in all children with Down syndrome. This might assist in preventing the long-term secondary problems of colonic expansion. More serious but rarer conditions should be considered and eliminated as appropriate, particularly constipation associated with gut anomalies coeliac disease and hypothyroidism.

MANAGEMENT OF CONSTIPATION

Providing an explanation and written information to parents about constipation, including the mode of action and safe use of medication, optimizes its effectiveness and leads to better results. Often the usual approach of increasing fibre content and ensuring adequate daily fluid intake can result in favourable changes to the bowel pattern, but the additional need to compensate for low activity/exercise levels and low abdominal tone needs to be factored into any care plan. The Bristol Stool Chart is a helpful pictorial reference for the parent, and the 'Tough Going' pack developed for Health Practitioners in Scotland is a valuable source of information and support. At school entry, it is important that those with responsibility for the child's care are just as knowledgeable and proactive in ensuring that the child drinks adequately through the day. A daily target of about 1L should be achieved, as well as ensuring that the child participates in physical activities.

Toddler diarrhoea

Parents may find that diarrhoea that can persist through the toddler stage is causing concern and complicating toilet training. The child concerned is well with a healthy weight gain and reassurance is often the best approach, but the possibility of constipation as an underlying cause should be eliminated by good history taking and clinical examination of the abdomen. The history may reveal an excessive intake of roughage in the diet or fruit juices, and dietary change will often resolve the situation.

Pathological conditions affecting gut motility can be present and should always be considered. The most common of these is Hirschsprung disease.

What is Hirschsprung disease and why is it more common in Down syndrome?

Children with Down syndrome have a 100-fold increased risk of Hirschsprung disease (HSCR), compared with the general population. Between 4% and 35% of children with HSCR have additional congenital conditions. By far the most common of these is Down syndrome, which is seen in 2–10% of cases. The incidence of HSCR in the general population is approximately 1 in 5000 live births, with a 4:1 male to female ratio (Amiel and Lyonnet 2001). The extent of aganglionosis is similar in sporadic HSCR and HSCR associated with Down syndrome.

In 80% of cases, HSCR only affects the rectosigmoid region, but in the remainder the aganglionosis extends more proximally (Amiel and Lyonnet 2001), and rarely may involve the entire colon (total colonic aganglionosis). In longer segment disease, the male to female ratio becomes progressively less pronounced, and in total colonic aganglionosis there is a 1.5:1 female predominance (Moore and Zaahl 2009).

Most cases of HSCR arise sporadically; up to 15% are familial, particularly longer segment disease. Epidemiological factors indicate a complex genetic basis for HSCR, with differing patterns of inheritance according to the extent of disease. Segregation analysis has suggested the presence of a dominant gene with incomplete penetrance in long-segment HSCR and involvement of one or more recessive genes with low, sex-dependent penetrance in short-segment HSCR (Amiel and Lyonnet 2001). Of the nine genes implicated in the pathogenesis of HSCR, the most important is *RET* (10q11), which codes for a tyrosine kinase receptor (Kenny et al. 2010). *RET* mutations are estimated to account for up to 50% of familial and 20% of sporadic HSCR. Mutations in the endothelin B receptor gene (EDNRB, 13q22) are found in up to 5% of those with short-segment HSCR. Other gene mutations more rarely identified in HSCR include those coding for the EDNRB ligands (endothelins) and the transcription factors SOX10 and PHOX2B (Kenny et al. 2010).

In Down syndrome-associated HSCR, specific *EDNRB* polymorphisms have been identified at an increased frequency. More recently, a chromosome 21 dose-dependent interaction with an *RET* enhancer polymorphism has been described (Arnold et al. 2009). However, the genetic basis of the trisomy 21/HSCR association and how it relates to under-development of the myenteric plexus remains uncertain.

HOW DO CHILDREN WITH HIRSCHSPRUNG DISEASE PRESENT?

The classic history is a failure to pass meconium within 24 hours of birth, often associated with abdominal distension and subsequent vomiting, due to the progressive dilatation of the unaffected bowel proximal to the contracted aganglionic segment which has no peristalsis. Although less common, presentation in the later neonatal period with symptoms of enterocolitis (explosive diarrhoea, fever, abdominal distension) does occur. Occasionally, children present more insidiously with symptoms of chronic constipation and failure to thrive during infancy. Rarely, the diagnosis is made in older children who have a long history of refractory constipation. The strong association with HSCR mandates a high index of suspicion when investigating constipation in children with Down syndrome. Rectal biopsy to exclude HSCR should be considered in all cases, including those presenting outside the neonatal period.

APPROACH TO MANAGEMENT

Confirmation of the diagnosis of HSCR requires rectal biopsy showing aganglionosis of the distal bowel. Additionally, hypertrophied nerve fibres projecting into the aganglionic bowel from normal ganglia outside the gut can be detected on acetylcholinesterase staining.

Initial management of suspected HSCR comprises decompression of the bowel by rectal washouts, in combination with antibiotic treatment for enterocolitis. The surgical management is similar to any child presenting with Hirschsprung disease, which involves resection of the aganglionic bowel with anastomosis of the proximal normo-ganglionic gut to the anal canal.

OUTCOMES

Complications following surgery for HSCR include anastomotic leak and stricture, perineal excoriation (due to more liquid stool following colon resection), wound infections and enterocolitis. Of these, enterocolitis is the most difficult to manage, and recurrent episodes may occur for several years despite complete resection of the aganglionic bowel. This is more common in children with Down syndrome. Mortality, although low overall, is also higher for children with associated congenital anomalies, including Down syndrome. In both instances, immune deficiency and the impact of other comorbidities, particularly cardiac lesions, are contributory factors (Minford et al. 2004).

Functional outcome assessments in HSCR focus on continence and constipation. Results indicate that children with longer-segment HSCR have worse outcomes than those with rectosigmoid disease. Symptoms tend to improve over time, although this may reflect changing expectations and lifestyle adaptation (Mills et al. 2008). Up to 12% of children with HSCR require further surgery or a permanent colostomy to manage their bowel function satisfactorily (Baillie et al. 1999, Mills et al. 2008). Outcomes may be even poorer for children with Down syndrome and HSCR, although results are conflicting, possibly due to the wide range of scoring tools employed (Menezes and Puri 2005, Morabito et al. 2006).

Future therapies using neural stem cells to colonize the aganglionic bowel have been proposed (Almond et al. 2007).

Absorption

When there is no structural or mucosal abnormality, the ability of the intestine to absorb nutrients should not be impaired. However, research in animal models has found some evidence for impaired mineral and nutrient absorption that could predispose people with Down syndrome to have poorer development in the early years and increase the risk of dementia in adulthood. A controlled study in the UK in children with Down syndrome has found no evidence to support this hypothesis (Ellis et al 2008). The continuing advice to parents should be that children with Down syndrome, given a normal healthy diet, do not require supplementation, unless they are proven to have specific allergies affecting their gastrointestinal function or autoimmune problems such as coeliac disease (see Chapter 19).

A small number of children with Down syndrome following surgery for major gut abnormalities requiring resection of a large portion of the bowel may require dietary supplementation, as for any child. The most common sign of malabsorption is iron deficiency anaemia as a presenting feature in coeliac disorder.

Coeliac disease and Down syndrome

Coeliac disease is a life-long autoimmune (T-cell mediated) systemic inflammatory condition seen in genetically predisposed individuals, primarily affecting the small intestine. It presents with a multitude of phenotypes, including classic malabsorption, monosymptomatic gastrointestinal presentations and extra-intestinal conditions.

The association of Down syndrome and coeliac disease was first described in 1975 (Bentley 1975) but is still not completely understood. At least 30 studies worldwide have looked at prevalence and different screening strategies, predominantly in Caucasian populations with rates varying widely but up to 19% (Bonamico et al. 2001; Pavlovic et al. 2010a, 2010b; Saadah et al. 2012; Bhat et al. 2013). Most recently, a Swedish group (where there is no formal screening policy) studied all those registered with coeliac disease and found Down syndrome comprised 1.4% of the total. This 'real world' prevalence was six times the background general population risk. They suggested a likely prevalence rate (if children with Down syndrome were tested) of at least 3.3% (Mårild et al. 2013). A recent Scottish national coeliac disease incidence study identified only one participant with Down syndrome out of a total of 91 (1.1%) but significant geographical differences emerged, and may well reflect varying awareness of the condition (White et al. 2013).

DQ2- and DQ8-positive T-cell mucosal exposure to epitopes of gliadin drives an inflammatory process that produces a rising antibody response to anti-tissue transglutaminase 2. This results in architectural changes (crypt hyperplasia and villous atrophy) primarily in the small bowel. The modified Marsh grading system allows accurate description of histological changes (Dickson et al. 2006). Gluten is required to maintain this process and strict removal usually normalizes serology and histology and reduces many long-term risks in the majority (Fasano and Catassi 2012).

Symptoms and degrees of malabsorption vary (Hunt and Van Heel 2009). The most common deficiency seen is iron deficiency, but folate, vitamin B12 and fat-soluble vitamin deficiencies are also seen. Accurate serology testing for anti-endomysial antibodies (since 1990), tissue transglutaminase antibodies, tTGA (since 1997) and confirmatory biopsy remains the mainstay of diagnosis (Rubio-Tapia et al. 2013).

Presentation

Presenting gastrointestinal symptoms of coeliac disease in Down syndrome is not significantly different from those in the general population (Book et al. 2001). Reflux and vomiting, recurrent abdominal pain, wind and variable bowel habit with diarrhoea or constipation, with or without growth issues may alert care providers. There might be a delay in testing as these symptoms are so common that they might be assumed to be 'just' part of the Down syndrome 'motility spectrum' (Bonamico et al. 2001).

The prevalence of coeliac disease in the general population is accepted to be around 1% (Fasano and Catassi 2012). Targeted, rather than formal, screening (with a low threshold to test) is generally practised in Down syndrome in the UK, and this may be the reason for the lower ascertainment rates than seen in published studies. A formal screening strategy may lead to earlier diagnosis.

To screen or not to screen?

Screening needs to be cost-effective and to prevent important complications (e.g. malignancy, other autoimmune conditions and osteoporosis). The NICE Guideline CG86 (supported by the British Society for Paediatric Gastroenterology Hepatology and Nutrition) for coeliac disease diagnosis suggests that screening should be considered in 'at-risk' groups including Down syndrome (NICE CG86 2009). The American Academy of Pediatrics recommends screening for coeliac disease in symptomatic children with Down syndrome (Bull et al. 2011). Nonetheless, there is currently no formal national UK strategy.

Coeliac disease-related malignancy risk is low, although it is not zero (Lohi et al. 2009a, 2009b; Elfström et al. 2011). There is little evidence for specific coeliac disease-related cancers in Down syndrome (Goldacre et al. 2004). Enteropathy-associated lymphomas present in middle to later life in Down syndrome are associated with a limited life expectancy (Kawatu and Leleiko 2006). Coeliac disease screening is expensive in preventing lymphoma, estimated at $5 million per case in Down syndrome in the US (Swigonski et al. 2006). Screening could be detrimental to the child and families' quality of life if the person was asymptomatic.

Osteoporosis is more common in Down syndrome and this may be a stronger reason for screening (McKelvey et al. 2013). Conversely, some studies have not shown a strong association (van Allen et al. 1999). Until better health economic and quality of life data are available, the screening debate may continue.

WHAT STRATEGY SHOULD BE USED FOR SCREENING?

HLA typing is increasingly important in assessing risk. A Dutch study suggests that using HLA DQ testing to exclude the need for any future testing may well offer positive reassurance for families (Csizmadia et al. 2000). (The human leukocyte antigen [HLA] complex is located on the short arm of chromosome 6. HLA-DQ (DQ) is a cell surface receptor type protein found on antigen-presenting cells. DQ is an αβ heterodimer of the MHC Class II type.) The recent European Society for Paediatric Gastroenterology, Hepatology and Nutrition (ESPGHAN) guideline aims to reduce the need for diagnostic biopsy, proposing two algorithms—one for those with symptoms and one for those who are asymptomatic but 'at-risk' (Husby et al. 2012, Murch et al. 2013). Down syndrome is an at-risk condition, and people with Down syndrome could be screened using DQ typing as the initial strategy. People who are DQ2 and DQ8 negative will generally not require further testing. This approach is being 'road-tested' worldwide including an EU-funded study, the ProCeDE study (www.procede2011.jimdo.com). Up to 30–40% of individuals may have DQ2 and/or DQ8. The prevalence in the population with Down syndrome is thought to be similar (Sollid and Lie 2005, Hunt and Van Heel 2009). Cost and availability of DQ testing in the UK may prevent this strategy from being implemented.

Families, and primary and secondary health care providers should be informed and aware that there is an increased risk of coeliac disease in Down syndrome. Testing should be easily accessed. Families need to be counselled regarding the consequences of testing and any concerns addressed. Most would argue that using a low threshold to test, with increased population awareness might be a more cost-effective strategy. The new ESPGHAN guidance seems a sensible step forward with early DQ testing. A negative test is very reassuring. If positive, then serology testing can be discussed and planned following parental counselling. The approach could easily be achieved with commencement of annual thyroid function testing.

MANAGEMENT OF COELIAC DISEASE IN DOWN SYNDROME

Once the diagnosis is made, it is necessary to exclude gluten from the diet completely and replace identified nutritional deficiencies, until the intestine recovers. Ensuring a totally gluten-free diet may be challenging for parents and carers, but it is achievable.

Summary

Children with Down syndrome should be managed essentially in the same way as any other child in relation to disorders of their gastrointestinal system. We have highlighted those less common disorders which occur more frequently in children with Down syndrome, which need to be actively considered in management of them. Table 13.1 offers a synthesis of what we have considered in a symptom-based approach to clinical practice.

TABLE 13.1
A symptom-based approach to gastrointestinal disorders in Down syndrome

Symptom/sign		Possible problem
Antenatal polyhydramnios	Detailed antenatal anomaly scan Postnatally pass broad N/G tube	Oesophageal atresia, duodenal atresia
Not passing meconium at birth	Check anal patency Examine for perineal fistula	Anorectal anomaly Hirschsprung disease
Regurgitation of clear secretions at birth Respiratory symptoms	Pass broad N/G tube	Oesophageal atresia, with or without fistula
Vomiting		Postural regurgitation Possible significant reflux GORD Gastroenteritis Possible partial gut obstruction
Vomiting with blood		GORD Gastroenteritis
Vomiting with bile		Gut obstruction, check for duodenal atresia, partial or complete.
Weight loss		Poor feeding Cardiac problem GORD Coeliac disease Thyroid problem Hirschsprung disease
Constipation	Check patency of anus Check fluid and dietary intake	Habitual poor bowel function with dilatation Coeliac disease Hypothyroid Hirschsprung disease
Abdominal pain		GORD Gastroenteritis Constipation Pain/disease out with the gut Appendicitis Hernia Partial bowel obstruction/atresia
Diarrhoea		Persistent toddler diarrhoea Gastroenteritis Constipation with overflow Coeliac disease

GORD, gastro-oesophageal reflux disorder.

A 10-month-old with Down syndrome presents with a history of poor growth and weight gain, constipation and occasional bouts of severe loose stools. There is an occasional appearance of some blood in the stool. She was born at 38 weeks' gestation, bottle fed and appeared to thrive well initially. She has no associated cardiac defect.

What might the differential diagnosis be?

Non-specific constipation due to poor abdominal muscle control

Possible bouts of gastroenteritis

Poor dietary intake

Food allergy

Hirschsprung disease

Hypothyroidism

Coeliac disease

What investigations might usefully be ordered?

Full physical examination of the infant including inspection of the perineum to check for anal patency

Check for increased distention of abdomen and presence of faeces in colon

Check records about passage of meconium (in the newborn infant!)

Record weight and height on Down syndrome growth charts

Take full dietary history, including possible food allergens and fluid intake

Send stool for culture

Arrange FBC, thyroid check and consider immune function testing

Consider testing for coeliac disease, if appropriate

Consider abdominal radiograph/ultrasound

Consider referral to surgical team if biopsy necessary to exclude Hirschsprung disease

REFERENCES

Almond S, Lindley RM, Kenny SE, Connell MG, Edgar DH (2007) Characterisation and transplantation of enteric nervous system progenitor cells. *Gut* 56: 489–496.

Amiel J, Lyonnet S (2001) Hirschsprung disease, associated syndromes, and genetics: A review. *J Med Genet* 38: 729–739.

Arnold S, Pelet A, Amiel J et al. (2009) Interaction between a chromosome 10 RET enhancer and chromosome 21 in the Down syndrome-Hirschsprung disease association. *Hum Mut* 30: 771–775.

Baillie CT, Kenny SE, Rintala RJ, Booth JM, Lloyd DA (1999) Long-term outcome and colonic motility after the Duhamel procedure for Hirschsprung's disease. *J Pediatr Surg* 34: 325–329.

Beasley SW, Allen M, Myers N (1997) The effects of Down syndrome and other chromosomal abnormalities on survival and management in oesophageal atresia. *Pediatr Surg Int* 44: 550–551.

Bentley D. (1975) A case of Down's syndrome complicated by retinoblastoma and celiac disease. http://www.ncbi.nlm.nih.gov/pubmed/?term=down+syndrome+celiac+bentley. *Pediatrics* 56:131–3.

Best KE, Tennant PW, Addor MC et al. (2012) Epidemiology of small intestinal atresia in Europe: A register-based study. *Arch Dis Child Fetal Neonat Ed* 97: F353–F358.

Bhat AS, Chaturvedi MK, Saini S et al. (2013) Prevalence of celiac disease in Indian children with Down syndrome and its clinical and laboratory predictors. *Indian J Pediatr* 80: 114–117.

Bianca S, Bianca M, Ettore G (2002) Oesophageal atresia and Down syndrome. *Down Syndr Res Pract* 8: 29–30.

Boechat MC, Silva KS, Llerena JC, Boechat PR (2007) Cholelithiasis and biliary sludge in Downs syndrome patients. *Sao Paulo Med J* 125: 329–332.

Bonamico M, Mariani P, Danesi HM et al. (2001) Prevalence and clinical picture of celiac disease in Italian Down syndrome patients: A multicenter study. *J Pediatr Gastroenterol Nutr* 33: 139–143.

Book L, Hart A, Black J, Feolo M, Zone JJ, Neuhausen SL (2001) Prevalence and clinical characteristics of celiac disease in Down's syndrome in a US study. *Am J Med Genet* 98: 70–74.

Bull MJ, the Committee on Genetics (2011) Health supervision for children with Down syndrome. *Pediatrics* 128: 393–406.

Carlsson A, Axelsson I, Borulf S et al. (1998) Prevalence of IgA-antigliadin antibodies and IgA-antiendomysium antibodies related to celiac disease in children with Down syndrome. *Pediatrics* 101: 272–275.

Choudhry MS, Rahman N, Boyd P, Lakhoo K (2009) Duodenal atresia: Associated anomalies, prenatal diagnosis and outcome. *Pediatr Surg Int* 25: 727–730.

Csizmadia CG, Mearin ML, Oren A et al. (2000) Accuracy and cost-effectiveness of a new strategy to screen for celiac disease in children with Down syndrome. *J Pediatr* 137: 756–761.

Dickson BC, Streutker CJ, Chetty R (2006) Coeliac disease: An update for pathologists. *J Clin Pathol* 59: 1008–1016.

Elfström P, Granath F, Ekström Smedby K et al. (2011) Risk of lymphoproliferative malignancy in relation to small intestinal histopathology among patients with celiac disease. *J Natl Cancer Inst* 103: 436–444.

Ellis JM, Tan KH, Gilbert RE et al. (2008) Supplementation with antioxidants and folinic acid for children with Down's syndrome: randomised controlled trial *BMJ* 336: 594–597. doi: 10.1136/bmj.39465.544028. AE.

Fasano A, Catassi C (2012) Clinical practice. Celiac disease. *N Engl J Med* 367: 2419–2426.

Frazier JB, Friedman B (1996) Swallow function in children with Down syndrome: A retrospective study. *Dev Med Child Neurol* 38: 695–703.

Gilbertson-Dahdal DL, Dutta S, Varich LJ, Barth RA (2009) Neonatal malrotation with midgut volvulus mimicking duodenal atresia. *Am J Roentgenol* 192: 1269–1271.

Goldacre MJ, Wotton CJ, Seagroatt V et al. (2004) Cancers and immune related diseases associated with Down's syndrome: A record linkage study. *Arch Dis Child* 89: 1014–1017.

Gupta DK, Sharma S (2008) Esophageal atresia: The total care in a high-risk population. *Seminars Pediatr Surg* 17: 236–243.

Hunt KA, van Heel DA (2009) Recent advances in coeliac disease genetics. *Gut* 58: 473–476.

Husby S, Koletzko S, Korponay-Szabó IR et al. (2012) European Society for Pediatric Gastroenterology, Hepatology, and Nutrition guidelines for the diagnosis of coeliac disease. *J Pediatr Gastroenterol Nutr* 54: 136–160.

Ioannides AS, Copp AJ (2009) Embryology of oesophageal atresia. *Semin Pediatr Surg* 18: 2–11.

Kallen B, Mastroiacovo P, Robert E (1996) Major congenital malformations in Down syndrome. *Am J Med Genet* 65: 160–166.

Kamisawa T, Yuyang T, Egawa N, Ishiwata J, Okamoto A (2001) A new embryologic hypothesis of annular pancreas. *Hepatogastroenterology* 48: 277–278.

Kawatu D, LeLeiko NS (2006) Screening for celiac disease in asymptomatic children with Down syndrome: Cost-effectiveness of preventing lymphoma. *Pediatrics* 118: 816–817.

Kenny SE, Tam PK, Garcia-Barcelo M (2010) Hirschsprung's disease. *Semin Pediatr Surg* 19: 194–200.

Levitt MA, Pena A (2007) Anorectal malformations. *Orphanet J Rare Dis* 2: 33.

Lohi S, Mäki M, Montonen J et al. (2009a) Malignancies in cases with screening-identified evidence of celiac disease: A long-term population-based cohort study. *Gut* 58: 643–647.

Lohi S, Mäki M, Rissanen H, Knekt P, Reunanen A, Kaukinen K (2009b) Prognosis of unrecognized coeliac disease as regards mortality: A population-based cohort study. *Ann Med* 41: 508–515.

Lopez PJ, Keys C, Pierro A et al. (2006) Oesophageal atresia: Improved outcome in high-risk groups? *J Pediatr Surg* 41: 331–334.

Mancchini F, Leva E, Torricelli M, Valade A (2011) Treating acid reflux disease in patients with Down syndrome: Pharmacological and physiological approaches. *Clin Exp Gastroenterol* 4: 19–22.

Mårild K, Stephansson O, Grahnquist L, Cnattingius S, Söderman G, Ludvigsson JF (2013) Down syndrome is associated with elevated risk of celiac disease: A nationwide case-control study. *J Pediatr* 163: 237–242.

McKelvey KD, Fowler TW, Akel NS et al. (2013) Low bone turnover and low bone density in a cohort of adults with Down syndrome. *Osteoporos Int* 24: 1333–1338.

Menezes M, Puri P (2005) Long-term clinical outcome in patients with Hirschsprung's disease and associated Down's syndrome. *J Pediatr Surg* 40: 810–812.

Mills JL, Konkin DE, Milner R, Penner JG, Langer M, Webber EM (2008) Long-term bowel function and quality of life in children with Hirschsprung's disease. *J Pediatr Surg* 43: 899–905.

Minford JL, Ram A, Turnock RR et al. (2004) Comparison of functional outcomes of duhamel and transanal endorectal coloanal anastomosis for Hirschsprung's disease. *J Pediatr Surg* 39: 161–165; discussion 161–165.

Minnes P, Steiner K (2009) Parent views on enhancing the health care for children with fragile X syndrome, autism, or Down syndrome. *Child Care Health Dev* 35: 250–256.

Moore SW, Zaahl M (2009) Clinical and genetic differences in total colonic aganglionosis in Hirschsprung's disease. *J Pediatr Surg* 44: 1899–1903.

Morabito A, Lall A, Gull S, Mohee A, Bianchi A (2006) The impact of Down's syndrome on the immediate and long-term outcomes of children with Hirschsprung's disease. *Pediatr Surg Int* 22: 179–181.

Murch S, Jenkins H, Auth M et al. (2013) Joint BSPGHAN and Coeliac UK guidelines for the diagnosis and management of coeliac disease in children. *Arch Dis Child* 98: 806–811. doi: 10.1136/archdis-child-2013-303996. Epub 2013 Aug 28. PubMed PMID: 23986560.

Pavlovic M, Radlovi N, Lekovi Z, Berenji K, Stojsi Z, Radlovi V (2010a) Coeliac disease as the cause of resistant sideropenic anaemia in children with Down's syndrome: Case report. *Srpski Arhiv za Celokupno Lekarstvo* 138: 91–94.

Pavlovic M, Radlovic N, Lekovic Z, Stojsic Z, Puleva K, Berenji K (2010b) When to screen children with Down syndrome for celiac disease? *J Trop Pediatr* 56: 443–445.

Rubio-Tapia A, Hill ID, Kelly CP, Calderwood AH, Murray JA (2013) ACG clinical guidelines: Diagnosis and management of celiac disease. *Am J Gastroenterol* 108: 656–676.

Saadah OI, Al-Aama JY, Alaifan MA, Bin Talib YY, Al-Mughales JA (2012) Prevalence of celiac disease in children with Down syndrome screened by anti-tissue transglutaminase antibodies. *Saudi Med J* 33: 208–210.

Saha N, Hasanuzaman SM, Chowdhury LH, Talukder SA (2012) Congenital duodenal web (wind-soak variety) in the fourth part of the duodenum causing obstruction in a female child. *Mymensingh Med J* 21: 745–748.

Sollid LM, Lie BA (2005) Celiac disease genetics: Current concepts and practical applications. *Clin Gastroenterol Hepatol* 3: 843–851. Review. PubMed PMID: 16234020.

Spitz L (2007) Oesophageal atresia. *Orphanet J Rare Dis* 2: 24. doi: 10.1186/1750-1172-2-24.

Swigonski NL, Kuhlenschmidt HL, Bull MJ et al. (2006) Screening for celiac disease in asymptomatic children with Down syndrome: Cost-effectiveness of preventing lymphoma. *Pediatrics* 118: 594–602.

Torres R, Levitt MA, Tovilla JM, Rodriguez G, Pena A (1998) Anorectal malformations and Down's syndrome. *J Pediatr Surg* 33: 194–197.

van Allen MI, Fung J, Jurenka SB (1999) Health care concerns and guidelines for adults with Down syndrome. *Am J Med Genet* 89: 100–110.

Van Trotsenburg AS, Heymans HS, Tijssen JG, de Vijlder JJ, Vulsma T, (2006). Comorbidity, hospitalisation, and medication use and their influence on mental and motor development of young infants with Down syndrome. *Paediatrics* 2006; 118 (4):1633–1639.

White LE, Bannerman E, McGrogan P, Kastner D, Carnegie E, Gillett PM (2013) Childhood coeliac disease diagnoses in Scotland 2009–2010: The SPSU project. *Arch Dis Child* 98: 52–56.

RESOURCES

The Bristol Stool Chart. http://www.eric.org.uk/assets/ choose Childrens Bristol Stool Form Scale (accessed 07 January 2015)

'Tough Going' pack developed for Health Practitioners in Scotland.

National Institute for Clinical Excellence: NICE CG86 (2009). http://www.nice.org.uk/CG86. Recognition and assessment of coeliac disease (accessed 30 December 2014).

ProCeDE study. www.procede2011.jimdo.com. (accessed 30 December 2014)

14
RENAL AND URINARY TRACT ABNORMALITIES

Christine Hardie and Rajiv Puri

Introduction

Renal and urinary tract anomalies are not generally considered to be a common problem in children or adults with Down syndrome. However, recent publications indicate that 3.2% of children with Down syndrome have renal and urinary tract abnormality compared with 0.7% prevalence in general population (Kupferman et al. 2009). The literature on renal and urinary tract disease in adults is sparse, although there are an increasing number of case reports documenting chronic renal failure in adults with Down syndrome secondary to a range of conditions, including glomerulonephritis and obstructive uropathy. Delayed identification of the underlying problem is a common theme, primarily due to delayed investigation, perhaps another example of diagnostic overshadowing.

What congenital abnormalities in the urinary system are reported?

Several congenital anomalies have been reported. The most common can be subdivided into the following three groups:

1. Upper renal tract anomalies
2. Lower renal and urinary tract anomalies and disorders, including obstructive uropathy
3. Anomalies involving the male genitalia

In a retrospective study, Kupferman et al. (2009), comparing a population of 3832 children with Down syndrome to 3 411 833 children in the general population, found the prevalence of ectopic kidney and ureteropelvic junction obstruction to be the same. However, the prevalence of renal tract anomalies, as listed in Table 14.1, was increased in children with Down syndrome.

How do renal and urological problems present in people with Down syndrome?

NEONATAL PERIOD

Significant congenital renal anomalies may be visualized at the 19–20 week fetal anomaly scan and should be managed accordingly. A thorough examination in the neonatal period will identify anomalies such as congenital undescended testes, hypospadias and epispadias. There is insufficient evidence to suggest any benefit in screening asymptomatic infants

TABLE 14.1
**The prevalence of renal tract anomalies in children with Down syndrome
and the general population**

	Down syndrome: rate of cases per 10 000 population	General population: rate of cases per 10 000 population
Renal agenesis	23.5	4.3
Cystic kidney	7.8	1.7
Hydronephrosis	180	21
Hydroureter	13	1.5
Anterior urethral obstruction	2.6	0.1
Posterior urethral valves	5.2	0.7
Hypospadias	80.9	39.6
Prune belly syndrome	2.6	0.2

Adapted from Kupferman et al. (2009).

with Down syndrome provided the infant has had an antenatal fetal anomaly scan. (Personal communication Mr. Patrick Malone, Consultant Paediatric Urologist at the annual Down Syndrome Medical Interest Group, UK and Ireland, June 2012.)

CHILDHOOD

Children with Down syndrome usually achieve continence by a mean age of 3 years 4 months, which is delayed compared with typically developing children. (Brown et al. 2013). After being toilet trained, 46% of children with Down syndrome developed secondary urinary incontinence. However, only 3.8% of the children with Down syndrome were investigated compared with 13.8% of the general population, despite similar rates of urinary tract infection rates in both groups.

Josh, a 6-year-old boy, presented with a 6-month history of daytime wetting. He had a long-standing history of constipation managed with the use of laxatives. Initially, his daytime wetting was considered to be a result of him starting school and an exacerbation of his constipation. However, a history of two urinary tract infections over the previous 6 months, treated by his general practitioner, was noted. He had always had a poor urinary stream. A renal and bladder ultrasound showed evidence of incomplete bladder emptying. There was no evidence of anatomical urethral obstruction. Video urodynamics revealed decreased bladder compliance, with bladder over activity suggestive of detrusor dyssynerngia. He responded to alpha blockers and bladder training. He will require long-term follow-up to ensure that he does not develop renal damage.

BLADDER DYSFUNCTION

Dysfunctional voiding is common in children with Down syndrome and should be investigated and managed appropriately to prevent long-term renal disease (Handel et al. 2003).

Hicks et al. (2007) in a three-part study in children with Down syndrome identified a high incidence (77%) of bladder dysfunction with 68% having a history of wetting. In the retrospective arm of the study over 16 years, seven children, one girl and six boys were identified as having significant bladder dysfunction with three children requiring surgical intervention due to the presence of renal injury.

A non-neurogenic neurogenic bladder is considered to be related to a functional bladder outlet obstruction due to detrusor sphincter dyssynergia. This is considered to be primarily an acquired condition. Hicks et al. (2007) also postulate that detrusor sphincter dyssynergia in Down syndrome may be a part of a congenital bladder dysfunction rather than an acquired phenomenon.

The authors recommend that all children with Down syndrome should have a history of bladder function taken. This is important, as children with Down syndrome may be late in acquiring toileting skills than typically developing children, so a high index of suspicion needs to be maintained. It is important to enquire about a history of urinary tract infections, a delay in acquiring daytime continence, urgency, frequency or urinary retention, weak urinary stream, or pain on voiding. Symptoms of cervical spine disorders should also be excluded as this may confuse matters. If there is evidence of possible bladder dysfunction, a urinary tract ultrasound scan should be performed.

Some children and adults with non-neurogenic neurogenic bladder may require intermittent self-catheterization or behavioural modification with or without alpha blockers. The management of obstructive uropathy may involve surgery to relieve the obstruction to prevent further renal damage. The surgical management of the underlying renal and genital anomalies may be complicated by the associated congenital cardiac defects and wound healing. Preoperative anaesthetic evaluation should include an evaluation of the airways and consideration of associated cervical spine instability.

Should we screen for renal disease in children with Down syndrome?

In 2012, Onal et al. indicated that there was little clinical evidence to support screening of asymptomatic children with Down syndrome for urological anomalies. In their sample study involving 237 participants, just 3% who were asymptomatic had urological anomalies, compared with 40% of those with renal symptoms.

Current guidelines from the American Academy of Pediatrics (Bull 2011) and the Down Syndrome Medical Interest Group UK and Ireland (DSMIG) do not recommend screening for renal or urological problems in Down syndrome; however, knowledge of these conditions is important for clinicians responsible for care of children with Down syndrome.

Adulthood

Glomerular renal disease was previously considered to be rare in people with Down syndrome. However, with increasing life expectancy, there are now more case series reporting acquired renal disease in Down syndrome (Lo et al. 1998, Said et al. 2012). This usually presents in the second and third decade. Renal disease accounts for 9% of the mortality of older adults with Down syndrome (Bittles et al. 2006).

Said et al. (2012) reported a case series of 17 people with Down syndrome over a 16-year period who underwent a renal biopsy. IgA nephropathy was present in 5 patients and focal glomerular sclerosis in 4 of the cohort. This distribution was similar to that found in the general population. However, 8 of the cohort had associated autoimmune disorder, in particular hypothyroidism. Five people in the cohort developed chronic kidney disease and 6 progressed to end-stage renal disease. One person had a successful renal transplant. They concluded that although renal disease is not common in Down syndrome it is not rare, and it should be considered as a part of the investigative work up for people with Down syndrome, presenting with renal or urinary symptoms.

Renal transplantation

A North American Pediatric Renal Transplant Cooperative study (Baqi et al. 1998) found that 14 people with Down syndrome over a nearly 9-year period had a renal transplant. The study group included six males and eight females and their age range was 6–21 years. Three people died during the study period as a result of complications of the transplant.

The following reasons were given for transplantation:

- Obstructive uropathy (4 patients)
- Hypoplastic/dysplastic renal disease (2 patients)
- Focal segmental glomerulosclerosis (2 patients)
- Chronic glomerulonephritis (2 patients)
- Unspecified (2 patients)

Testicular tumours

The lifetime risk of testicular germ cell tumour in the general population is approximately 0.3–0.7%, whereas in individuals with Down syndrome this risk is 6–50 times higher (Dexeus et al. 1988, Satge et al. 1997).

In a retrospective population-based study, Chew and Hutson (2004) found the incidence of undescended testis in children with Down syndrome to be 6.25% compared with 1.1% in the general population. Undescended testis are at risk of developing testicular cancer; a recent meta-analysis shows that there is a relative risk of 6.3 (95% CI, 4.30–9.31) in the ipsilateral and 1.7 (95% CI, 1.01–2.98) in the contralateral testis compared with controls (Akre et al. 2009).

Goede et al. (2012) report a 22.8% prevalence of testicular microcalcification with associated smaller testicular volumes in boys with Down syndrome as compared with a 4.2% incidence reported in boys without Down syndrome (Goede et al. 2009). Testicular microcalcification is a condition usually diagnosed on testicular ultrasound, where multiple small calcifications are present in the seminiferous tubules.

Although the exact correlation between testicular microcalcification and testicular tumour is unclear, in the general population males with testicular microcalcification with associated undescended testis or infertility are taught testicular self-examination from the age of 15 years. Regular follow-up is recommended (Tan et al. 2010) to allow for early detection of possible testicular tumours. As testicular self-examination may be less reliable in people with Down syndrome, Goede et al. (2012) recommend annual testicular ultrasound after the age of 15 in males with Down syndrome even in the absence of the risk factors. However, it is also recommended that men with Down syndrome need to learn testicular self-examination as their cognitive level permits (Elkins et al. 1987, Van Dyke et al. 1995).

Every undescended testis carries some risk for cancer. As a result, anyone with a history of cryptorchidism should be taught testicular self-examination. Parents should be made aware that orchidopexy enables early detection but does not necessarily decrease the cancer risk (Ashley et al. 2010). Input from urologists may be needed to manage testicular abnormality and to teach testicular self-examination.

Key points
- Renal disease is not a common condition in children or adults with Down syndrome but yet it is not rare.
- Presentation of renal disease can be non-specific, and may result in diagnostic overshadowing as symptoms can be attributed to underlying behavioural issues and not investigated promptly.
- Children with Down syndrome presenting with urinary tract infections, at any age, should be investigated with a renal ultrasound scan.
- Both girls and boys presenting with symptoms of a dysfunctional bladder should be investigated with an initial ultrasound of the urinary tract.
- Regular testicular examination should be undertaken with a low threshold to investigate after the age of 15 years.
- There is, as yet, little evidence to embark on a surveillance program and more research needs to be undertaken before this can be advocated.

REFERENCES

Akre O, Pettersson A, Richiardi L (2009) Risk of contralateral testicular cancer among men with unilateral undescended testis: A meta-analysis. *Int J Cancer* 124: 687–689.

Ashley RA, Barthold JS, Kolon TF (2010) Cryptorchidism: pathogenesis, diagnosis, treatment and prognosis. *Urol Clin North Am.* 37: 183–193. doi: 10.1016/j.ucl.2010.03.002.

Baqi N, Tejani A, Sullivan EK (1998) Renal transplantation in Down syndrome: A report of the North American Pediatric Renal Transplant Cooperative Study. *Pediatr Transpl* 2: 211–215.

Bittles AH, Bower C, Hussain R, Glasson EJ (2006) The four ages of Down syndrome. *Eur J Public Health* 17: 221–225. doi: 10.1093/eurpub/ckl103.

Brown E, Hogan R, Zhang J, Dinh K, Langston S, Roth C (2013) Urologic health in children with Down syndrome. *J Urol* 189: e75–e76.

Bull M, the Committee on Genetics (2011) American Academy of Paediatrics, Health supervision for children with Down syndrome. *Pediatrics* 128: 393–406.

Chew G, Hutson JM (2004) Incidence of cryptorchidism and ascending testes in trisomy 21: A 10 year retrospective review. *Pediatr Surg Int* 20: 744–747. doi: 10.1007/s00383-004-1290-8.

Dexeus FH, Logothetis CJ, Chong C, Sella A, Ogden S (1988) Genetic abnormalities in men with germ cell tumors. *J Urol* 140: 80–84.

Elkins TE, McNeeley SG, Punch M, Kope S, Heaton C (1990) Reproductive health concerns in Down syndrome. A report of eight cases. *J Reprod Med.* 35: 745–50. PubMed PMID: 2142964.

Goede J, Hack WW, van der Voort-Doedens LM (2009) Prevalence of testicular microlithiasis in asymptomatic males 0 to 19 years old. *J Urol* 182: 1516.

Goede J, Weijerman ME, Broers CJ (2012) Testicular volume and testicular microlithiasis in boys with Down syndrome. *J Urol* 187: 1012–1017. doi: 10.1016/j.juro.2011.10.167. Epub 20 January 2012.

Handel LN, Barqawi A, Checa G, Furness PD, Koyle MA (2003) Males with Down syndrome and non-neurigenic neurogenic bladder. *J Urol* 169: 646–649. doi: 10.1097/01.ju.0000047125.89679.28.

Hicks JA, Carson C, Malone PSJ (2007) Is there an association between functional bladder outlet obstruction and Down syndrome? *J Pediatr Urol* 3: 369–374.

Kupferman JC, Druschel CM, Kupchik GS (2009) Increased prevalence of renal and urinary tract anomalies in children with Down syndrome. *Pediatrics* 124: 615–621.

Lo A, Brown HG, Fivush BA, Neu AM, Racusen LC (1998) Renal disease in Down syndrome: Autopsy study with emphasis on glomerular lesions. *Am J Kidney Dis* 31: 329.

Malone P. Urinary tract anomalies in Down syndrome – to screen or not to screen? *Lecture to Down Syndrome Medical Interest Group UK and Ireland, Winchester.* Consultant Paediatric Urologist, Southampton, 29 June 2012.

Onal B, Oliveira CM, Chow JS, Rowe CK, Nguyen HT (2012) *J Urol* 187: e184–e185.

Said SM, Cornell LD, Sethi S, Fidler ME, Al Masri O, Marple J, Nasr SJ (2012) Acquired glomerular lesions in patients with Down syndrome. *Human Pathology* 43: 81–88. doi:10.1016/j.humpath.2011.04.009.

Satge D, Sasco AJ, Cure H (1997) An excess of testicular germ cell tumors in Down syndrome: Three case reports and a review of the literature. *Cancer* 80: 929.

Tan IB, Ang KK, Ching BC, Mohan C, Toh CK, Tan MH (2010) Testicular microlithiasis predicts concurrent testicular germ cell tumors and intratubular germ cell neoplasia of unclassified type in adults. A meta-analysis and systematic review. *Cancer* 116: 4520–4532.

Van Dyke DC, McBrien DM, Sherbondy A (1995) Issues of sexuality in Down syndrome. *Down Syndr Res Pract* 3: 65–69.

15
MUSCULOSKELETAL MANIFESTATIONS

Janet Gardner-Medwin, Maureen Todd, Sally Tennant and Shiela Puri

Introduction

Hypotonia, ligamentous laxity and hypermobility are key features in Down syndrome which interact cumulatively to add to the burden of musculoskeletal disability (see Fig. 15.1). It is probably due to an increase in Type VI collagen genes, COL6A1 and COL6A2 mapped to the 21q22.3 (Karousou et al. 2013). Musculoskeletal complications attributed to hypotonia, hyper laxity and hypermobility include cranio-vertebral instability, along with a floppy larynx, difficulties in mastication (Faulks et al. 2008) (see also Chapter 18a) hip instability, scoliosis and foot problems (Jacobsen and Hansson 2000, Caird et al. 2006).

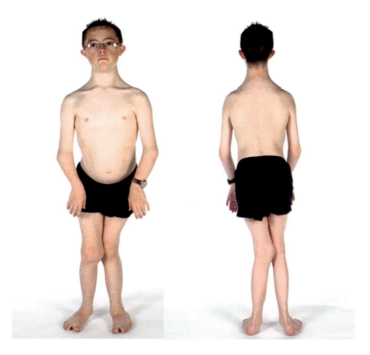

Fig. 15.1. Photograph showing 15-year-old boy with widespread joint destruction at presentation to paediatric rheumatology services after a decade of unrecognized inflammatory arthritis.

Hypotonia and lax ligaments also lead to differences in posture and mechanics in loco-motion (Jover et al. 2010; Rigoldi et al. 2011a, 2011b), with slower performance (Galli et al. 2010), and lower levels of physical activity associated with increased energy require-ments (Agiovlasitis et al. 2009), with the potential to become a negative feedback cycle of decreased levels of physical activity contributing to lower bone mass (Hawli et al. 2009, Gonzalez-Aguero et al. 2010) and a failure to develop or maintain maximum possible muscle strength. Inappropriately low expectations of physical activity from family, health care workers and self, feed into this cycle. Conversely over-attributing motor difficulties to hypotonia and hypermobility may lead to missed pathology and misdiagnoses (Cruikshank et al. 2008, Juj and Emery 2009).

In addition an increased prevalence of autoimmune disorders (e.g. hypothyroidism) and an increased body mass index commonly encountered in Down syndrome may predispose to, or exacerbate motor impairment and orthopaedic conditions and make treatment difficult.

Several studies have suggested that low bone mineral density may be relatively common in Down syndrome (McKelvey et al. 2013, Wu 2013) predisposing to fractures. Osteopoenic bone frequently makes fixation with orthopaedic implants very challenging.

The commonly used scales for recording hypermobility are outdated and are designed for use in adults (Juul-Kristensen et al. 2007) with little relevance to paediatric populations where joint movement ranges are more mobile, widely variable and alter with age and puberty. They are of little value in children with Down syndrome. We undertook a study in Glasgow in 2011 looking at the prevalence of musculoskeletal disorders in a population of

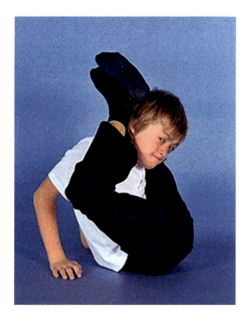

Fig. 15.2. Hypermobile hips in Down syndrome (Courtesy of M Todd 2013).

188

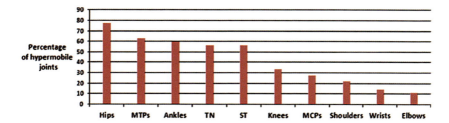

Fig. 15.3. The distribution of hypermobile joints in a study of 73 children with Down syndrome demonstrating the preponderance of hypermobile joints in the lower limb weight bearing joints (Courtesy of M Todd 2013); MTPs, metatarsals; TN, talonavicular; ST, subtalar; MCPs, metacarpals.

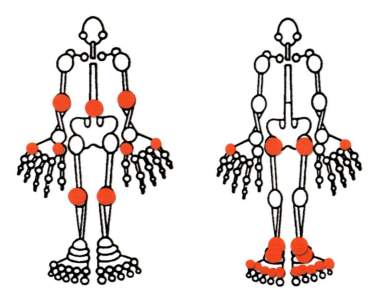

Fig. 15.4. Left drawing shows the joints assessed by the Beighton hypermobility scoring criteria, right drawing shows the most frequently hypermobile joints within the Down syndrome study cohort (M Todd, personal communication, 2013).

143 children with Down syndrome. We recruited 73 children, the study involved examining their joints, anthropometric measurements and parental history regarding joint problems (Todd and Gardner-Medwin, personal communication, 2013). Hypermobility was present in at least one joint in 97%, most commonly the hip joint (77% of children; 76% of hips) (see Fig. 15.2). Beighton scores poorly identified only 25% of children as hypermobile, underestimating the level of hypermobility because of the mismatch of the joints actually scored and those most likely to be hypermobile in Down syndrome, as well as failing to identify the severity of hypermobility characteristic in these children (see Fig. 15.3). A condition-specific score would address these issues (Fig. 15.4).

189

A 15-year-old boy with Down syndrome was referred to paediatric rheumatology services: 'His knee has been synovitic with marked crepitus for some time; would intra-articular steroids help'? He had extensive clinical and radiographic features of a widespread polyarthritis and florid synovitis on a background of widespread joint hypermobility and extensive joint damage. He used a wheelchair for mobility. His father had ankylosing spondylitis.

He did not vocalize pain, but his adapted postures which reduced mechanical forces through his joints were highly suggestive of it. His hips maintained an extreme range of movement (ROM) without pain and magnetic resonance imaging (MRI) with gadolinium confirmed long-standing synovitis. He had a long-standing microcytic anaemia (haemoglobin 6.0–9.5g/dl), despite repeated courses of iron, associated with persistent thrombocytosis (590–729×109/l) supportive of chronic inflammation.

He had long-standing symptoms dating back 9 years, initially hip pain, and then an 'odd gait' with the emergence at 12 years of fixed flexion knee deformities and limited walking ability distance. Diagnostic opportunities were missed by his general practitioner, paediatrician, orthopaedic surgeon and physiotherapist. Despite crepitus and a warm, swollen joint being noted along the way the original radiograph diagnosis of multiple epiphyseal dysplasia had been retained for years. The family members were considered anxious in expressing concern over his pain and told to expect a gradual deterioration in mobility.

Treatment with methylprednisolone was dramatic. He no longer relied on his wheelchair. He tolerated methotrexate poorly but on etanercept had a sustained clinical response, with no active synovitis and normal bloods. He played golf, and was relaxed and happy. However, extensive joint damage in conjunction with hyper-mobility leaves him with residual significant functional loss (see Fig. 15.1).

Inflammatory arthritis

Inflammatory arthritis in children with Down syndrome is more common than juvenile idiopathic arthritis in the general population. It is characterized by particular clinical features but continues to be poorly recognized by clinicians. This results in late diagnosis often with established joint damage and a significantly worsened prognosis (see Fig. 15.5, one of Dr Langdon Down's original photos).

Descriptions of musculoskeletal features associated with Down syndrome over the last 25 years have omitted to report inflammatory arthritis in children (Weijerman and de Winter 2010) or suggest arthritis might be less common than in the general population (Kinnell 1984). This contributes to the continuing lack of awareness amongst medical professionals including those performing regular health checks in this population. Inflammatory arthritis in children with Down syndrome is not included in the clinical synopsis for Online Mendelian Inheritance in Man (OMIM 2013).

Yancey et al. (1984) first described an inflammatory arthritis with a high prevalence occurring in Down syndrome, closely resembling the clinical features of juvenile idiopathic arthritis, the modern umbrella term for the inflammatory arthritides of childhood. Considering this a new 'arthropathy of Down syndrome' rather than an increased incidence of juvenile

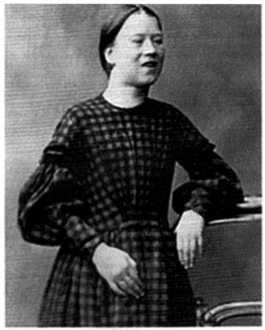

Langdon Down began to take clinical photographs in 1862. His first photograph of an Earlswood resident with Down's syndrome was this unnamed girl in the 1865 series. She was probably the first ever Down's syndrome patient to be photographed.

Fig 15.5. John Langdon Down's original photograph showing changes of longstanding inflammatory arthritis in the hands (C Ward 2002). Photograph used with kind permission of the Down's syndrome Association and the Down's Syndrome Medical Interest Group (www.intellectualdisability.info).

idiopathic arthritis, they started a debate about the aetiology that is likely to be resolved by further immunological and genetic study. Subsequent case series recognized that children with Down syndrome were overrepresented in populations of juvenile idiopathic arthritis, described the clinical features and repeatedly reported delayed diagnosis (Olson et al. 1990, Padmakumar et al. 2002, Cruikshank et al. 2008, Juj and Emery 2009).

EPIDEMIOLOGY

There are no published population surveys establishing the prevalence and incidence of inflammatory arthritis in children with Down syndrome. Crude estimates from case series consistently report a higher incidence than juvenile idiopathic arthritis (see Table 15.1). A population survey in Scotland identified a prevalence of 2.87% (Lynn R and Todd M, personal communication, 2013), approximately 100 times the prevalence of juvenile idiopathic arthritis. A survey in progress in Ireland (similar population size to Scotland) has identified a much larger population of children with Down syndrome (1300 vs 300), and has already identified many instances of inflammatory arthritis (Foley C and Killeen O, personal communication, 2013).

Table 15.1
Estimated incidence and prevalence, and delay in diagnosis of
IADS compared to JIA in the same population from published case series, and
the reasons for delay identified by authors.

Reference	Estimated incidence/ prevalence	Number of cases with delayed diagnosis/ total cases	Mean delay in diagnosis (years)		Cited reasons for delay in diagnosis
			IADS	JIA	
Olson et al., 1990	Three fold increase in incidence compared to JIA in normal population.	8/9	3.3	0.7	Functional change attributed to behavioural problems Lack of awareness of IADS
Padmakumar et al., 2002	Incidence 3.3/10 000/y	-	-		Challenges assessing joints due to hypermobility and unusual hand shapes.
Cruikshank et al., 2008	Prevalence 2.8/1000	8/9	2.2	0.3	Incorrect diagnostic label (soft tissue injury, skeletal dysplasia, behavioural problems) Hypermobility led to failure to recognise loss of ROM Lack of expression of pain Falsely attributing delay in motor development to intellectual disability Gradual functional loss without acute presentation
Juj and Emery, 2009	Incidence 3.3/10 000/y Prevalence 8.7/1000 (six fold increase)		2 y	-	Lack of awareness IADS Challenges around diagnosis Falsely attributing delay in motor development to intellectual disability Hypermobility

IADS, inflammatory arthritis in children with Down syndrome; JIA, juvenile idiopathic arthritis.

CLINICAL FEATURES

The pattern of joint involvement in inflammatory arthritis in children with Down syndrome is broadly consistent in all case reports. The majority have polyarthritis and a high proportion have involvement of the small joints of the hands and feet (Padmakumar et al. 2002; Cruikshank et al. 2008; Juj and Emery 2009; Foley C, personal communication, 2013). The clinical features match the juvenile idiopathic arthritis subgroups 'rheumatoid factor negative polyarthritis' or the asymmetrical small joint involvement typical of 'psoriatic arthritis'. The joints most commonly affected by arthritis correlate to those most likely to be hypermobile (Todd M, personal communication, 2013) (see Figs. 15.3 and 15.7).

In the west of Scotland five of eight children with Down syndrome and inflammatory arthritis fulfilled the criteria for psoriatic arthritis, compared with children with juvenile

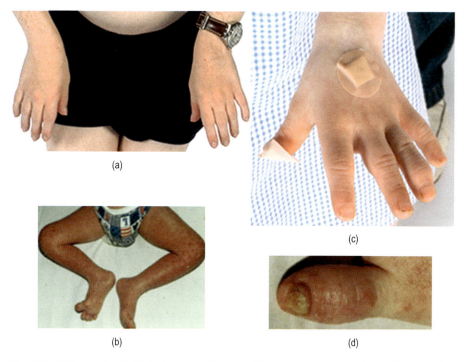

(a)

(c)

(b)

(d)

Fig. 15.6. Patterns of arthritis in the hands in three children with Down syndrome. From top left clockwise: (a) Polyarthritis with ulnar deviation at the wrists, swollen MCP, PIP and DIPs; (b) swelling of the fourth DIP in a pattern consistent with psoriatic arthritis; (c) psoriatic nail changes and rash with a sausage finger of psoriatic arthritis, and in the same child (d) widespread psoriasis and multiple joint involvement.

idiopathic arthritis from the same population of whom only 5.5% had psoriatic arthritis. Moreover, all five of these children had aggressive widespread joint involvement seen in only 41% of the cohort of juvenile idiopathic arthritis, and 22% of those in the cohort with psoriatic arthritis in the general population. The children with Down syndrome were more disabled by their condition. Two of the eight children with Down syndrome had a pattern consistent with polyarticular juvenile idiopathic arthritis and one had an oligo-articular presentation (the most common presentation of juvenile idiopathic arthritis, affecting 59% of juvenile idiopathic arthritis cases). Other reports in Down syndrome have not classified the arthritis by juvenile idiopathic arthritis criteria, but comment on the high proportion with a polyarticular pattern of joint involvement (Padmakumar et al. 2002, Juj and Emery 2009). Where sufficient detail is reported asymmetrical finger involvement is common (Padmakumar et al. 2002, Cruikshank et al. 2008, Juj and Emery 2009). Foley and Killeen (personal communication, 2013) describe 21 children with Down syndrome and a rheumatoid factor negative polyarthritis presentation with finger involvement, particularly proximal interphalangeal joints and distal inter-phalangeal joints.

Chronic anterior uveitis is not reported in association with the inflammatory arthritis in children with Down syndrome in the current literature, and neither is an increased incidence of isolated uveitis (Liza-Sharmini et al. 2006). Regular eye screening in this population suggest the diagnosis is not being missed. This may be important in defining its aetiology because chronic anterior uveitis occurs in around 10% of juvenile idiopathic arthritis as a significant complication. Nonetheless the case for continuing ophthalmological screening throughout life made in Chapter 6 remains particularly pertinent for those with inflammatory arthritis.

INFLAMMATORY ARTHRITIS IN CHILDREN WITH DOWN SYNDROME AND PAIN RESPONSE

Pain in juvenile idiopathic arthritis often has an indolent onset, improves with movement, is reported as stiffness and is a difficult for children to vocalize. People with Down syndrome take longer still to express pain and make more errors localizing the stimulus (Martinez-Cue et al. 1999, Hennequin et al. 2000). Failure to express pain leads to delay and misdiagnosis of inflammatory arthritis in children with Down syndrome (see Table 15.1), although there are other clues with children showing functional loss and adaption to pain and reported observations such as slowing mobility, reluctance to hold a parental hand (Cruikshank et al. 2008) or behavioural change (Padmakumar et al. 2002, Cruikshank et al. 2008, Juj and Emery 2009). Thoughtful consideration of possible interpretations of the history, careful observation and detailed clinical examination are important in reaching a diagnosis.

INFLAMMATORY ARTHRITIS IN CHILDREN WITH DOWN SYNDROME AND HYPERMOBILITY

Losses of ROM with end of ROM pain are taught as characteristic features of arthritis. Hips are particularly difficult to assess because of their depth, and examination relies heavily on these two features. In children with Down syndrome both these features are extremely difficult to assess. The even more extreme ranges of movement than most children combined with the absence of the usual guarding caused by end of ROM pain contribute to overlooking hip arthritis in the inflammatory arthritis of Down syndrome. Gait is difficult to assess in Down syndrome because of hypotonia and hypermobility. As we have already noted, the joints most likely to be affected by arthritis are the most mobile (see Fig. 15.4).

INVESTIGATIONS

Inflammatory arthritis is a clinical diagnosis supported by appropriate investigations. Rheumatoid factor, antinuclear antigen and HLA B27 are neither sensitive nor specific, remaining negative in most cases of inflammatory arthritis in children with Down syndrome. Acute phase responses are not consistently raised. Clinicians should not be falsely reassured by negative tests. Where present, diagnostic clues suggesting chronic inflammation may be identified, from chronically raised acute phase responses, often not excessively high but persistently present, and the anaemia of chronic disease (Cruikshank, personal communication). Plain radiographs may show non-specific soft tissue swelling or bony overgrowth, although high proportions with erosive disease are currently being described indicative of late diagnosis (C Foley, personal communication, 2013). MRI with gadolinium contrast

(Sheybani et al. 2013) is the criterion standard for identifying synovitis often requiring a general anaesthetic in a child with Down syndrome. Ultrasound performed by a musculoskeletal expert is also sensitive for the identification of synovitis (Sheybani et al. 2013). However, clinical consideration of inflammatory arthritis and initiating the appropriate referral is the key step for diagnosis, which is too often delayed (Olson et al. 1990, Padmakumar et al. 2002, Cruikshank et al. 2008, Juj and Emery 2009).

MANAGEMENT

With no clinical trials in inflammatory arthritis in children with Down syndrome, management currently follows therapeutic regimes for juvenile idiopathic arthritis (Stoll and Cron 2013). Early reports suggesting a poor response to therapy, with high levels of drug intolerance (Olson et al. 1990, Padmakumar et al. 2002), have not been borne out with newer therapies with responses largely similar to those in juvenile idiopathic arthritis (Cruikshank et al. 2008, Juj and Emery 2009). Inflammatory arthritis in Down syndrome requires the same approach and standard of care as juvenile idiopathic arthritis (Davies et al. 2010) within specialist paediatric rheumatology services, with access to clinical nurse specialists, intra-articular steroid injections under general anaesthetic, using the same range of disease modifying and biologic agents. The expertise of the multidisciplinary paediatric rheumatology team offers benefit with skills different from the neurological and non-inflammatory focus of community and school health teams. The use of methotrexate is often associated with recurrent episodes of mild neutropenia identified on routine blood monitoring, which may or may not be due to the methotrexate in this patient group. The resulting recurrent interruptions to therapy are associated with loss of disease control. Moving up the therapeutic ladder to a biologic agent or resisting interruptions to treatment despite mild neutropenia is often a successful tactics in maintaining good disease control.

PROGNOSIS

The prognosis in inflammatory arthritis in children with Down syndrome is much poorer than juvenile idiopathic arthritis (Padmakumar et al. 2002; Cruikshank et al. 2008; Juj and Emery 2009; C Foley personal communication, 2013). Significant delay in diagnosis and barriers to care are highlighted as a key reason for worse outcomes (see Table 15.1).

BONE HEALTH IN DOWN SYNDROME

Osteoporosis and bone quality are affected by the following factors: level of exercise, dietary intake of vitamin D and calcium, exposure to sunshine, use of antiepileptic drugs, diabetes, autoimmune diseases (coeliac disease and thyroid disorder), height and age at menopause. Many of these risk factors are applicable to people with Down syndrome. Bastiaanse et al. (2014) report a prevalence of low bone quality of 49.5% in women and 38.7% in men in people with an intellectual disability and Down syndrome. Further studies have suggested that Down syndrome is an independent risk factor for osteoporosis compared with the general population with or without a learning disability (Baptista et al. 2005, Geijer et al. 2014). Recent studies suggest that in Down syndrome there is a significant decrease in bone formation markers with a reduction in osteoblastic bone formation and low bone quality and mass (McKelvey et al. 2013) and there may be a role for intermittent parathyroid hormone treatment (Fowler et al. 2012).

Wu (2013) demonstrated that boys with Down syndrome in the age group 7–10 years have a lower bone mineral density in the pelvis, but not in the spine or femoral neck, suggesting that osteoporosis starts early in life. However, it is encouraging that the findings of low bone mineral density may be preventable and reversible as shown in a study by Gonzalez-Aguero et al. (2012), which demonstrated that a 21-week physical exercise programme enhanced the bone mass density in young people with Down syndrome between the ages of 10 and 19 years. It is therefore imperative to encourage regular physical activity and optimum intake of calcium and vitamin D from a young age and to promote optimum bone health. Adults with Down syndrome should be offered screening for osteoporosis and treated appropriately.

Spinal disorders

The main spinal abnormalities described in Down syndrome are

- instability of the occipito-cervical junction (cranio-vertebral instability);
- scoliosis;
- cervical arthropathy; and
- lumbar spondylolysis and spondylolisthesis.

As there is considerable concern amongst professionals and carers around cranio-vertebral instability this will be discussed in detail.

Cranio-vertebral instability

The reported incidence of asymptomatic cranio-vertebral instability in people with Down syndrome is between 10 and 24%; however, the incidence of symptomatic instability is much less and is around 1%. Symptomatic cranio-vertebral instability may present at any age and needs urgent medical evaluation.

Eleanor is a 7-year-old girl with Down syndrome with learning difficulties and significant behaviour challenges. She had reasonably good general health although she had an atrioventricular septal defect operated at 4 months and a subaortic stenosis operated 4 months prior to presentation and long-standing chronic constipation.

She presented initially to her General Practitioner with a limp. She was well in herself and examination was unremarkable. She was prescribed analgesia and reassured. Three weeks on she presented to her local accident and emergency department with reluctance to walk and her gait had changed. She developed daytime enuresis.

She had normal radiograph hips and both legs and blood tests to exclude infections and arthritis. Her parents were reassured. Cardiological assessment was unremarkable (she had been operated upon 4 months previously).

Ten weeks after her initial presentation she attended for an annual medical review with her local community paediatrician. She entered in a wheelchair and had daytime enuresis. Her neurological examination was a challenge due to behavioural difficulties. A change in gait was noted with an increased tightness of both tendo-achilles. A working diagnosis of cranio-vertebral subluxation was made. Cervical spine-radiograph in the flexion and extension were of poor quality. Following neurosurgical review an MRI scan of the brain and spine showed an os odontoideum and cervicomedullary junction compression due to the presence of an interposing transverse ligament.

Twelve weeks after Eleanor's initial presentation she underwent surgery to reduce and stabilize the atlanto-occipital instability. Three months' post-operative immobilization followed with a good outcome.

Cranio-vertebral instability in Down syndrome is likely to result from the associated hypotonia and ligamentous laxity leading to repeated shearing stress in the area between the centrum of C-1 and the articular surfaces of C-2 resulting in an abnormal ossification and development of the os odontoideum (Crockard and Stevens 1995). In addition, the odontoid process may be hypoplastic with delayed ossification of the arch of C-1 and C-2 and occipito-atlas instability (Menezes 2008). The association of these anomalies may complicate surgical management (Nader-Sepahi et al. 2005).

Symptomatic cranio-vertebral instability in Down syndrome usually has an insidious onset, except if there is trauma which may be iatrogenic in nature, e.g., at the time of anaesthesia.

The presenting symptoms may include the following:

- Mechanical neck or occipital pain with an extended neck position
- Torticollis
- Myelopathy/weakness
- Change in gait or manipulative skills
- Recent onset incontinence

In the presence of symptoms, a full clinical evaluation must be undertaken. There should be a low threshold to undertake lateral view radiographs of the occipito cervical region both in full flexion and extension. Requesting the person to look up to the ceiling and to look down to their shoes is a useful technique to facilitate flexion and extension and demonstrate any restriction in the occipito cervical region. An Atlanto-Dental Interval ADI (distance between the posterior surface of the anterior arch of C-1 and the anterior surface of the dens) of more than 5 mm and a Posterior Atlanto-Dental Interval (PADI) of less than 14 mm is abnormal and specialist opinion should be sought. The neural canal width (NCW) is a good predictor of spinal cord compression. (see Figure 15.7) MRI should accompany any residual doubt.

Radiological screening for asymptomatic cranio-vertebral instability is not recommended as:

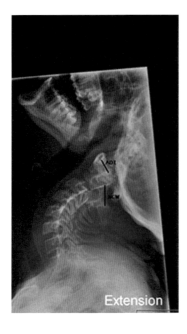
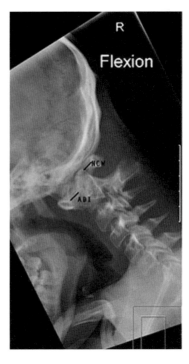

Fig. 15.7. Flexion and extension views of the cervical spine demonstrating a significant increased atlanto dental interval (ADI) and decreased neural canal width (NCW) in flexion.

- radiographs have a very poor predictive value (Ferguson 1997)
- measurement of occipito-atlanto subluxation can be very difficult
- the long term natural history of asymptomatic cranio-vertebral instability is very variable (Morton et al. 1995)

The definitive management of cervico-vertebral instability is surgery, the aim is to reduce subluxation and provide both translational and rotational stability. However as surgery is associated with significant morbidity and mortality, it is not recommended in asymptomatic individuals. Surgery should only be undertaken in neurosurgical units with the appropriate expertise and experience. Occiput fixation may also be warranted, particularly if there is evidence of occipito-atlanto instability (Nader-Sepahi et al. 2005). Additional surgical risk factors include associated osseous abnormalities, and young age (due to a relatively large head, small spine and immature bones).

Any general anaesthetic procedures in people with Down syndrome holds risk. A full history and neurological examination should be undertaken pre-operatively but screening radiographs are not required in the absence of symptoms. However even in the absence of symptoms, peri-operatively it is important to keep the neck in a neutral position, avoiding extreme flexion, extension and rotational movements. The use of a soft collar during and after the general anaesthetic is sometimes advocated to prevent inadvertent extreme neck movements.

People with Down syndrome should not be barred from sporting activities, as there is no evidence to suggest that asymptomatic individuals with cranio-vertebral instability have ever come to harm by participation in sports. The British Gymnastic Association (2012) have developed a clinical screening criteria to detect symptomatic individuals. However, radiological screening continues to be a requirement for participation in high risk sporting activities at the Special Olympics.

SCOLIOSIS

The prevalence of adolescent idiopathic scoliosis in the general population is reported to be between 1.5% and 3% (Lonstein 1994). Milbrandt and Johnston (2005) reported an incidence of 8.7% in Down syndrome from a case series of 379 people with Down syndrome attending their institution over a 50-year period. Forty-nine percent had previously undergone thoracotomy for congenital heart defects. Bracing was ineffective for the majority of the young people, surgery was only undertaken in 21.2% and was associated with a 57% complication rate. The authors recommend evaluation for scoliosis particularly in children who have undergone surgery.

CERVICAL ARTHROPATHY

Accelerated ageing, ligamentous laxity and hypermobility of the cervical segments predispose people with Down syndrome to an increased incidence of cervical arthropathy.

Alison, a 35-year-old woman with Down syndrome was referred because of increasing difficulty with daily living activities and occasional episodes of falling with associated dizziness. Her systemic and neurological examination was unremarkable, although it was difficult to undertake an objective assessment of her fine motor skills because of lack of documentation of previous assessments. She was diagnosed with labyrinthitis and was given general advice and exercises. In addition she was referred for an eye check and found that she had bilateral cataracts. After successful cataract surgery with intraocular lens implants, her fine motor skills improved marginally but her gait continued to deteriorate. She was reassessed 3 years later as she became unable to walk. She was noted to have marked spasticity, hyperreflexia and upgoing plantars. An MRI of the spine examination revealed marked compression of the spinal cord extending from C-2 to C-4. However despite Alison undergoing a laminectomy her neurological symptoms did not improve and she remains unable to walk.

Fidone (1986) reported that in 41 adults with Down syndrome, cervical arthopathy was found in 50% of adults between the ages of 30–40 years and universally present in those over the age of 40 years. The cervical segments between C-5 and C-6 are most commonly involved and the degenerative changes in Down syndrome tend to be more severe (Maclachlan et al. 1993).

Bosma et al. (1999) described five cases of cervical spondyloarthritic myelopathy in adults with Down syndrome between the ages of 27 and 52 years. All adults presented with progressive walking difficulties and ataxia. However, symptoms were attributed to other causes, e.g., visual difficulties and cognitive decline resulting in a delayed diagnosis of 2 years in four out five cases and by 6 years in a 31-year-old. The authors highlight the importance of being aware of the increased prevalence of cervical arthropathy in people with Down syndrome to enable early identification and management to prevent irreversible damage.

LUMBAR SPONDYLOLYSIS AND SPONDYLOLISTHESIS
Lumbar spondylolysis is reported to present in 3% to 6% of the general population with 2.7 to 8.4% affected by spondylolisthesis. Hansdorfer et al. (2013) in a case series of 110 people with Down syndrome reported that 18.2% had spondylolysis and 34.6% had spondylolisthesis. In addition, in contrast to the general population, lower back pain and leg pain correlated well ($p = 0.006$) with spondylolisthesis. They postulated that an increased body mass index and an immature skeletal system in people with Down syndrome may predispose them to both. It is important to consider lumbar spondylolisthesis as a cause of lower lumbar back pain and leg pain in people with Down syndrome.

The hip
Capsular insufficiency, ligamentous laxity and muscle hypotonia produce hip instability in Down syndrome with a reported incidence of between 2% and 5% (Diamond et al. 1981, Shaw and Beals 1992). Under the age of 2 years, it is thought that hips are often stable but hypermobile, but may then pass through phases of subluxation and dislocation, leading eventually to fixed dislocation and osteoarthritis.

The underlying bony morphology of the hip in Down syndrome, including a deep and horizontal acetabulum, would be expected to confer increased stability; but capsular laxity dominates and recurrent posterior dislocations can affect the growth and shape of the acetabulum (dysplasia), contributing to tendency to dislocate.

Dislocations may be acute, or habitual. An acute episode of dislocation presents with the sudden onset of a limp or refusal to walk. Relocation is possible under general anaesthetic. Habitual dislocation describes hips that dislocate easily without trauma but reduce spontaneously. This occurrence can look dramatic and be of concern for the family but only requires reassurance, unless there is evidence of functional abnormality or pain.

Up to 28% of adults with Down syndrome have a hip abnormality, the instability worsening with time and correlating with walking ability (Hresko et al. 1993). Occasionally instability begins after skeletal maturity. With life expectancy in Down syndrome increasing, this relatively high incidence of long-term problems is concerning.

MANAGEMENT
Very occasionally in the young child with Down syndrome, it has been reported that treatment of the unstable hip is possible with closed reduction and prolonged casting (Greene 1998). While capsular reefing is possible, any such tightening procedure tends to stretch

out, and more permanent solutions attempt to stabilize the joint by altering the alignment of the proximal femur or the acetabulum by osteotomies. Once there is a fixed dislocation, a total hip replacement (THR) is usually required.

The decision to perform major reconstructive surgery should balance the likely benefits and risks. The aims of surgery need to be clear, and all these issues need to be discussed with parents or carers. Healing and rehabilitation take several months, the complication rate is high, and the success rate is variable. Depending on the age of the child, a hip spica cast may need to be worn for 6 to 12 weeks postoperatively which can severely hinder mobility and personal care. Complications include recurrent subluxation, dislocation and infection amongst others (Bennet 1982, Katz et al. 2005). In addition, there is some controversy about the best procedure to perform. In general, if the acetabulum appears normal, then a femoral osteotomy is advocated (Beguiristain et al. 2001, Knight et al. 2011) with the addition of acetabular surgery if the acetabulum is deficient (Woolf and Gross 2003, Katz et al. 2005, Sankar et al. 2011).

For these reasons management should be individualized, with functional impairment the most important indication for surgery. The underlying pathology and altered bony anatomy in each patient should be carefully considered, with 3D computed tomography of the acetabulum to aid in surgical planning (Woolf and Gross 2003, Sankar et al. 2011).

Slipped upper femoral epiphysis

Slipped upper femoral epiphysis (SUFE—Fig. 15.8) occurs most commonly during puberty when hormonal changes weaken the growth plate, with a strong association with obesity and hypothyroidism. Both these risk factors are increased in Down syndrome, and contribute to its increased incidence. Bosch et al. (2004) describe 11 slipped hips in eight children (aged 7–13 years) with Down syndrome, all of whom had an increased body mass index and six of the eight had hypothyroidism.

SUFE may present acutely with hip or knee pain, with or without a background history of chronic pain. Sometimes this may be acute enough to prevent weight bearing, even with crutches. Diagnosis is often delayed in the general population, particularly since hip pathology frequently manifests as knee pain only: Radiographs of the pelvis and hip are frequently not done. Diagnosis is likely to be even more delayed in Down syndrome, where there may be communication difficulties, or previous and coexisting joint complaints. Delay in treatment risks progression of the slip, compromising outcome and makes treatment more complex.

Conventional treatment involves passing a screw across the growth plate to stabilize the femoral head and prevent further slip. However, the complication rate in Down syndrome is high, with slip progression despite pinning, avascular necrosis and infection (Bosch et al. 2004, Dietz et al. 2004).

Perthes disease and avascular necrosis

Perthes disease is characterized by an avascular process affecting the skeletally immature femoral head. The head gradually collapses and deforms and then proceeds through a period

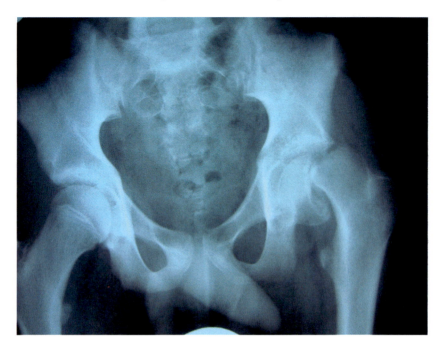

Fig. 15.8. Radiograph of pelvis showing slipped upper femoral epiphysis of the left hip.

of repair, regeneration and remodelling, which takes several years (Fig. 15.9). Perthes disease usually presents as episodes of recurrent pain and limping.

The incidence of Perthes disease or avascular necrosis is thought to be increased in children with Down syndrome but there have been no studies to corroborate this. The aim of treatment is to keep the hip gently moving during this process, and to 'contain' it within the acetabulum, to aid the repair process, to prevent stiffness and fixed deformity, and to avoid high-impact activities. The outcome of Perthes disease in any child is highly dependent on the age at onset, with young children doing much better (having a greater period of time in which the femoral head can remodel). There is no evidence that the disease process in children with Down syndrome is any different from the general population and treatment principles are the same.

Total hip replacement in Down syndrome

As the end result of any hip condition, pain and osteoarthritis may adversely affect function and independence. THR may then be considered. Theoretical concerns regarding THR in Down syndrome include a higher than normal potential risk of dislocation (due to capsular laxity and muscle hypotonia), and a higher than normal risk of infection. Obesity makes surgery technically more difficult, and can prejudice outcome.

Zywiel et al. (2013) elegantly summarized the evidence, and suggest that these risks may not necessarily be as high as once considered. In 42 patients from four studies, standard

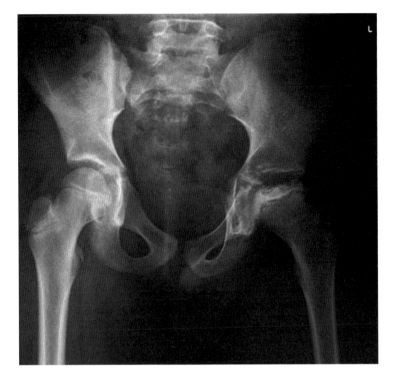

Fig. 15.9. Radiograph of pelvis showing avascular necrosis of the left femoral head.

components were used, although constrained liners and extra acetabular screws were often needed to enhance stability of components. Survival rates varied between 81% and 100% at a mean follow up of 105 months. This review suggested that 'while THR in patients with Down syndrome does present some unique challenges, the overall clinical results are good, providing these patients with reliable pain relief and good function', which is encouraging for a population of patients in whom life expectancy is increasing.

Patellofemoral instability
Patellofemoral instability can commonly develop whereby the patella dislocates out of its position in front of the knee. Diamond et al. (1981) found that 108 knees in 68 people out of 97 examined showed evidence of excessive mobility of the patella, ranging from subluxation to habitual dislocation to fixed dislocation. Capsular laxity, muscle hypotonia and in theory, genu valgum (knock knees) are probable contributing factors in Down syndrome, although in Diamond's series this was present in only two.

The degree of patella-femoral instability is not related to walking ability (Dugdale and Renshaw 1986, Mendez et al. 1988). The main indication for surgical treatment is functional impairment limiting independence but this should be considered very carefully, and treatment should be individualized. Although results are encouraging, only small case series describing a variety of different procedures are reported in the literature (Bettuzzi et al. 2009, Kocon et al. 2012).

The foot in Down syndrome

The main foot problems encountered in the foot in Down syndrome are hallux valgus, flat feet and congenital talipes equino varus (CTEV 'clubfoot').

High proportions of children with Down syndrome have bony deformities in the fore-foot and increased joint laxity of a severity warranting early detection and management to improve posture, and quality of life which are underestimated and neglected (Prasher et al. 1995, Concolino et al. 2006). Screening by a paediatric podiatrist experienced in Down syndrome would help prevent later foot deformity and pain, improve gait and maximize mechanical advantage (compensating for instability due to lax ligaments and hypotonia), and encourage a more 'normal' foot posture through podiatric interventions and good footwear (Selby-Silverstein et al. 2001; Galli et al. 2008; Chang et al. 2009; Rigoldi et al. 2011a, 2011b; Watt and Todd, personal communication, 2013). Out of 66 children with Down syndrome the majority had adequate footwear (64%), 39% had foot orthoses fitted although the need for orthoses and those who had received them were not well matched (Todd and Watt, personal communication, 2013). The majority had foot types predisposing to deformity and challenges for shoe fitting, with short, broad feet with an adducted first ray, hypermobility and a low arch with pes plano valgus as the most frequent pattern. The great variability in foot types was notable with few having the classic features of a Down syndrome foot (triangular shape with a narrow heel compared with forefoot width, and a plantar cleft between the first and second metatarsophalangeal joint). Hypermobility in the feet at ankle, subtalar and talonavicular joints was associated with pes plano valgus, and subtalar joint pronation, a complication of hypotonia (see Fig. 15.10).

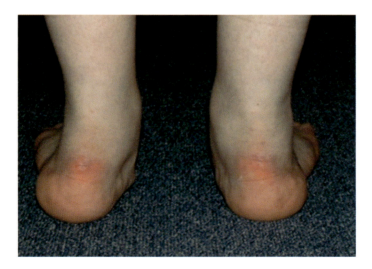

Fig. 15.10. Subtalar pronation with hypermobility (Courtesy of G Watt Gordon Watt).

Metatarsus primus varus and hallux varus

Metatarsus primus varus describes a deformity where the first metatarsal deviates towards the midline. This can produce a hallux valgus or bunion deformity or a hallux varus deformity if the big toe also deviates towards the midline. Either of these deformities can cause problems with shoe fitting and pain across the front of the foot, which can often be treated with appropriate shoe wear. Symptoms of pain may require surgical correction. This will usually involve resection of any bunion, with first metatarsal osteotomy to correct the varus.

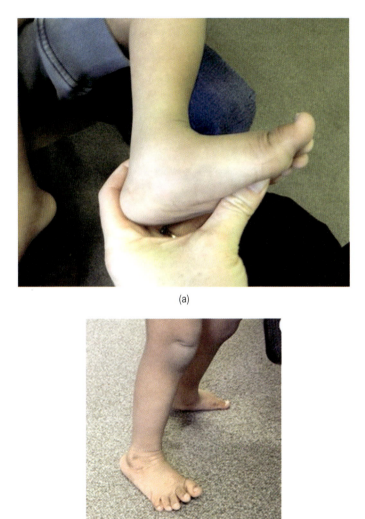

(a)

(b)

Fig. 15.11a and b. Demonstrating the good surgical outcome post congenital talipes equino varus surgery.

There are currently no studies documenting outcome or recurrence rates in people with Down syndrome.

Congenital talipes equino varus

CTEV (clubfoot) occurs in the UK general population with an incidence of approximately 2–3 per 1000 live births and is believed to occur more commonly in Down syndrome; however, there is very little literature to support this. Miller et al. (1995) described 15 cases of CTEV eight children with Down syndrome, all of whom underwent surgical correction, with an 'acceptable' result. The majority of clubfeet nowadays are treated using the Ponseti technique, describing a particular method of serial manipulation and casting, followed by night-time bracing for the first 5 years of life (Moroney et al. 2012).

Children with Down syndrome respond extremely well to the Ponseti technique. The associated ligamentous laxity probably contributes to the good outcome and can prompt an early removal of the night-time brace in children with Down syndrome (Tennant S, personal communication, 2013) (Fig. 15.11a and b).

Summary

Musculoskeletal examination remains a neglected and poorly maintained skill in most non-specialists. The additional challenges in people with Down syndrome, of identifying gradual functional deterioration in those who find it difficult to vocalize pain and who have a different ROM contributes to diagnostic delay. An increased expectation of motor function with encouragement to maintain and maximize motor potential and a better ability to identify deterioration in motor function and its cause are needed. Understanding the genetic basis of inflammatory arthritis in children with Down syndrome will lead to specific clinical trials. Physical approaches to develop and maintain maximum muscle strength requires further research.

Key points

- Hypotonia, ligamentous laxity and associated autoimmune disorders may predispose to, or exacerbate musculoskeletal conditions and make treatment more difficult.
- Early identification of musculoskeletal problems can be a challenge and often diagnosis is delayed due to diagnostic overshadowing.
- Incorporating a targeted musculoskeletal assessment within routine health screening would improve speed and quality of diagnosis of musculoskeletal problems, including inflammatory and degenerative arthropathy.
- Symptomatic cranio-vertebral instability is rare occurring in less than 1% of individuals.
- There is no role for radiological screening for asymptomatic cranio-vertebral instability. Asymptomatic individuals should not be barred from normal sporting activities.
- Often there are increased rates of infection and associated health problems orthopaedic surgical intervention and postoperative care should be carefully considered. Regular physical activity and optimum intake of calcium and vitamin D from a young age should be encouraged to prevent poor bone mineral density.

REFERENCES

Agiovlasitis S, McCubbin JA, Yun J, Pavol MJ, Widrick JJ (2009) Economy and preferred speed of walking in adults with and without Down syndrome. *Adapt Phys Activ Q* 26: 118–130.

Atlanto-Axial Information Pack. www.british-gymnastics.org/.../3636-atlanto-axial-information-pack (last updated 17 December 2012; accessed 1 January 2015).

Baptista F, Varela A, Sardinha LB (2005) Bone mineral mass in males and females with and without Down syndrome. *Osteoporos Int* 16: 380–388. Epub 9 September 2004.

Bastiaanse LP, Mergler S, Evenhuis HM, Echteld MA (2014) Bone quality in older adults with intellectual disabilities. *Res Dev Disabil* 35: 1927–1933. doi: 10.1016/j.ridd.2014.04.018. Epub 21 May 2014.

Beguiristain JL, Barriga A, Gent RA (2001) Femoral anteversion osoteomy for treatment of hip dislocation in Down syndrome: Long term evolution. *J Pediatr Orthop B* 10: 85–88.

Beighton P, Horan F (1969) Orthopaedic aspects of the Ehlers-Danlos syndrome. *J Bone Joint Surg Br* 51B: 444–453.

Bennet GC, Rang M, Royde DP, April H (1982) Dislocation of the hip in trisomy 21. *J Bone Joint Surg Br* 64: 289–294.

Bettuzzi C, Lampasi M, Magnani M, Donzelli O (2009) Surgical treatment of patellar dislocation in children with Down syndrome: A 3–11 year follow up study. *Knee Surg Sports Traumatol Arthrosc* 17: 334–340.

Bosch P, Johnston CE, Karol L (2004) Slipped capital femoral epiphysis in patients with Down syndrome. *J Pediatr Orthop* 24: 271–277.

Bosma GP, van Buchem MA, Voormolen JH, van Biezen FC, Brouwer OF (1999) Cervical spondylarthrotic myelopathy with early onset in Down's syndrome: Five cases and a review of the literature. *J Intellect Disabil Res* 43: 283–288.

Caird M, Wills B, Dormans J (2006) Down syndrome in children: The role of the orthopaedic surgeon. *J Am Acad Orthop Surg* 14: 610–619.

Chang C, Kubo M, Ulrich B (2009) Emergence of neuromuscular patterns during walking in toddlers with typical development and with Down syndrome. *Hum Movement Sci* 28: 283–296.

Concolino D, Pasquzzi A, Capalbo G, Sinopoli S, Strisciuglio P (2006) Early detection of podiatric anomalies in children with Down syndrome. *Acta Paediatr* 95: 17–29.

Crockard HA, Stevens JM (1995) Cranio-vertebral junction anomalies in inherited disorders: Part of the syndrome or caused by the disorder? *Eur J Pediatr* 154: 504–512.

Cruikshank M, Tunc A, Walsh J, Galea P, Davidson J, Gardner-Medwin J (2008) Arthritis in Down's syndrome is still being missed. *Pediatr Rheumatol* 6: 54.

Davies K, Cleary G, Foster H, Hutchinson E, Baildam E (2010) British Society of Paediatric and Adolescent Rheumatology. Standards of care for children and young people with juvenile idiopathic arthritis. *Rheumatology (Oxford)* 49: 1406–1408.

Diamond LS, Lynne D, Sigman B (1981) Orthopedic disorders in patients with Down's syndrome. *Orthop Clin North Am* 12: 57–71.

Dietz FR, Albanese SA, Katz DA et al. (2004) Slipped capital femoral epiphysis in Down syndrome. *J Pediatr Orthop* 24: 508–513.

Dugdale TW, Renshaw TS (1986) Instabiltiy of the patellofemoral joint in Down syndrome. *J Bone Joint Surg Am* 68: 405–413.

Faulks D, Collado V, Mazlle MN, Veyrune JL, Hennequin M (2008) Masticatory dysfunction in persons with Down's syndrome. Part 1: Aetiology and incidence. *J Oral Rehabil* 35: 854–862.

Ferguson RL, Putney ME, Allen BL Jr. (1997) Comparison of neurologic deficits with atlanto-dens intervals in patients with Down syndrome. *J Spinal Disord* 10: 246–252.

Fidone GS (1986) Degenerative cervical arthritis and Down's syndrome. *N Engl J Med* 314: 320.

Fowler TW, McKelvey KD, Akel NS et al. (2012) Low bone turnover and low BMD in Down syndrome: Effect of intermittent PTH treatment. *PLoS One* 7: e42967. doi: 10.1371/journal.pone.0042967. Epub 14 August 2012.

Galli M, Cimolin V, Patti P et al. (2010) Quantifying established clinical assessment measures using 3D-movement analysis in individuals with Down syndrome. *Disabil Rehabil* 32: 1768–1774.

Galli M, Rigoldi C, Brunner R, Virji-Babul N, Giorgio A (2008) Joint stiffness and gait pattern evaluation in children with Down syndrome. *Gait Posture* 28: 502–506.

Geijer JR, Stanish HI, Draheim CC, Dengel DR (2014) Bone mineral density in adults with Down syndrome, intellectual disability, and nondisabled adults. *Am J Intellect Dev Disabil* 119: 107–114. doi: 10.1352/1944-7558-119.2.107.

Gonzalez-Aguero A, Vicente-Rodriguez G, Moreno LA, Guerra-Balic M, Ara I, Casajus JA (2010) Health-related physical fitness in children and adolescents with Down syndrome and response to training. *Scand J Med Sci Sports* 20: 716–724.

González-Agüero A, Vicente-Rodríguez G, Gómez-Cabello A, Ara I, Moreno LA, Casajús JA (2012) A 21-week bone deposition promoting exercise programme increases bone mass in young people with Down syndrome. *Dev Med Child Neurol* 54: 552–556. doi: 10.1111/j.1469-8749.2012.04262.x. Epub 13 March 2012.

Greene WB (1998) Closed treatment of hip dislocation in Down syndrome. *J Pediatr Orthop B* 18: 643–647.

Guijarro M, Valero C, Paule B, Gonzalez-Macias J, Riancho JA (2008) Bone mass in young adults with Down syndrome. *J Intellect Disabil Res* 52: 182–189. doi: 10.1111/j.1365-2788.2007.00992.x.

Hansdorfer MA, Mardjetko SM, Knott PT, Thompson SE (2013) Lumbar spondylolysis and spondylolisthesis in Down syndrome: A cross-sectional study at one institution. *Spine Deformity* 1: 382–388.

Hawli Y, Nasrallah M, El-Hajj Fuleihan G (2009) Endocrine and musculoskeletal abnormalities in patients with Down syndrome. *Nat Rev Endocrinol* 5: 327–334.

Hennequin M, Morin C, Feine J (2000) Pain expression and stimulus location in individuals with Down's syndrome. *Lancet* 356: 1882–1887.

Hresko MT, McCarthy JC, Goldberg MJ (1993) Hip disease in adults with Down's syndrome. *J Bone Joint Surg Br* 75-B: 604–607.

Jacobsen FS, Hansson G (2000) Orthopaedic disorders in Down's syndrome. *Curr Orthop* 14: 215–222.

Jover M, Ayoun C, Berton C, Carlier M (2010) Specific grasp characteristics of children with trisomy 21. *Dev Psychobiol* 52: 782–793.

Juj H, Emery H (2009) The arthropathy of Down's syndrome: An underdiagnosed and under-recognized condition. *J Pediatr* 154: 234–238.

Juul-Kristensen B, Røgind H, Jensen D, Remvig L (2007) Inter-examiner reproducibility of tests and criteria for generalized joint hypermobility and benign joint hypermobility syndrome. *Rheumatology* 46: 1835–1841.

Karousou E, Stachtea X, Moretto P et al. (2013) New insights into the pathobiology of Down syndrome—hyaluronan synthase-2 overexpression is regulated by collagen VI α2 chain. *FEBS J* 280: 2418–2430. doi: 10.1111/febs.12220. Epub 28 March 2013.

Katz DA, Kim YJ, Millis MB (2005) Periacetabular osteotomy in patients with Down's syndrome. *J Bone Joint Surg Br* 87: 544–547.

Kinnell H (1984) Arthritis in Down's syndrome. *Br J Radiol* 57: 1162.

Knight DM, Alves C, Wedge JH (2011) Femoral varus derotation osteotomy for the treatment of habitual subluxation and dislocation of the pediatric hip in trisomy 21: A 10-year experience. *J Pediatr Orthop B* 31: 638–643.

Kocon H, Kabacyj M, Zgoda M (2012) The results of the operative treatment of patellar instability in children with Down's syndrome. *J Pediatr Orthop B* 21: 407–410.

Liza-Sharmini AT, Azlan ZN, Zilfalil BA (2006) Ocular findings in Malaysian children with Down syndrome. *Singapore Med J* 47: 14–19.

Lonstein JE (1994) Adolescent idiopathic scoliosis. *Lancet* 344: 1407–1412. doi: 10.1016/S0140-6736(94)90572-X.

Maclachlan RA, Fidler KE, Yeh H, Hodgetts PG, Pharand G, Chau M (1993) Cervical spine abnormalities in institutionalized adults with Down's syndrome. *J Intellect Disabil Res* 37: 277–285. doi: 10.1111/j.1365-2788.1993.tb01284.x.

Martinez-Cue C, Baamonde C, Angeles Lumbreras A, Vallina I, Dierssen M, Florez J (1999) A murine model for Down syndrome shows reduced responsiveness to pain. *NeuroReport* 10: 1119–1122.

McKelvey KD, Fowler TW, Akel NS et al. (2013) Low bone turnover and low bone density in a cohort of adults with Down syndrome. *Osteoporos Int* 24: 1333–1338. doi: 10.1007/s00198-012-2109-4.

Mendez AA, Keret D, MacEwen GD (1988) Treatment of patellofemoral instability in Down's syndrome. *Clin Orthop Relat Res* 234: 148–158.

Menezes AH (2008) Specific entities affecting the craniocervical region: Down's syndrome. *Childs Nerv Syst* 24: 1165–1168.

Milbrandt TA, Johnston CE II. (2005) Down syndrome and scoliosis: A review of a 50-year experience at one institution. *Spine* 30: 2051–2055.

Miller PR, Kuo KN, Lubicky JP (1995) Clubfoot deformity in Down's syndrome. *Orthopaedics* 18: 449–452.

Moroney PJ, Noel J, Fogarty EE, Kelly PM (2012) A single centre prospective evaluation of the Ponseti method in non-iodiopathic congenital talipes equinovaurus. *J Pediatr Orthop* 32: 636–640.

Morton RE, Khan MA, Murray-Leslie C, Elliott S (1995) Atlantoaxial instability in Down's syndrome: A five year follow up study. *Arch Dis Child* 72: 115–119.

Nader-Sepahi A, Casey AT, Hayward R, Crockard HA, Thompson D (2005) Symptomatic atlantoaxial instability in Down syndrome. *J Neurosurg* 103: 231–237.

Olson J, Bender J, Levinson J, Oestreich A, Lovell D (1990) Arthropathy of Down syndrome. *Pediatrics* 86: 931–936.

Online Mendelian Inheritance in Man National Center for Biotechnology Information, U.S. National Library of Medicine, Bethesda MD. http://www.ncbi.nlm.nih.gov/omim, Down Syndrome, http://omim.org/entry/190685 (last updated 25 October 2013, accessed 1 January 2015).

Padmakumar B, Evans Jones LG, Sills JA (2002) Is arthritis more common in children with Down's syndrome? *Rheumatology* 41: 1191–1193.

Prasher V, Robinson L, Krishnan V, Chung M (1995) Podiatric disorders among children with Down syndrome and learning disability. *Med Child Neurol* 37: 131–134.

Rigoldi C, Galli M, Albertini G (2011a) Gait development during lifespan in subjects with Down syndrome. *Res Dev Disabil* 32: 158–163. doi: 10.1016/j.ridd.2010.09.009.

Rigoldi C, Galli M, Mainardi L, Crivellini M, Albertini G (2011b) Postural control in children, teenagers and adults with Down syndrome. *Res Dev Disabil* 32: 170–175.

Sankar WN, Millis MB, Kim YJ (2011) Instability of the hip in patients with Down syndrome. Improved results with complete re-directional acetabular osteotomy. *J Bone Joint Surg Am* 93: 1924–1933.

Selby-Silverstein L, Hilstrom H, Palisano R (2001) The effect of foot orthoses on standing foot posture and gait of young children with Down syndrome. *Neuro Rehabil* 16: 183–193.

Shaw ED, Beals RK (1992) The hip joint in Down's syndrome: A study of its structure and associated disease. *Clin Orthop* 278: 101–107.

Sheybani EF, Khanna G, White AJ, Demertzis JL (2013) Imaging of juvenile idiopathic arthritis: A multi-modality approach. *Radiographics* 33: 1253–1273.

Stoll ML, Cron RQ (2013) Treatment of juvenile idiopathic arthritis in the biologic age. *Rheum Dis Clin North Am* 39: 751–766.

Weijerman ME, de Winter JP (2010) Clinical practice: The care of children with Down syndrome. *Eur J Pediatr* 169: 1445–1452.

Woolf SK, Gross RH (2003) Posterior acetabular wall deficiency in Down syndrome. *J Pediatr Orthop* 23: 708–713.

Wu J (2013) Bone mass and density in preadolescent boys with and without Down syndrome. *Osteoporos Int* 24: 2847–2854. doi: 10.1007/s00198-013-2393-7. Epub 17 May 2013.

Yancey C, Zmijewski C, Athreya B, Doughty R (1984) Arthopathy of Down's syndrome. *Arthritis Rheum* 27: 929–934.

Zywiel MG, Mont MA, Callaghan JJ et al. (2013) Surgical challenges and clinical outcomes of total hip replacement in patients with Down's syndrome. *Bone Joint J* 95-B: 41–45. doi: 10.1302/0301-620X.95B11.32901.

16
DERMATOLOGICAL MANIFESTATIONS

Sheila M Clark and Laura Savage

Introduction

Down syndrome is associated with an increased frequency of some common dermatoses, and specifically with some of the rarer dermatological disorders. The literature primarily refers to the dermatoses seen in children and data concerning adults are mostly case reports. There is, therefore, a need for further research to understand the pathophysiology of the dermatological manifestations of Down syndrome.

Why are skin conditions more common in Down syndrome?

This is probably due to a combination of factors, including inefficient physiological processes and immune and genetic dysregulation.

Defective innate and cell-mediated immunity (see Chapter 7) may predispose to alopecia areata and vitiligo. Serum levels of Interferon-gamma (IFN-gamma) producing $CD4^+$ and $CD8^+$ T-cells are elevated in Down syndrome (Marmon et al. 2012). IFN-gamma has been implicated as a key cytokine in the pathogenesis of psoriasis, leading to postulation of a link between psoriasis and Down syndrome. However, no significant increased prevalence of psoriasis is reported in several large case series evaluating the frequency of mucocutaneous problems in Down syndrome.

IFN-gamma dysregulation may explain the increased reported prevalence of skin infections. Reduced in vitro killing of *Candida albicans* and *Staphylococcus aureus* has been described. Xu et al. (2013) identified dysregulated microRNAs in children with Down syndrome, which may be involved in T- or B-cell activation, as well as haemopoietic and lymphoid cell and thymus development.

Collagen VI is an extracellular matrix protein, which is important in maintaining muscle and skin integrity and function. It is formed by the assembly of three chains: $\alpha1$, $\alpha2$ and $\alpha3$. The COL $\alpha1$ (VI) and $\alpha2$ (VI) chains are encoded by genes *COL6A1* and *Col6A2* which are located on chromosome 21. The $\alpha3$ (VI) chain is encoded by the *COL6A3*, located on chromosome 2. Overexpression of *COL6A1* and *COL6A2* genes, therefore, occurs in Down syndrome. Overexpression of *COL6A2* is linked to increased levels of hyaluronan and hyaluronan synthase-2; and increased levels have been detected in Down syndrome fetal skin fibroblasts (Karousou et al. 2013). The distribution for collagen type VI is different from normal in fetal skin in Down syndrome, and there is overexpression of *COL6A1* compared with *COL6A3*. Immunohistochemistry has demonstrated that in trisomy 21 fetuses, collagen type VI formed a dense network extending from the epidermal basement

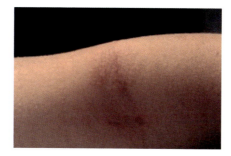

Fig. 16.1. Icthyosis with atopic eczema at the elbow flexure.

membrane to the subcutis, whereas in normal fetuses dense staining was confined to the upper region of the dermis. It is likely that these effects may link to skin conditions affecting connective tissue in Down syndrome.

Skin abnormalities, including predisposition to keratosis pilaris (exaggerated keratinization of the hair follicles) and abnormal scarring, have been described in people carrying mutations in *COL6A1* and *COL6A2* (Sabatelli et al. 2002). Keratosis pilaris is a feature of icthyosis vulgaris, the most common type of the icthyoses (very dry skin), which itself is associated with significantly increased atopic risk (see Fig. 16.1).

There is increased interest in the link between atopy and autoimmunity, and the possibility of a common immunological determinant between the two has been suggested as a cause of an increased incidence of these conditions in Down syndrome.

How do physiological differences in Down syndrome contribute to the dermatological manifestations?

ACROCYANOSIS

Poor peripheral circulation is often more pronounced in Down syndrome, particularly if there is an underlying cardiac disorder. This leads to acrocyanosis of the hands and feet, a common observation in the newborn period (Schepis et al. 2002). No treatment is required.

CUTIS MARMORATA AND LIVEDO RETICULARIS

Cutis marmorata is a lacey mottled discoloration of the skin due to altered flow in small blood vessels supplying the skin so that adjacent vessels dilate to compensate. It is most marked when the skin is cool. It is common in all infants in the first few weeks of life, but it is more common in Down syndrome where it persists for longer.

Parents need to be reassured that this is usually a harmless phenomenon. Skin warming can help.

Livedo reticularis looks similar to cutis marmorata but less marked and is also seen in increased frequency in Down syndrome. It occurs most commonly on the legs but may also occur on the arms and trunk. It is more pronounced in cold weather. It too is harmless, only requiring reassurance.

Preterm changes consistent with advancing age constitute part of the Down syndrome phenotype (Kusters et al. 2011). Changes include greying and thinning of the hair, generalized skin atrophy and the early development of rhytides (wrinkles) and lentigines.

What dermatological manifestations in Down syndrome are associated with an immune dysfunction?

ATOPIC DERMATITIS

The association between atopic eczema and Down syndrome may be explained both in terms of immune dysregulation and the increased incidence of xerosis/skin dryness. There is controversy on whether there is an increased frequency of atopic dermatitis in Down syndrome. Schepis et al. (1997) using the Hanifin and Rajka (1980) specific diagnostic criteria for atopic dermatitis found a 3% prevalence of atopic dermatitis in 100 people with Down syndrome compared with 5% in the general population. Daneshpazhooh et al. (2007) in a study on 100 children with Down syndrome did not report any children with atopic eczema, though they found an 11% prevalence of xerosis. However, xerosis is a key feature in atopic dermatitis, making the distinction difficult. Skin dryness increases itching and the risk of skin infection, and can be sufficient to trigger inflammation and therefore eczema. A dry skin is also more prone to reacting to irritants and may be more at risk of developing secondary contact allergies, for example, to nickel and fragrance (see Fig. 16.2a and b).

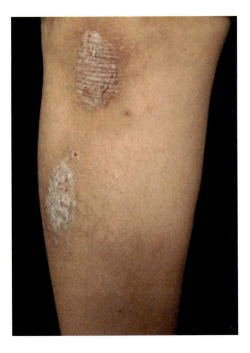

Fig. 16.2a. Localized discoid atopic eczema.

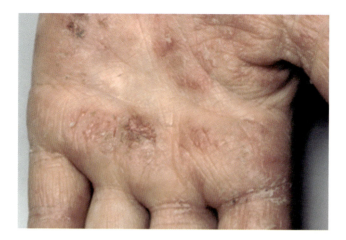

Fig. 16.2b. Chronic hand eczema with xerosis and surface erosions.

The principles of treatment of atopic dermatitis in Down syndrome are similar to the treatment in the general population. The mainstay of the treatment involves preventing skin dryness and avoiding irritants. Soaps and bubble baths should be avoided; emollients should be used as a substitute for bathing. Cream-based emollients are cosmetically less messy; however, they have an increased preservative content, which can cause irritation and occasionally exacerbation. Ointment-based emollients are more hydrating and usually less irritant, though they can occasionally cause follicular irritation/folliculitis, especially in warmer weather or if used under occlusion. Occluding the skin with prescription garments (silk or cotton), bandages or local dressings can reduce transepidermal water loss and therefore dryness, increase treatment penetration and reduce itching and infection from scratching.

Topical steroids should always be used alongside, not instead of, an emollient and only applied to inflamed skin. The preparation containing the least potent steroid, at the lowest strength, which is effective, is the one of the choices. The detailed appropriate management of atopic dermatitis is documented in the UK NICE Guidelines (2007).

Autoimmune-related conditions

ALOPECIA AREATA

The prevalence of alopecia areata in Down syndrome has been reported to be approximately 9% compared with under 2% in the general population (Carter and Jegasothy 1976). The disorder tends to be more extensive and persistent than in the general population. Alopecia totalis and universalis have been reported in up to 2.5% and are often refractory to standard treatment (Madan et al. 2006). Alopecia areata in people with Down syndrome is reported to occur in association with other autoimmune pathologies, including vitiligo, hypothyroidism and trachyonychia (Norton and Demidovich 1993). Alopecia areata usually presents with discrete areas, often annular, of non-inflammatory hair loss. This usually affects scalp

213

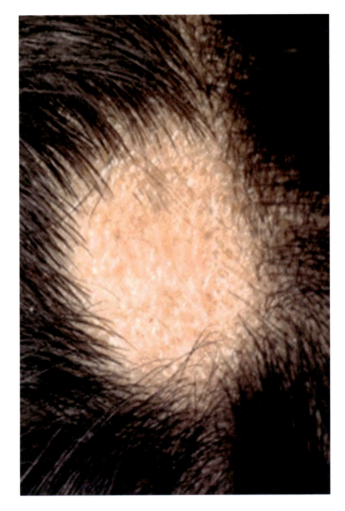

Fig. 16.3. Alopecia areata—showing exclamation mark hairs.

hair, but may also affect the eyebrows, eyelashes, facial and body hair. The autoimmune T-cell inflammatory reaction against the hair bulb results in a weakened and damaged hair that breaks off above the scalp surface. Broken or 'exclamation mark' hairs may be seen when the process is active (see Fig. 16.3).

Signs of inflammation are not seen, although some people report altered scalp sensation (e.g. itching) when the process is active. There is occasionally a link with trichotillomania (Daneshpazhooh et al. 2007).

A new candidate gene, *Mx1*, may be implicated in the pathogenesis of alopecia areata. MxA, the product of the *Mx1* gene, is an interferon-inducible p78 protein, which is highly expressed in lesional anagen hair bulbs from people with alopecia areata, but not in normal

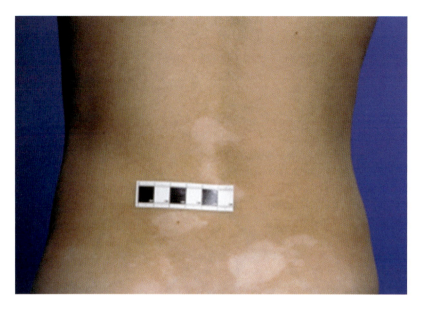

Fig. 16.4. Vitiligo of lower back.

follicles (Tazi-Ahnini et al. 2000). Interestingly, the *Mx1* gene maps to the distal part of the Down syndrome critical region on chromosome 21. The trisomy for chromosome 21 offers a greater chance of having the alopecia areata variant gene, which could explain the higher incidence of alopecia areata and a poorer prognosis.

The majority (up to 80%) of people with limited patches of alopecia areata will regrow hair spontaneously and do not specifically require treatment. Evidence-based research on management of alopecia areata is lacking. Investigations are unnecessary in most cases, though for those with more extensive problems, an autoimmune screen (including thyroid peroxidase antibodies) and serum ferritin is recommended. Though not specifically linked to alopecia areata, low iron reserves may affect hair regrowth. Where the diagnosis is in doubt, additional investigations may include a scalp skin biopsy, fungal culture and trace element levels (e.g. zinc). Psychological support and a wig prescription for more extensive hair loss are all important. Steroids, either potent topical or intralesional, are widely used; however, evidence for effectiveness is limited. Contact immunotherapy (e.g. with diphencyprone) is available only in a few UK secondary care dermatology centres. It requires long-term regular application of treatment and has produced very variable results.

Vitiligo

Vitiligo is a loss of skin pigmentation, this may occur anywhere in the body (see Fig. 16.4). An increased prevalence of vitiligo has been reported in people with Down syndrome, in many cases associated with alopecia areata. Carter and Jegasothy (1976) found a prevalence of 1.9% in their series of 213 people with Down syndrome compared with 1% in the general population and a study of 100 children with Down syndrome reported a prevalence of 3% (Daneshpazhooh et al. 2007).

Management is similar to that in the general population. The initial approach may be no active treatment other than sunscreen and cosmetic camouflage. Topical steroids and calcineurin inhibitors can be helpful in triggering repigmentation. Phototherapy may be considered for older people with darker skin types. For those with extensive vitiligo requiring significant regular sun protection, vitamin D levels should be checked periodically.

Cutaneous infections and infestations

People with Down syndrome are more prone to developing infections caused by bacteria and fungi, and appear more susceptible to ectoparasite infestations (Kavanagh et al. 1993, Scully et al. 2002, Ram and Chinen 2011).

FOLLICULITIS

Folliculitis, either bacterial or fungal, is reported as the most common non-phenotypic dermatological manifestation of Down syndrome (Schepis et al. 2002). Bacterial skin infections occur with greater frequency in Down syndrome and are often more widespread and/or prolonged in their course (Kavanagh et al. 1993, Schepis et al. 2002, Sureshbabu et al. 2011). This is probably a reflection of the lowered immunity in Down syndrome (see Chapter 7). Gram-positive folliculitis due to *S. aureus* is more common and frequently associated with xerosis, for example, lower legs (see Fig. 16.5a and b), whilst gram-negative folliculitis is more common in moist and seborrhoea areas, for example, face.

Folliculitis due to commensal yeasts, such as *Malassezia furfur/Pityrosporum ovale*, also usually affects seborrhoeic areas such as the scalp, face and upper trunk. A higher prevalence of pityrosporum folliculitis is reported in males with Down syndrome (Kavanagh et al. 1993).

Check swabs from involved skin and the nares from the person (and if recurrent infection, also from close carers) to exclude staphylococcal or streptococcal carriage. Treat with antiseptic bath emollients and topical antiseptics (or if indicated, antifungal preparations) for mild infection or oral antibiotics for more significant infections. Folliculitis in the perineal region is often improved with extra attention to hygiene, wearing cotton underwear and improved aeration (avoiding excessive friction and occlusion).

SEBORRHOEIC DERMATITIS

Seborrhoeic dermatitis is an eczematous disorder affecting the sebum-rich, greasy areas of the scalp, face and upper trunk and has a worldwide prevalence of 3–5% (Schwartz et al. 2006). Seborrhoeic dermatitis is believed to be an inflammatory reaction related to proliferation of *Malassezia furfur* and/or *Pityrosporum ovale*. In addition, it is hypothesized that the pathogenesis of seborrhoeic dermatitis has an immune component, which is supported by the increased incidence in people with impaired cellular immunity and immunosuppressive disorders (Prohic 2010).

Antifungal topical preparations, including ketoconazole shampoo (used both as a shampoo and as a body wash), are helpful. If inflammation is significant, topical combined steroid/antifungal agents can be used to good effect, either once or twice daily.

DERMATOPHYTE FUNGAL INFECTION

Schepis et al. (2002) reported 4.4% prevalence for onychomycosis and 2% for tinea corporis (fungal infection of trunk, legs and arms) in a cohort of 203 people with Down syndrome. For localized skin involvement, topical antifungal creams for 2–4 weeks are often sufficient. However, for scalp (Tinea capitis) or nail involvement, a course of oral antifungal treatment is required (see Fig. 16.5a and b).

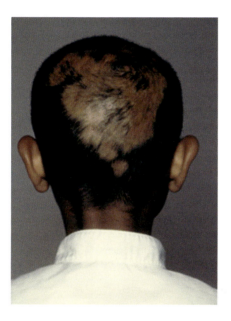

Fig. 16.5a. Tinea capitis—showing scaling, erythema and alopecia.

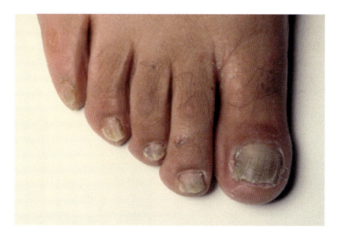

Fig. 16.5b. Tinea ungium and pedis.

CANDIDIASIS

Orofacial Candida infections occur with an increased frequency in people with Down syndrome. Lip cheilitis often begins after the age of 5 years. It is reported to occur in about 25% people with Down syndrome compared with 0.5% of the general population and can be associated with a fissured tongue (Scully et al. 2002).

SCABIES

People with Down syndrome appear to be more predisposed to crusted (Norwegian) scabies, and not only within the institutional setting (Scherbenske et al. 1990) (see Fig. 16.6). Poor cutaneous sensation, leading to a decreased likelihood of mites being mechanically scratched from the skin, may also contribute to increased infestation rates (Scherbenske et al. 1990). The treatment for scabies in Down syndrome is similar to that in the general population. For Norwegian crusted scabies, a single dose of oral ivermectin may be curative (Fig 16.6).

What skin disorders are linked to a defect in keratinization?

XEROSIS

Xerosis is associated with skin dryness, scaling and itching; it occurs in about 10% of people with Down syndrome. The reason for the increased prevalence is not clear. There may be a link to keratosis pilaris (see below). Treatment is similar to atopic dermatitis (see above). Urea-based emollients can be particularly helpful, although are occasionally not tolerated because of stinging.

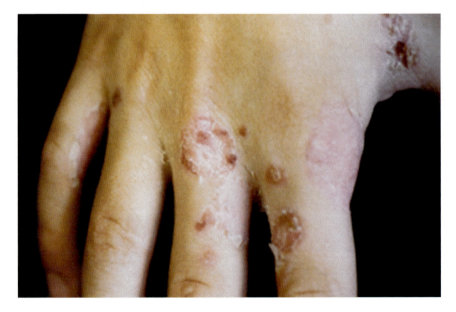

Fig. 16.6. Bullous impetigo with scabies infection of the hand.

KERATOSIS PILARIS

Keratosis pilaris is characterized by rough pin-point spots (which may contain twisted hair), with varying degrees of red or brown pigmentation (see Fig. 16.7). It usually appears in adolescence but may also be present in infants and continuing into adulthood. It most commonly occurs symmetrically on the upper outer arms but may also be seen on the thighs, outer cheeks, trunk, buttocks and occasionally forearms and lower legs. No treatment is necessary and it does not respond particularly well to treatment; however, a regular emollient with or without a keratolytic or urea can be used.

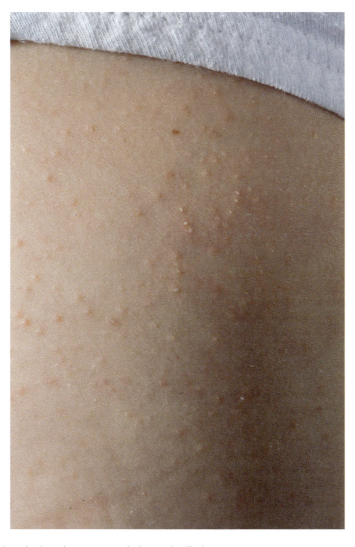

Fig. 16.7. Rough pin-point spots seen in keratosis pilaris.

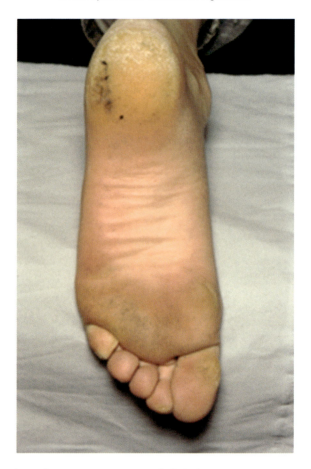

Fig. 16.8. Plantar keratoderma on pressure areas of whole foot.

PALMOPLANTAR HYPERKERATOSIS/KERATODERMA

Palmoplantar hyperkeratosis (marked thickening of the skin of the palms and soles; see Fig. 16.8) has been reported in between 10% and 40% in Down syndrome in two large case series of 100 and 71 participants, respectively (Ercis et al. 1996, Daneshpazhooh et al. 2007, Sureshbabu et al. 2011).

Treatment is as for skin xerosis. For significant hyperkeratosis, topical keratolytics (such as topical salicylic acid and urea-based preparations) can be helpful. If skin fissuring is significant, occluding with adherent dressings can help to soften the skin, reduce pain and the risk of secondary infection.

PSORIASIS

The literature on an association between Down syndrome and psoriasis is linked to a few case reports with no obvious significant increased prevalence in Down syndrome.

OTHER DISORDERS OF KERATINIZATION

There are individual case reports of pityriasis rubra pilaris in Down syndrome (Kusters et al. 2011). This is a rare skin disorder characterized by well-defined areas with hyperkeratotic erythematous follicular papules often associated with palmoplantar keratoderma or hyperkeratosis. Treatment is with emollients and for more severe cases oral retinoids or methotrexate.

What dermatological manifestations of Down syndrome are associated with alterations in connective tissue?

ELASTOSIS PERFORANS SERPIGINOSA

Elastosis perforans serpiginosa is a rare skin disorder in which abnormal elastic fibres pass from the dermis/deeper skin layer to the epidermis/superficial layer in a process termed 'transepidermal elimination'. It presents as clusters of small, red, 2–5mm papules, sometimes with a scaly central plug, often in groups, that may be in a circular, linear or snake-like pattern. Changes are most commonly seen on the neck, less frequently on the arms, face, trunk and legs. It is usually asymptomatic though can be itchy. It usually appears in the second decade of life and is more common in males. Diagnosis is made clinically and on skin histology.

Up to 1% of individuals with Down syndrome are reported to have reactive elastosis perforans serpiginosa and are predisposed to developing a generalized form of the disorder (O'Donnell et al. 1992). There are many features of Down syndrome that suggest connective tissue dysplasia (preterm ageing, joint hyperlaxity), which may offer a potential explanation, and it may also link to overexpression of *COL6A1* and *COL6A2* collagen genes (see above). Espinosa et al. (2008) postulated that elastosis perforans serpiginosa may serve as a biological marker in Moyamoya disease associated with Down syndrome. Elastosis perforans serpiginosa usually resolves spontaneously after several years. No treatment is needed or helpful, but there are case reports on the use of retinoids, cryotherapy and topical imiquimod.

ANETODERMA

Anetoderma is a benign condition with focal loss of dermal elastic tissue, resulting in localized areas of atrophic, flaccid or herniated sack-like skin. In Down syndrome, it can be primary, that is, due to a congenital malformation of elastic fibres (Barankin and Guenther 2001), or secondary due to local inflammation, often as a result of a localized infection such as folliculitis (Schepis and Siragusa 1999). It presents as asymptomatic, well-defined, annular, often pale or white areas, which wrinkle more easily than normal skin. They are usually several millimetres and occasionally up to 1–2cm in size. Lesions may look flat, raised or depressed. However, on palpation there is a palpable depression, termed the 'button-hole sign'. They are most commonly found on the chest, back, neck and arms, but any site can be affected.

If in clinical doubt, the diagnosis can be confirmed with skin biopsy; histology shows loss of elastic fibres in the upper and mid-dermis. Early recognition and treatment of skin infections such as folliculitis may prevent the development of anetoderma (Schepis and Siragusa 1999). Unfortunately, no treatment is helpful.

COLLAGENOMA

Collagenomas are benign connective tissue naevi that exhibit increased collagen deposition in the dermis. There are reports of multiple connective tissue naevi occurring in people with Down syndrome (Togawa et al. 2003). As with milia-like calcinosis cutis and anetoderma, they may occur at sites of recurrent trauma and/or friction, such as the feet, knees or dorsal joints of the hands. Collagenomas in people with Down syndrome have been reported in association with other cutaneous changes including multiple syringomas, milia-like calcinosis cutis and ichthyosis. They are usually asymptomatic and no treatment is necessary.

MULTIPLE ERUPTIVE DERMATOFIBROMAS

The development of five to eight dermatofibromas appearing over the period of a few months is usually linked to immunodeficiency-associated conditions (transplant, HIV, malignancy and autoimmunity) and there are isolated case reports in Down syndrome (Monteagudo et al. 2009).

Other dermatological manifestations of Down syndrome

SYRINGOMAS

Syringomas are benign adnexal tumours, formed by well-differentiated ductal elements. They appear as asymptomatic, small (<3mm), flesh-coloured or translucent dermal papules/bumps, typically in a periorbital/palpebral distribution (Schepis et al. 1994b) (see Fig. 16.9). Axillary, chest, abdominal and genital syringomas may coexist. The incidence of syringomas in Down syndrome is reported to be 30 times that of the general

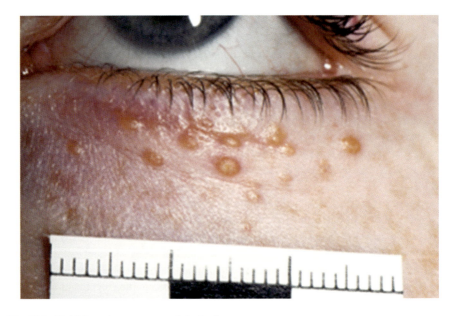

Fig. 16.9. Multiple syringomas upper left cheek.

population and rare cases of eruptive syringomas associated with Down syndrome have been reported (Urban et al. 1981, Schepis et al. 2001, Ong et al. 2010). There appears to be a female preponderance, for unknown reasons, with 26–42% of females being affected compared with 3–13% of males with Down syndrome (Schepis et al. 2001). They may be seen in association with milia-like calcinosis cutis. They are asymptomatic and treatment is cosmetic only, for example, with electro-surgery (diathermy) or lasers.

MILIA-LIKE CALCINOSIS CUTIS

Milia-like calcinosis cutis is a distinct subtype of idiopathic calcinosis cutis, with characteristic clinical and histological features. Clinically, they present as small, white papules, like classic milia, but have a more firm consistency and can eliminate a chalky substance, particularly when manipulated. They occur most commonly on the hands and feet, are largely asymptomatic and have a frequent association with syringomas (Maroon et al. 1990, Schepis et al. 1994a, Schepis et al. 2001) (see Fig. 16.10a and b). Histologically, discrete calcium deposits with a fibrous rim are seen within the papillary dermis (Madan et al. 2006).

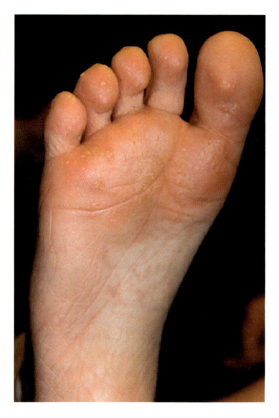

Fig. 16.10a. Milia-like calcinosis cutis on the soles of the feet with associated almost confluent syringomas on the neck.

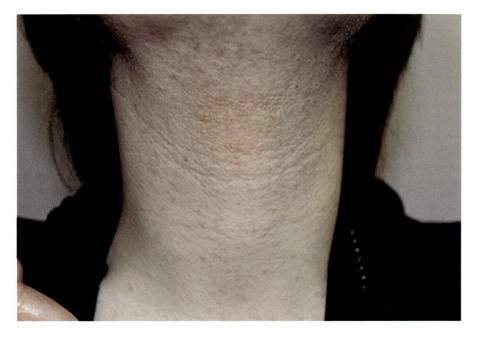

Fig. 16.10b. Milia-like calcinosis cutis on the soles of the feet with associated almost confluent syringomas on the neck.

Whilst calcium metabolism appears to be normal, higher concentrations of calcium in sweat have been reported in Down syndrome, which could lead to sweat duct calcification (Maroon et al. 1990). Increased calcium levels have also been found in fibroblast cultures in Down syndrome (Ceder et al. 1982). Although unconfirmed, it is possible that this high calcium state may predispose to the formation of milia-like calcinosis cutis.

This is a benign condition. The majority of these lesions resolve spontaneously, and heal without sequelae and require no treatment. The condition should be differentiated from epidermal cysts, warts and molluscum contiagosum (see Fig. 16.11a–c).

What dermatological conditions are associated with an underlying systemic disorder?

Leukaemia cutis

Leukaemia cutis is the infiltration of neoplastic leukocytes or their precursors into the epidermis, dermis, and/or subcutis from any type of leukaemia. Clinically, this manifests typically as blue, firm, indurated papules and nodules. Histology demonstrates a diagnostic nodular, perivascular and/or periadnexal dermal infiltrate of leukaemic cells. Unusual vesiculopustular eruptions have also been described in children with Down syndrome in association with leukaemoid reactions and myeloproliferative disorders. Hence, it is important for children with vesiculo-proliferative eruptions to consider an urgent blood count to rule out haematological abnormalities (Patel et al. 2012).

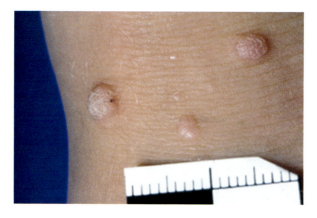

Fig. 16.11a. Viral warts on the trunk and periungal warts.

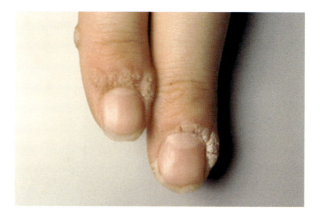

Fig. 16.11b. Viral warts on the trunk and periungal warts.

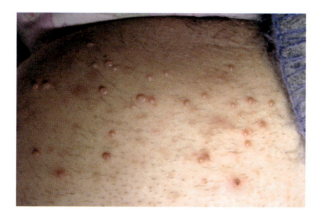

Fig. 16.11c. Molluscum contiagosum with umbilicated centre.

ACANTHOSIS NIGRICANS

A retrospective study that included 51 non-diabetic people with Down syndrome found acanthosis nigricans in 26 (50.9%) (Munoz-Perez and Camacho 2001). Of note, all 51 people were obese—it is therefore probable that the acanthosis nigricans was due to relative insulin resistance. However, in addition to commonly affected sites, in people with Down syndrome the acanthosis nigricans was reported in a distinct distribution affecting the flexor aspect of the elbows and knees and the dorsal surfaces overlying the interphalangeal and metacarpal joints.

CAROTENAEMIA

Carotenaemia is the benign yellow/orangey hue of the skin commonly involving the naso-labial folds, pinna, palms and soles of the feet but sparing the mucous membranes and sclera (see Fig.16.12). Carotenemia is commonly caused by an increased consumption of

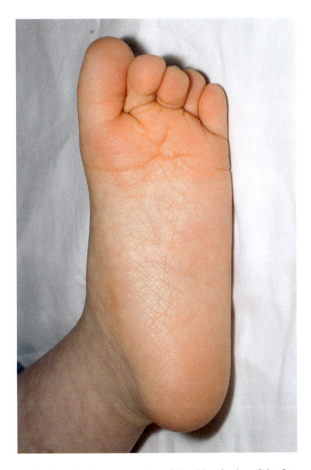

Fig. 16.12. Carotenaemia showing the orangey hue of the skin of soles of the feet.

β-carotene, for example, carrots and green beans. The bioavailability of carotene is increased by heat and small particle size, for example, in pureed and commercially prepared food. Storm (1990) identified asymptomatic carotenaemia in 14 out 44 children with Down syndrome. It has been postulated that increased consumption of a pureed food may account for the increased prevalence of carotenaemia in people with Down syndrome (Patel et al. 1973). However, there have been case reports of carotenemia in people with Down syndrome being associated with systemic conditions, for example, hypothyroidism (Aktuna et al. 1993), diabetes (Lin 2006) and myelodysplasia (Hurley et al. 2011); it is therefore important to investigate carotenaemia to exclude possible associated comorbidities.

Key points

- Dermatoses are commonly encountered in individuals with Down syndrome, and may be a specific association or be coincidental.
- Many common skin disorders, such as xerosis, seborrhoeic dermatitis and alopecia areata, are seen with increased frequency and sometimes greater severity in Down syndrome. The treatment of these disorders is similar to that in the general population.
- Many of the specific cutaneous associations with Down syndrome are benign and largely cosmetic (e.g. syringomas, milia-like calcinosis cutis, anetoderma). Some may be representative of a serious systemic abnormality (e.g. leukaemia cutis) and should prompt further investigation.

REFERENCES

Aktuna D, Buchinger W, Langsteger W, Aktuna D, Meister E, Sternad H, Lorenz O, Eber O (1993) Beta-carotene, vitamin A and carrier proteins in thyroid diseases. *Acta Med Austriaca.* 20(1–2): 17–20.

Barankin B, Guenther L (2001) Dermatological manifestations of Down's syndrome. *J Cutan Med Surg* 5: 289–293.

Carter DM, Jegasothy BV (1976) Alopecia areata and Down syndrome. *Arch Dermatol* 112: 1397–1399.

Ceder O, Roomans GM, Hosli P (1982) Increased calcium content in cultured fibroblasts from trisomy patients: Comparison with cystic fibrosis fibroblasts. *Scan Electron Microsc.* (Pt 2): 723–30.

Daneshpazhooh M, Nazemi TM, Bigdeloo L, Yoosefi M (2007) Mucocutaneous findings in 100 children with Down syndrome. *Pediatr Dermatol* 24: 317–320.

Ercis M, Balci S, Atakan N (1996) Dermatological manifestations of 71 Down syndrome children admitted to a clinical genetics unit. *Clin Genet* 50: 317–320.

Espinosa PS, Baumann RJ, Vaishnav AG (2008) Elastosis perforans serpiginosa, Down syndrome, and moyamoya disease. *Pediatr Neurol* 38: 287–288.

Hanifin, JM and Rajka, G (1980) Diagnostic features of atopic dermatitis. *Acta Derm Venereol Suppl* (Stockh). 92: 44–47.

Hurley M, Martin K, Marder E (2011) Hypercarotenaemia in children with Down syndrome. *Down Syndr Q* 13: 52–54.

Karousou E, Stachtea X, Moretto P et al. (2013) New insights into the pathobiology of Down syndrome—hyaluronan synthase-2 overexpression is regulated by collagen VI alpha2 chain. *FEBS J* 280: 2418–2430.

Kavanagh GM, Leeming JP, Marshman GM, Reynolds NJ, Burton JL (1993) Folliculitis in Down's syndrome. *Br J Dermatol* 129: 696–699.

Kusters MA, Verstegen RH, de Vries E (2011) Down syndrome: Is it really characterized by precocious immunosenescence? *Aging Dis* 2: 538–545.

Lin JN (2006) Images in clinical medicine. Yellow palms and soles in diabetes mellitus. *N Engl J Med.* 355: 1486.

Madan V, Williams J, Lear JT (2006) Dermatological manifestations of Down's syndrome. *Clin Exp Dermatol* 31: 623–629.

Marmon S, De Souza A, Strober BE (2012) Psoriasis and Down syndrome: A report of three cases and a potential pathophysiologic link. *Dermatol Online J* 18: 13.

Maroon M, Tyler W, Marks VJ (1990) Calcinosis cutis associated with syringomas: A transepidermal elimination disorder in a patient with Down syndrome. *J Am Acad Dermatol* 23: 372–375.

Monteagudo B, Suarez-Amor O, Cabanillas M, Leon-Mateos A, Perez-Valcarcel J, de las Heras C (2009) Down syndrome: Another cause of immunosuppression associated with multiple eruptive dermatofibromas? *Dermatol Online J* 15: 15.

Munoz-Perez MA, Camacho F (2001) Acanthosis nigricans: A new cutaneous sign in severe atopic dermatitis and Down syndrome. *J Eur Acad Dermatol Venereol* 15: 325–327.

NICE UK (2007) National Institute for Health and Clinical Excellence. Atopic eczema in children: Full guideline CG57. http://www.nice.org.uk/guidance/CG57 (accessed 1 January 2015).

Norton SA, Demidovich CW, 3rd (1993) Down syndrome, alopecia universalis, and trachyonychia. *Pediatr Dermatol* 10: 187–188.

O'Donnell B, Kelly P, Dervan P, Powell FC (1992) Generalized elastosis perforans serpiginosa in Down's syndrome. *Clin Exp Dermatol* 17: 31–33.

Ong GC, Lim KS, Chian LY (2010) Eruptive syringoma in a patient with trisomy 21. *Singapore Med J* 51: e46–e47.

Patel H, Dunn HG, Tischer B, McBurney AK, Hach E (1973) Carotenemia in mentally retarded children: I. Incidence and etiology. *Canadian Med Assoc J* 108: 848–852.

Patel LM, Maghari A, Schwartz RA, Kapila R, Morgan AJ, Lambert WC (2012) Myeloid leukemia cutis in the setting of myelodysplastic syndrome: A crucial dermatological diagnosis. *Int J Dermatol* 51: 383–388.

Prohic A (2010) Distribution of Malassezia species in seborrhoeic dermatitis: Correlation with people' cellular immune status. *Mycoses* 53: 344–349.

Ram G, Chinen J (2011) Infections and immunodeficiency in Down syndrome. *Clin Exp Immunol* 164: 9–16.

Sabatelli P, Gara SK, Grumati P et al. (2002) An updated survey on skin conditions in Down syndrome. *Dermatology* 205: 234–238.

Schepis C, Barone C, Siragusa M, Romano C (1997) Prevalence of atopic dermatitis in people with Down syndrome: A clinical survey. *J Am Acad Dermatol* 36: 1019–1021.

Schepis C, Siragusa M (1999) Secondary anetoderma in people with Down's syndrome. *Acta Dermato-Venereol* 79: 245.

Schepis C, Siragusa M, Palazzo R, Batolo D, Romano C (1994a) Perforating milia-like idiopathic calcinosis cutis and periorbital syringomas in a girl with Down syndrome. *Pediatr Dermatol* 11: 258–260.

Schepis C, Siragusa M, Palazzo R, Ragusa RM, Massi G, Fabrizi G (1994b) Palpebral syringomas and Down's syndrome. *Dermatology* 189: 248–250.

Schepis C, Torre V, Siragusa M et al. (2001) Eruptive syringomas with calcium deposits in a young woman with Down's syndrome. *Dermatology* 203: 345–347.

Scherbenske JM, Benson PM, Rotchford JP, James WD (1990) Cutaneous and ocular manifestations of Down syndrome. *J Am Acad Dermatol* 22: 933–938.

Schwartz RA, Janusz CA, Janniger CK (2006) Seborrheic dermatitis: An overview. *Am Family Physician* 74: 125–130.

Scully C, van Bruggen W, Diz Dios P, Casal B, Porter S, Davison MF (2002) Down syndrome: Lip lesions (angular stomatitis and fissures) and *Candida albicans*. *Br J Dermatol* 147: 37–40.

Storm W (1990) Prevalence and diagnostic significance of gliadin antibodies in children with Down syndrome. *Eur J Pediatr* 149: 833–834.

Sureshbabu R, Kumari R, Ranugha S, Sathyamoorthy R, Udayashankar C, Oudeacoumar P (2011) Phenotypic and dermatological manifestations in Down syndrome. *Dermatol Online J* 17: 3.

Tazi-Ahnini R, di Giovine FS, McDonagh AJ et al. (2000) Structure and polymorphism of the human gene for the interferon-induced p78 protein (MX1): Evidence of association with alopecia areata in the Down syndrome region. *Hum Genet* 106: 639–645.

Togawa Y, Nohira G, Shinkai H, Utani A (2003) Collagenoma in Down syndrome. *Br J Dermatol* 148: 596–597.

Urban CD, Cannon JR, Cole RD (1981) Eruptive syringomas in Down's syndrome. *Arch Dermatol* 117: 374–375.

Xu Y, Li W, Liu X et al. (2013) Identification of dysregulated microRNAs in lymphocytes from children with Down syndrome. *Gene* 530: 278–286.

17
ORAL AND DENTAL HEALTH

Liz Marder and June Nunn

Do people with Down syndrome have specific issues with dental health?

People with Down syndrome have head and neck features of relevance to oral/dental health including muscle hypotonia and mid-face hypoplasia, as well as specific intraoral features. The flattened nasal bridge together with a generally smaller nose and mid-face can create difficulties with airway patency for inhalation sedation and endotracheal intubation (Sureshbabu et al. 2011). Obesity can lead to cervical accumulations making visualization of the laryngeal area difficult, thus posing risks for general anaesthesia (Kieser et al. 2003). A small mid and lower face may predispose to sleep-disordered breathing (see Chapter 9).

Specific intraoral features are a mouth open posture, sometimes accompanied by drooling and a protrusive tongue often with deep fissuring (Fig. 17.1), a challenge for oral hygiene. Other oral features are relative prognathism, hypodontia, microdontia (Fig. 17.2), enamel hypoplasia, aggressive periodontal disease (Fig. 17.3), reduced root length, delayed eruption in both dentitions, delayed exfoliation of primary teeth and tooth wear (Kieser et al. 2003).

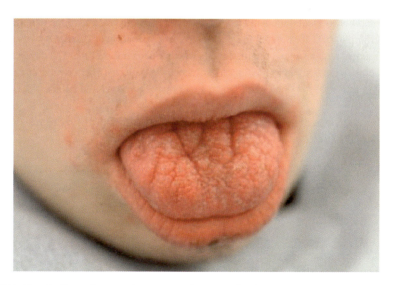

Fig. 17.1. Deeply fissured, protrusive tongue; plaque and food may become stagnant in fissures and lead to halitosis.

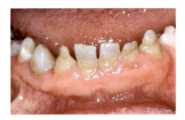

Fig. 17.2. Enamel defects: Hypoplasia, microdontia (coeliac disease related); retained 'baby' teeth, missing permanent teeth and enamel hypoplasia (ridges/grooves on teeth) that act as plaque traps.

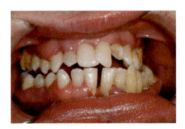

Fig. 17.3. Missing teeth and advanced periodontal disease with bone loss and mobile lower front teeth that have started to drift.

There is evidence that growth retardation in Down syndrome reduces the amounts of enamel and dentine in permanent incisors but not the earlier-forming primary tooth predecessors. Bell et al. (2001) conclude that this is evidence of the concept of an amplified developmental instability for dental traits in Down syndrome. Specific features of the dentition, such as altered morphology, are thought to be indicative of a reduction of cellular activity of tooth germs consistent with a general retardation in growth in Down syndrome. The different shape of the lower incisors is thought possibly to influence the pattern of periodontal disease seen, especially in this area, in people with Down syndrome (Townsend and Brown 1983).

What impact do other medical conditions associated with Down syndrome have on dental health?

CARDIAC

People with cardiac defects are at increased risk of developing infective endocarditis. In the past, it was standard practice in the UK to recommend prophylactic antibiotics prior to dental treatment. This is no longer recommended (NICE 2008) as

(1) there is no consistent association between a dental procedure and development of infective endocarditis, and
(2) regular toothbrushing undoubtedly poses a greater risk of infective endocarditis than a single dental procedure because of the repeated exposure to bacteraemia with oral flora.

In addition, it is felt, on the basis of evidence, that there is no proof of the effectiveness of antibiotic prophylaxis and the risk of anaphylaxis may, in fact, lead to a greater number of deaths.

HYPOTHYROIDISM

There is a purported link between the autoimmune manifestation of thyroid disease, Hashimoto thyroiditis and periodontal (gum) disease (Scardina and Messina 2008). Hypothyroidism and cardiac anomalies are linked with hypodontia (Reuland-Bosma et al. 2010). Hypothyroidism may result in hypotonia and anaemia, both relevant in dental care.

OTHER AUTOIMMUNE EFFECTS

The higher prevalence and severity of periodontal disease seen in Down syndrome, in the absence of significant deposits of the initiating factor of plaque, may be as a consequence of differential modulation of expression of genes resulting in an attenuation of anti-inflammatory and increase of pro-inflammatory mediators (Cavalcante et al. 2012). Phagocytic activity has been recorded as more intense in individuals with demonstrably greater periodontal attachment loss (Khoct et al. 2012). Other factors implicated in the pathophysiology of the extensive periodontal effects seen in people with Down syndrome are enhanced PGE_2 production and increased activity of plasminogen activators, and thus collagenase activity.

Kathleen has gradually lost teeth since adolescence because of periodontal (gum) disease. This started with her lower incisors and then gradually molar teeth loosened and eventually fell out. More recently, one of her remaining upper incisors was very loose and her mother was concerned that if it went, the gap at the front would look awful. The dentist discussed at length the pros and cons of taking it out before it fell out and fitting a denture. Kathleen's mum was unsure how she would cope with a denture. In the end, it was decided that it was better to take Kathleen through the stages of having a denture made, using nitrous oxide sedation ('Happy air') to make it easier for her to tolerate the appointments, rather than wait for the tooth to fall out and have a crisis on their hands. Kathleen tolerated the removal of the loose front tooth under sedation well and is delighted with her new tooth. As she loses more teeth, they can be added to the denture so that she is not left with gaps and she can still bite and chew. Kathleen's mum helps with cleaning the denture and ensuring it is stored safely overnight when it is not worn to give a chance for the soft tissues to recover.

GASTROINTESTINAL DISEASE

Down syndrome is associated with increased prevalence of both coeliac and gastro-oesophageal reflux disease (GORD). Atypical, silent or even latent forms of coeliac disease may be responsible for the malformation (hypoplasia) of enamel (Fig. 17.2) seen in Down syndrome (Admou et al. 1999) and may manifest with aphthous ulcers (Cheng et al. 2010). GORD, if sufficiently severe, can lead to dental erosion (Wallace 2007) (Fig. 17.4).

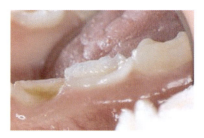

Fig. 17.4. Tooth wear (erosion) with sharp cusps that irritate the tongue or cheeks. The teeth may also be sensitive to cold foods/drinks.

Peter presents with tooth wear related to reflux disease. The constant regurgitation of acid has worn his retained 'baby' teeth and some permanent teeth. Irritation from a sharp tooth was constant and eventually produced an ulcer on his tongue. The dentist took a biopsy, in case the ulcer was more sinister. It was not. The dentist made sure that the worn and sharp tooth surfaces were covered with dental cement so that they did not irritate the tongue or cheek, also making cleaning easier and reducing sensitivity to cold things.

What oral/dental conditions commonly occur in Down syndrome?
The hypotonia, altered morphology and dental anomalies seen in Down syndrome impact on feeding and swallowing. Masticatory function affects the nutrition as well as the social integration of affected children and adults (Faulks et al. 2008). The tendency for a prognathic lower jaw and mid-face hypoplasia results in an Angles class III malocclusion, which may be complicated by any of the dental anomalies listed above. This may not be amenable to orthodontic treatment on its own, requiring surgical correction in combination with more complex orthodontic intervention.

Drooling in children with Down syndrome is common. It can be excessive, necessitating several changes of clothing/bibs per day and lead to alienation from peers because of wet play areas, keyboards and so on. Constant drooling in cold weather leads to excoriation of the chin. Surgery to divert salivary flow from the submandibular glands more posteriorly may alleviate the problem, but may not be successful and carries the risk of increasing caries prevalence due to greatly diminished salivary volume. A more sustainable approach is the use of oral screens, followed by, if indicated, acrylic training plates that encourage the formation of an oral seal, as well as promoting a more active swallowing mechanism so that saliva does not pool and dribble out from an open mouth (Fig. 17.5). This approach requires a multidisciplinary team of dentists, paediatricians and speech therapists working with the family to support the necessary home therapy. This is fundamental to success. Anecdotal case reports support the use of these plates, but few studies have offered objective data (Kelly et al. 2013). An alternative, less invasive method of reducing saliva flow is using hyoscine hydrobromide which blocks parasympathetic transmission to the salivary glands. It is applied as a patch behind the ear and changed every 3 days. The use of botulinum neurotoxin type A injected

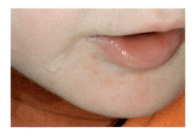

Fig. 17.5. Saliva dribbling from open mouth.

into the parotid gland is now the preferred management in some centres. It needs to be performed as a day case procedure under guided ultrasonography, with a general anaesthetic to avoid the risk of escape from the gland capsule and resultant paralysis of pharyngeal muscles.

Hypodontia has been reported in approximately half of people with Down syndrome (Suri et al. 2011). Some studies report a relationship between craniofacial, especially mandibular, differences and hypodontia. Other dental anomalies such as extra teeth (supernumerary or supplemental), conical teeth and impaction of teeth as well as a general delay in tooth eruption/retention of primary teeth (Fig. 17.2) are more commonly seen (de Moraes et al. 2007).

The smaller teeth observed in Down syndrome are thought to be the result of an early transitory acceleration in mitotic activity of developing enamel organs, which endures through the initial stages of mineralization of the primary teeth. This is followed by growth retardation, resulting in smaller permanent teeth (Peretz et al. 2013).

A recent sibling-controlled study has again concluded that dental caries is less prevalent in young people with Down syndrome (Macho et al. 2013). This may be related to the delay in eruption and/or the reduced number of teeth or possibly a reduced prevalence of mutans streptococci, the intraoral commensal acidogenic bacteria (Areias et al. 2012).

Tooth wear described above in relation to GORD may also be seen where there is excessive consumption of, for example, carbonated beverages (Fig. 17.4). Tooth sensitivity to sweet or cold foods/drinks may result especially at the stage when excessive loss of tooth substance is found by the dental team. Tooth wear is also seen where there is tooth grinding or bruxism. This can be very distressing for family members and nocturnal bruxism may disrupt their sleep (Miamato et al. 2011; Uong et al. 2001). Splints can be fitted to minimize tooth damage but this can be an intractable problem (Waldman et al. 2009).

Susan's family complain about the noise she makes when she grinds her teeth. Her teeth are getting quite worn, especially the 'baby' ones, still present as she is missing some permanent teeth. As grinding was more obvious at night, a splint was proposed to use during sleep. Susan was apprehensive about having the impression of her teeth taken to make the splint but some inhalation sedation ('Happy air') helped her cope. The next week she returned to have the splint fitted (like a sports mouthguard usually fitting over the top teeth). Susan manages the splint easily, fitting it, rinsing it each morning and storing it in her special case.

How should we approach dental management?

ORAL HYGIENE

Oral hygiene is of paramount importance for people with Down syndrome because rapidly progressive periodontal disease is prevalent. It can be challenging to perform because of difficulty understanding, poor attention span or manual dexterity of the individual, along with resistance to assistance .There may also be reluctance on the part of carers to intervene because of the feeling of the need to respect the autonomy of the individual and/or unfamiliarity with correct oral hygiene methods. The physical limitations imposed by a small upper jaw and a large tongue present barriers. Relative hypomotility of the oral soft tissues allows for food stagnation. All of these can be overcome by appropriate training, suitable oral hygiene aids such as finger brushes and special brushes (Collis Curve©, [www.colliscurve.co.uk]; and Dr Barman© 'Superbrushes' [http://mun-h-center.se/en/Mun-H-Center/Mun-H-Center-E/Hjalpmedel/Produktlista/]) (Fig. 17.6a–c). Powered brushes may be an alternative but are often not well tolerated.

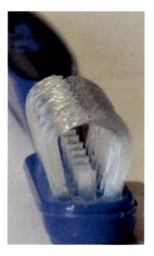

Fig. 17.6a. Collis Curve brush.

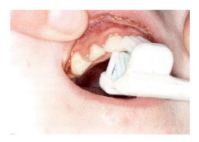

Fig. 17.6b. Dr Barman's 'Superbrush'.

234

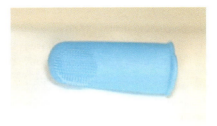

Fig. 17.6c. Fingerbrush.

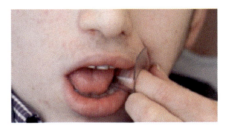

Fig. 17.7. Mouth prop to aid access for tooth brushing and to avoid being bitten.

The dental team may undertake a risk assessment to decide the most appropriate agent to use on the toothbrush. If both dental caries and periodontal risks are high, an agent including both fluoride and chlorhexidine (900ppm fluoride and 0.1% chlorhexidine) will be recommended. This variant on chlorhexidine is often better tolerated than the more conventional product as it tastes better and does not stain teeth. Where periodontal risk is highest and dental caries not a risk, then a chlorhexidine-containing gel (0.2%) may be advocated. This is also available as a spray. Children at high risk of developing dental caries can be prescribed high concentration toothpastes containing either 2800ppm fluoride (over 10y of age) or 5000ppm fluoride (over 16y of age). In addition, such high-risk individuals may have concentrated fluoride varnishes (22 600ppm fluoride) applied at dental visits, every 3–4 months. Fluoride-containing daily mouthwashes (250ppm fluoride) are more difficult for some people with intellectual disabilities to use routinely and should only be used at a different time of day to fluoride toothpaste use.

A mouth prop can be helpful in maintaining an open mouth posture for toothbrushing, as well as protecting the operator's fingers from being bitten (Fig. 17.7).

DIET

Young people with Down syndrome benefit from a diet low in non-milk extrinsic sugars, not only to protect against dental caries but also to prevent obesity. Retained primary teeth, especially where there is not a permanent successor, are more vulnerable to dental caries and tooth wear.

Children assessed at risk of developing dental caries should have susceptible pits and fissures sealed as soon as the risk is identified and the surface is erupted sufficiently for the sealant to be applied. Worn primary teeth that may be sensitive can be protected with sealants or more usually glass ionomer cements. These materials leach fluorides and thus confer additional dental caries protection.

Challenges in providing treatment

Children and adults with any degree of intellectual disability may be fearful of new experiences and dentistry is no exception. Whilst early intervention is the ideal, allowing familiarity to be established before any dental intervention is required, this does not always happen. Appropriately trained dental teams can deliver care in such circumstances using clinical Holding, provided consent/assent has been obtained (Kerr et al. 2013). A patient who finds dental care difficult may react with challenging behaviour. Time and patience may overcome this. If this approach fails, oral sedation can be prescribed prior to a visit or have dental care can be provided under conscious sedation—either with nitrous oxide inhalation sedation or intravenous benzodiazepines, usually midazolam. Treatment under general anaesthesia is usually a final resort. It should not be assumed that adolescents and adults with Down syndrome cannot consent for dental care but the clinician needs to judge on an individual basis each person's capacity to give consent for dental care (Jones et al. 2010).

Health surveillance
GENERAL OR SPECIAL DENTAL CARE SERVICES
There is no justification for a child, or adult, with Down syndrome to be referred automatically for special dental care services (Oliver and Nunn 1995). Routine check-ups can be with the rest of the family. If there are behaviour management or other dental issues beyond the competence of the general dental practitioner, then referral to a special care dentist will be appropriate.

Key points
- Dental anomalies are common in people with Down syndrome.
- Children and young people may not experience as much dental decay as their non-affected peers.
- People with Down syndrome are more prone to gum disease.
- Treatment may be challenging, requiring general anaesthetic.
- Dental disease may pose a particular challenge for those with other health issues. Prevention is important.
- Tooth grinding is a common problem and can be improved by using splints.

REFERENCES

Areias C, Sampaio-Maia B, Pereira Mde L et al. (2012) Reduced salivary flow and colonization by mutans streptococci in children with Down syndrome. *Clinics (Sao Paulo)* 67: 1007–1011.

Bell E, Townsend G, Wilson D, Kieser J, Hughes T (2001) Effect of Down syndrome on the dimensions of dental crowns and tissues. *Am J Hum Biol.* 13:690–8.

Cavalcante LB, Tanaka MH, Pirees JR et al. (2012) Expression of the interleukin-10 signaling pathway genes in individuals with Down syndrome and periodontitis. *Oral Dis* 18: 346–352.

Cheng J, Malahias T, Brar P, Minaya MT, Green PH (2001) The association between celiac disease, dental enamel defects, and aphthous ulcers in a United States cohort. *Am J Respir Crit Care Med* 163: 731–736.

De Moraes ME, De Moraes LC, Dotto GN, Dotto PP, dos Santos LR (2007) Dental anomalies in patients with Down syndrome. *Brazilian Dent J* 18: 346–350.

Faulks D, Collado V, Mazille MN, Veyrune JL, Hennequin M (2008) Masticatory dysfunction in persons with Down's syndrome. Part 1: Aetiology and incidence. *J Oral Rehabil* 35: 854–862.

Jones EL, Ballard CG, Prasher VP, Arno M (2010) An intron 7 polymorphism in APP affects the age of onset of dementia in Down syndrome. *Int J Alzheimer's Dis* 2011: 929102. doi: 10.4061/2011/929102.

Kelly G, Pritchard M, Thompson S (2013) The use of orofacial regulation therapy including palatal plate therapy, in the management of orofacial dysfunction in patients with Down syndrome. *J Disabil Oral Health* 14: 15–24.

Kerr B, Edwards JA, Moosajee S, Shehabi Z, Rafique S (2013) Audit of clinical holding in Special Care Dentistry. *J Disabil Oral Health* 14: 29–33.

Khoct A, Russell B, Cannon JG, Turner B, Janal M (2007) Phagocytic cell activity and periodontitis in Down syndrome. *J Intellect Dev Disabil* 32: 45–50.

Kieser J, Townsend G, Quick A (2003) The Down syndrome patient in dental practice, part I: Pathogenesis and general and dental features. *N Z Dent J.* 99:5–9.

Mach V, Palha M, Macedo AP, Ribeiro O, Andrade C (2013) Comparative study between dental caries prevalence of Down syndrome children and their siblings. *Special Care Dentistry* 33: 2–7.

Miamato CB, Pereira LJ, Ramos-Jorge ML, Marques LS (2011) Prevalence and predictive factors of sleep bruxism in children with and without cognitive impairment. *Brazilian Oral Res* 25: 439–445.

National Institute for Health and Clinical Excellence (2008) Prophylaxis against infective endocarditis antimicrobial prophylaxis against infective endocarditis in adults and children undergoing interventional procedures. http://www.nice.org.uk/nicemedia/pdf/CG64NICEguidance.pdf (accessed 1 January 2015).

Oliver H, Nunn J (1996) The accessibility of dental treatment to adults with physical disabilities aged 16–64 in the North-East of England. *Special Care Dentistry* 15: 97–101.

Peretz B, Katzenel V, Shapira J (2013) Comparative study between dental caries prevalence of Down syndrome children and their siblings. *Special Care Dentistry* 33: 2–7.

Reuland-Bosma W, Reuland MC, Bronkhorst E, Phoa KH (2010) Patterns of tooth agenesis in patients with Down syndrome in relation to hypothyroidism and congenital heart disease: An aid for treatment planning. *Am J Orthodont Dentofac Orthoped* 137: 584. doi: http://dx.doi.org/10.1016/j.ajodo.2009.10.032.

Scardina GA, Messina P (2008) Modifications of interdental papilla microcirculation: A possible cause of periodontal disease in Hashimoto's Thyroiditis? *Ann Anat* 190: 258–263.

Suri S, Tompson BD, Atenafu E (2011) Prevalence and patterns of permanent tooth agenesis in Down syndrome and their association with craniofacial morphology. *Angle Orthod* 81: 260–269.

Townsend GC, Brown RH (1983) Tooth morphology in Down's syndrome: evidence for retardation in growth. *J Ment Defic Res.* 27:159–69.

Uong EC, McDonough JM, Tayag-Kier CE et al. (2001) Magnetic resonance imaging of the upper airway in children with Down syndrome. *Am J Respir Crit Care* 163: 731–736.

Van-Garneren-Oosterom HB, van Dommelen P, Schonbeck Y, Oudesluys-Murphy AM, van Wouwe JP, Buitendijk SE (2012) Prevalence of overweight in Dutch children with Down syndrome. *Pediatrics* 130: 1520–1526.

Waldman HB, Hasan FM, Perlman S (2009) Down syndrome and sleep-disordered breathing: The dentist's role. *Am J Dent Assoc* 140: 307–312.

Wallace RA (2007) Clinical audit of gastrointestinal conditions occurring among adults with Down syndrome attending a specialist clinic. *J Intellect Dev Disabil.* 32:45–50.

18
NEUROPSYCHIATRY OF DOWN SYNDROME

Part 1: Neurological Disorders

Richard Newton

Introduction

In Chapter 2, we saw how a variety of biological mechanisms, most of which are poorly understood, lead to neurodevelopmental impairment in trisomy 21. This may be a reflection of the underdevelopment of neural circuits or abnormal neural signalling, or both. One consequence of trisomy 21 is Alzheimer disease. The underlying biology, presentation and management of this disorder are dealt with in a separate section in this chapter. Here, we shall consider other common neurological presentations.

From about 18 weeks' gestation onwards, in Down syndrome there is a reduction of brain size compared to that of the average person. This disparity continues into adult life. Volumetric studies matching specific brain areas demonstrate a reduction in size in the frontal and temporal lobes. The brain is foreshortened (brachycephalic) with a small cerebellum, simplified gyral appearance and narrow superior temporal gyrus. Paradoxically, the parahippocampal gyrus may be larger than in the average person.

Histological studies have demonstrated a reduced number of neurons, decreased neuronal densities and an abnormal neuronal distribution most marked in cortical layers II and IV. There is reduced production of synapses and synaptic length. Contact zones between neurons are abnormal. Deceleration in neurogenesis probably begins after 22 weeks' gestation. Alongside this reduced neurogenesis, an increase in apoptosis is also seen. Having said that, children with Down syndrome can have greater dendritic branching and total dendritic length may be increased relative to children with typical development up to the age of 6 months but dendritic arborization is reduced during childhood and into adult life (Lott 2012). The net result of all of this is the underdevelopment of neural circuits probably coupled with inefficient signalling patterns.

What is the developmental potential in Down syndrome for cognitive, language and social ability?

There have been a number of cohort studies on developmental attainment in Down syndrome. In 2006, Cliff Cunningham reviewed the results of studies available at that time (Cunningham 2006). Different studies used different assessment tools but mean developmental quotients of about 80 were seen in infancy, which fell to about 60 by the age of 5 years. Often by this age, they are being measured as mean intelligence quotients (IQs). A fall in IQ does not indicate loss of skills but rather a slowing of assimilation of skills, relative to children with typical development. These IQ scores appear to be stable from around the age of 5 years until the 20s. There are no cohort data beyond this age until those captured around the subject of ageing and dementia. The distribution of the data indicates that about 40% have IQs in the range of 50–70 (mild learning disability), 35% between 30 and 70 (moderate learning disability), around 1% above 70 and around 25% below 30 (severe/profound learning disability). Many in the latter range have comorbidities including an autistic spectrum disorder. These results are concordant with the study of Guéant et al. (2005). They determined the IQs of 131 people with Down syndrome (age unspecified). They found the 25th centile IQ to be 30 and the 75th centile IQ to be 60.

The mean age equivalent (MAE) of these scores indicates a spread of ability in adulthood from less than 3 years for about 6%, less than 5 years for 50%, less than 6 years for 85% with 10% with an MAE over 7 years. The spread of ability is from very low to over 9 years. We need to be mindful that an IQ measure is never more than an approximation of an individual's strengths and weaknesses; it says little about an individual. Couzens et al. (2004) collected longitudinal assessments of IQ using the fourth version of the Stanford-Binet test in 191 individuals with Down syndrome. The study highlighted the major pitfalls in the interpretation of test scores for this population. Despite obvious divergent abilities illustrated by age equivalent scores, 37% of the assessments were at the 'floor level' IQ of 36. MAE scores were also problematic as they failed to represent either the range or divergence of abilities adequately. There is more to a person than an IQ score.

These data demonstrate that there are large differences in abilities between individuals with Down syndrome and that a one approach for all is unlikely to suffice. The more difficult learning is for an individual, the more important it becomes to provide an education that takes advantage of the person's learning strengths and minimizes confrontation with learning barriers. Understanding cognitive strengths and weaknesses for individuals at lower levels of functioning is important if optimal support is to be provided. For individuals scoring at the floor of an assessment, the large discrepancies between subtest scores are generally masked by low domain scores. Age equivalent scores are more successful in discriminating between abilities at this level. They serve a more useful function for these individuals, if a true picture of their developmental strengths and weaknesses is to be attained.

Couzens et al. (2012) in a longitudinal study assessed associations between cognitive development, intrapersonal and environmental characteristics in 89 participants with Down syndrome so as to understand developmental patterns and cognitive strengths and weaknesses. Early cognitive advantage and opportunities to learn academic rather than life skills content facilitated cognitive development, although ability and maternal education were confounding variables in the study. (The positive association between maternal education and cognitive development is considered more in Chapter 19.) These data indicate that interventions that enhance verbal and problem-solving environments throughout early and middle childhood along with efforts to reduce negative, over-pessimistic influences can enhance cognitive development. Most children with Down syndrome are good at learning visually; if they see it done, they usually understand what is required. If they hear it explained, they have more trouble. Working memory function, particularly verbal short-term memory, is often impaired.

There are subtle differences in how children with Down syndrome approach and understand the social world around them. These differences might well have an impact on the development of later, more complex, sociocognitive abilities such as emotion recognition, theory of mind and empathy (Cebula et al. 2010). Differences in these early interpersonal responses may also influence language development. This, in turn, plays a central role in the development of successful interpersonal functioning at later ages. Research suggests that development across domains in Down syndrome may not be as well integrated as in typical development. This suggests that fundamentally different approaches to intervention may be required. Encouragingly, the wide individual variation in level and ages of acquisition of sociocognitive abilities indicate that the syndrome itself does not necessarily constrain social development in any predetermined way. More detailed study of sociocognitive development in Down syndrome could lead to more effective interventions. The use of new technologies and innovative paradigms, used already in the field of autism research such as eye tracking, functional magnetic resonance imaging, event-related potentials, electroencephalography and magnetoencephalography techniques, may prove of value.

Is there a central motor disorder in Down syndrome and how does it present?

The term 'central motor disorder' is usually reserved for instances where 'hard' neurological signs can be attributed to dysfunction in corticospinal, extrapyramidal or cerebellar movement control systems. We shall consider the following:

- Central hypotonia which resolves to a certain extent with age.
- A developmental coordination disorder usually broadly speaking anyway commensurate with a child's developmental age.
- Speech dysfluency.

A cardinal feature of the majority of children with an intellectual disability is low muscle tone, particularly in infancy which tends to improve with age, poor dexterity and poor balance and coordination. Tone describes the resting activity in a muscle. That is the resistance shown to passive muscle stretching. The stability of any joint depends on the tone of the muscles that control movement in the joint and the elasticity of the ligaments. Unfortunately, people with Down syndrome are in double jeopardy as a degree of ligamentous laxity usually accompanies the low tone.

From the neonatal period onwards, the low tone tends slowly to improve (this generally applies to any form of intellectual disability). The improvement in tone tends to spread caudally over months and years. Truncal stability precedes the emergence of better leg tone, with the distal leg being the last to improve. The result of this is that it is very common for young people with Down syndrome to be walking on a wobbly base with pes planus and valgus at the ankle persisting long after it has usually disappeared in typically developing children and often into adult life.

This poor base for movement coupled with longer processing times (Galli et al. 2010) often leads to different strategies (Rigoldi et al. 2011) being adopted for movement. One example is atypical finger grasping patterns (Jover et al. 2010). This cross-sectional study compared 35 young people with Down syndrome aged 4 years 3 months–18 years 4 months, with 35 age-matched controls. They noted significantly that fewer fingers were used when the participants grasped a small object with a tendency to extend those fingers uninvolved in the grip. With increasing age, the strategy slowly waned starting to approach that of the typically developing children, but nonetheless persisted in many. This finding is in keeping with what we have already discussed. If you are poorly coordinated with poor proximal fixation and low tone, you will try to find a strategy that allows you to offer a firm base for fine distal movement. Any parent observing their child with Down syndrome will also report a tendency to tire more easily. It is easy to see how any child with a poor base for movement and coordination difficulties is likely to have to expend more energy than the average person for the simplest of tasks and this has been demonstrated by Agiovlasitis et al. (2009) (see also Chapter 15).

The cognitive impairment in Down syndrome is accompanied by language impairment as with most children with intellectual disability. However, in Down syndrome there is an additional impairment of speech which proves to be deeply frustrating to those affected. We should note there is a lack of correlation between speech and cognition. All language measurements strongly suggest the speech disorder in Down syndrome is not simply due to cognitive impairment (Cleland and colleagues 2010). We take it for granted but the very fine movements of the tongue and lips that produce the pockets of sound we call speech, intelligible by others, represent the most intricate skill controlled by the brain. It is this alongside fine finger movement that separates us from the great apes. These fine movements are governed by the motor cortex and it is no surprise that the area of cortex in the precentral gyrus governing this volition occupies a large area. However, speech production involves good liaison with other areas including processing of much sensory data via the thalamus, cerebellum and sensory cortex in the postcentral gyri, the collation of auditory data (including memory function) in the temporal lobe and feedback on motor performance through the auditory apparatus. In viewing the performance of a brain that we know has reduced computing power, it is no surprise to note that some of these processes are inefficient.

Our current knowledge in this area with suggestions for the focus of future research has been well reviewed by Kent and Vorperian (2013). Their review highlights four main areas of disorder.

VOICE

Dysphonia clearly plays a part, though the prevalence is not clear from published studies. Inherent low tone in pharyngeal muscles and the resulting greater effort required to make them work both contribute to the slightly husky voice often heard in Down syndrome (even without thyroid dysfunction).

SPEECH SOUNDS

A note is made here of both developmental (slow normal) and deviant (non-developmental) phenomena. The production of babbling and non-speech sounds is very similar to that seen in typically developing children, though some delay may be seen from the age of 6 months onwards. However, once speech sounds are made, errors with both consonant and vowel production start to appear with substitution of the incorrect consonant and inaccurate vowel sounds. The latter is often produced by limitation of regulation of tongue height and advancement. A tendency to this may reflect anatomical variants (e.g. large tongue). Most of the errors would seem to be due to motor planning. Abnormalities observed in Down syndrome have included both excessive and reduced areas of articulatory contact, moving contact, extended closure durations for occlusive consonants and lengthened consonant transition times within clusters. All this is seen alongside data suggestive of greater respiratory pressures generated to produce speech, no doubt part of the overall sequencing problem. These phenomena are often linked with hypernasality often seen in association with variation in craniofacial anatomy. This can include ossified nasal bones, a compact mid and lower face skeleton accompanied by a high and often shelf-like pallet.

FLUENCY AND PROSODY

Speech dysfluency (a term used to include stuttering, cluttering and stammering) is seen with an incidence of between 10% and 45% in studies of people with Down syndrome. This compares to an incidence of about 1% in the general population. Problems initiating speech are often observed followed then by poor annunciation of vowels and consonants with a lack of rhythm reflecting the poor motor performance described above.

INTELLIGIBILITY

The scoring of intelligibility brings methodological difficulty but usually represents the proportion of complete and intelligible utterances over total utterances. Studies in Down syndrome generally give an average of 80%, largely influenced by the length of the utterance and how familiar the listener is to the person speaking. Problems with intelligibility continue throughout life for many individuals with a clear negative impact on social and vocational advancement. Clearly, all the things we have discussed so far contribute to this.

Other factors will influence speech production. Speech is likely to be poorer in a person with hearing impairment who is not wearing his or her hearing aids. People with Down syndrome also have a poor short-term auditory memory (Jarrold et al. 2002) so that in any social interaction they are disadvantaged. They may hear what is said and then be unable to recall a significant part of that before they formulate a reply. Here again we see how sensory input is influencing the difficulty with praxis.

Kent and Vorperian's review (2013) indicates how intervention studies may bring some short-term gain, the benefit of coaching. No one has demonstrated sustained improvement in resolution of these combined confounding difficulties. That is not to say that continuing common sense interventions including encouragement to wear a hearing aid, when appropriate, or to try to speak more slowly should not be pursued.

The epilepsies and other paroxysmal events; is epilepsy more common in Down syndrome and what types of epilepsy are seen?

The approach to paroxysmal episodes in people with Down syndrome should be the same as with any other person. The diagnosis of an epilepsy syndrome is hard; false-positive rates are high even in specialist centres. The starting point is always the history and the detail in the history. Never accept third-party descriptions. Always keep an open mind.

Remember that autonomic disturbance is often prominent in a nervous system with inefficient control systems. Remember also that the most common cause of a tonic or tonic clonic seizure is syncope rather than an epilepsy syndrome. This is where the story of a precipitant (pain or standing up) followed by a story of pallor and loss of tone followed by tonic or tonic clonic movement can be particularly revealing. In children with a paroxysmal event where the diagnosis is uncertain, fewer than 10% will ultimately prove to have an epilepsy syndrome. Just to tax us even more, it is common for one child to have epileptic and non-epileptic events.

Always adopt a four-level approach to the diagnosis of an epilepsy syndrome:

1. Does the historical detail make it more likely than not this is an epilepsy syndrome? Is there supportive evidence from an electroencephalogram (EEG)?
2. What seizure types are occurring?
3. Do the child's symptoms fit in with a particular epilepsy syndrome?
4. What is the aetiology?

Once you have arrived at a diagnostic formulation, then look at the associated social, educational or psychological aspects that might benefit from an intervention.

The EEG can be helpful but it is not central to the diagnostic issue. You are looking to the EEG for evidence supportive of a diagnosis of epilepsy. Repeat standard recordings may be helpful if the index of suspicion is high, supplemented at times by a sleep-deprived EEG. Ambulatory EEGs may be helpful but only if the episodes are occurring reliably on a daily basis. EEGs may also help define an epilepsy syndrome.

A decision to use an antiepileptic drug or not should be based on how intrusive the episodes are in that person's life (young or old). A case has been made in the past to avoid drugs which might have a negative effect on folate metabolism. In general, the choice of medication should be the same in Down syndrome as for the general population. Nonetheless, phenytoin should probably be avoided.

Studies on seizure incidence and prevalence in Down syndrome are drawn from secondary or tertiary medical centres, the prevalence figures varying between 5% and 13%. It is likely that a community-based study would reveal an incidence significantly lower than this. It is clear there is a bimodal distribution of seizure onset in Down syndrome. Forty percent of those going to develop an epilepsy syndrome present in infancy with West syndrome. Another 40% will present after the third decade with the onset of neurodegenerative disease. Senile myoclonic epilepsy appears to be a common manifestation of dementia in Down syndrome. Although the response of children with West syndrome to antiepileptic drugs in the form of steroids or vigabatrin is often good, there is a strong association between this infantile encephalopathy presentation and the emergence of marked autistic features. Eisermann et al. (2003) showed (unsurprisingly) an interesting correlation between treatment delay and delay in control of spasms with a higher tendency to the emergence of autistic features. Clearly, awareness of the condition with a need to intervene early is important but clinical evaluation can be difficult.

Ahmed is 14 months old and has Down syndrome. He was leaving his notable neonatal hypotonia behind him and beginning to feed well when, at the age of 7 months, his parents noted a change in his development. His head and truncal control deteriorated somewhat. During the day, he would have short episodes in which they found it difficult to get eye contact and indeed his eyes would roll up at times. Then, as he went off to sleep he would have short runs of low-amplitude twitching of his hands and feet. The family's GP offered reassurance saying that it was to be expected but the bouts persisted for 3 weeks or so and then there was a change. Ahmed began having wakeful episodes involving extension of the arms with sudden flexion of the head and trunk. Alarmed by these, his parents took him to the Accident and Emergency Department. The paediatric service arranged further tests, the most helpful of which was an EEG which confirmed the diagnosis as an epilepsy syndrome. The EEG showed the chaotic background activity of hypsarrhythmia. Ahmed's seizures went into remission on prednisolone, but now at 14 months he shows significant developmental impairment with poor-quality eye contact and no imitative gesture. His postural control also remains poor.

Ferlazzo et al. (2009) indicate how children with Down syndrome may present much later than typically developing children with the Lennox Gastaut syndrome. This is characterized by a diffuse epileptic encephalopathy associated with a number of seizure types often initially tonic clonic seizures, slow spike and wave discharge on the EEG and the emergence of a high level of cognitive impairment. In typically developing children, this usually presents between 3 and 5 years of age but in Ferlazzo's series of 13 children it was between the ages of 5 and 16 years. Interestingly, 9 of the 13 had reflex seizures mostly precipitated by sudden unexpected sensory stimulations including sound. As in the general population, their epilepsy proved to be resistant to treatment.

In adults with Down syndrome, the onset of seizures is often associated with rapid cognitive decline (Lott and Dierssen 2010).

How might cranio-vertebral instability and myelopathy present?
This is dealt with in more detail in Chapter 15. It is appropriate to restate in this section that if a person with Down syndrome presents with a gait deterioration or the new emergence of difficulty with bladder or bowel control, neck pain or limitation of neck movement, then cranio-vertebral instability with an associated myelopathy should be considered. Appropriate investigations should be carried out.

Cerebrovascular disease and Moyamoya syndrome; what is the stroke risk in Down syndrome?

Arterial ischaemic stroke in Down syndrome carries the same range of aetiologies as in the general population. Given that cystathionine synthase is encoded on chromosome 21, it is likely that homocystinuria-associated strokes are rare. We could also hypothesize, given the increased levels of interferon in Down syndrome, that viral (in particular varicella) associated stroke would be less common but this remains unresolved. We can be certain that congenital heart disease associated embolic stroke is more common, at times associated with subacute bacterial endocarditis present in a heart with abnormal anatomy.

Moyamoya syndrome is a condition involving progressive stenosis of the intracranial internal carotid arteries and their proximal branches. This is associated with progressive growth of collateral vessels so as to overcome (in part) the obstruction. It involves predominantly the anterior circulation but may involve the posterior circulation. The term 'Moyamoya syndrome' is usually applied to the condition when it is associated with a well-known risk factor (e.g. neurofibromatosis, thrombophilia or indeed Down syndrome). Moyamoya disease is usually applied when there is no known cause (Scott and Smith 2009).

Jea et al. (2005) described 181 patients with Moyamoya syndrome presenting over a 20-year period to 2004 at Boston Children's Hospital. Sixteen of these children (10 females and 6 males) had Down syndrome; a significant increase in number observed over expected. Other commentators have cited a risk three times over the background risk for Down syndrome. Clearly, these estimates can be very inaccurate.

The incidence of Moyamoya syndrome peaks in two age groups: in children around the age of 5 years and in adults in their mid-40s. Predisposition to Moyamoya is not well understood. The background risk of 3 cases per 100 000 is noted in Japan with only a 10th of this incidence observed in Europeans. Affected vessels are occluded by hyperplasia of smooth muscle cells with a secondary luminal thrombosis. The media is attenuated with an irregular elastic lamina. Caspase-dependent apoptosis has been implicated as a contributory mechanism in the associated arterial wall degradation (Scott and Smith 2009). Associations have been found with abnormal loci on chromosome 3, 6 and 8 and 17 (but not 21 so far!). Familial cases appear to be polygenic in origin. An increase in growth factors, enzymes and peptides have been identified including fibroblast growth factor, transforming growth factor beta-1, hepatic growth factor, vascular endothelial growth factor, matrix metalloproteinases, intracellular adhesion molecules and hypoxia-inducing factor 1 alpha levels. There is also an association with hyperthyroidism. It may then be that the Moyamoya syndrome is an endpoint/final common pathway in a number of linked processes.

The presentation of either arterial ischaemic stroke or Moyamoya syndrome in Down syndrome will be indistinguishable on clinical grounds. There may be a prodromal period involving transient ischaemic attacks or the sudden onset of stroke in either. Lenticulostriate arteries may be involved in either and involuntary movements have been rarely reported in Moyamoya syndrome. Headache may precede either stroke or Moyamoya syndrome.

245

Melody is a 6-year-old girl with Down syndrome. She was enjoying settling in for her second term at her local primary school. She had some early literacy skills, was just learning to count 1:1 up to about 7 and starting to prefer quite a few single words rather than using her Makaton. She had made some good friends and they enjoyed using Makaton too. Her parents, and then her teachers started to notice occasional (every 10 days or so) episodes of her appearing blank and seemingly unaware. These would persist for 2–3 minutes and afterwards she would appear unsteady and confused. Between times, she was her usual self.

Then one day such an event progressed to involve right-sided weakness, including her face. This persisted for 30 minutes but recovered.

Urgent hospital assessment included an MRI scan with MR angiography. This showed that Melody had Moyamoya syndrome. She was prescribed aspirin. She is now being considered for an intracranial extracranial anastomosis which her parents know is likely to stabilize her condition foreseeably.

Clinical examination should pay particular attention to the heart, nails and the retina looking for evidence of embolization, signs of splenomegaly that might reflect subacute bacterial endocarditis, features of hyperthyroidism and the presence of cranial bruits.

Management should always include astute awareness of these diagnostic possibilities with appropriate imaging to include MRI and MRA. The natural history is variable, the condition stabilizing in many but deteriorating steadily in a sizable minority. Initial intervention should be with the prescription of low-dose aspirin, and increasingly this is complemented by a surgical approach which either involves direct revascularization, whereby a branch of the external carotid artery (usually the superficial temporal artery) is anastomosed to a cortical artery. Alternatively, an indirect technique can be used involving the placement of vascularized tissue supplied by the external carotid artery (e.g. dura or temporalis muscle or the superficial temporal artery itself) in direct contact with the brain. Growth of new blood vessels then follows after a period to the underlying cerebral cortex. Long-term clinical and radiological follow-up data from the Boston study (mean: 67.6 months; range: 6–146 months) showed no deterioration in all but one, with no clinical or radiological evidence of a new infarction.

When should we think of other conditions?
Professionals attending to people with Down syndrome of any age must be aware that neuropsychiatric presentations in Down syndrome may reflect other underlying conditions dealt with in other chapters in this book. These would include obstructive sleep apnoea, viral infection, immune conditions and, of course, dementia. Vigilance and imagination are required in being aware of these possibilities.

Key points
- The brain in Down syndrome has some underdeveloped circuitry and inefficient signalling patterns.
- The resulting motor impairment presents as slowly resolving central hypotonia, a developmental coordination disorder and speech dysfluency.

- The speech dysfluency is confounded by a poor short-term auditory memory.
- The enhanced prevalence of epilepsy in Down syndrome is bimodal. In infancy, a common presentation is West syndrome; senile myoclonic epilepsy appears to be a common manifestation of dementia.
- Myelopathy associated with cranio-vertebral instability may present with gait disturbance of bladder or bowel dysfunction.
- Transient ischaemic attacks in Down syndrome are often caused by Moyamoya syndrome.

REFERENCES

Agiovlasitis S, McCubbin JA, Yun J, Mpitsos G, Pavol MJ (2009) Effects of Down syndrome on three-dimensional motion during walking at different speeds. *Gait Posture* 30: 345–350. doi: 10.1016/j.gaitpost.2009.06.003.

Cebula KR, Moore DG, Wishart JG (2010) Social cognition in children with Down's syndrome: Challenges to research and theory building. *J Intellect Disabil Res* 54: 113–134. doi: 10.1111/j.1365-2788.2009.01215.x.

Cleland C, Wood S, Hardcastle W, Wishart J, Timmins C (2010) Relationship between speech, oromotor, language and cognitive abilities in children with Down's syndrome. *Int J Lang Comm Dis* 45: 83–95. doi: 10.3109/13682820902745453.

Couzens D, Haynes M, Cuskelly M (2012) Individual and environmental characteristics associated with cognitive development in Down syndrome: A longitudinal study. *J Appl Res Intellect* 25: 396–413. doi: 10.1111/j.1468-3148.2011.00673.x.

Couzens D, Cuskelly M, Jobling A (2004) The Stanford Binet Fourth edition and its use with individuals with Down syndrome: Cautions for clinicians. *Int J Disabil Dev Educ* 51: 39–56. doi: 10.1080/103491 2042000182193.

Cunningham C (2006) *Intelligence, Development and Attainments. In Down Syndrome an Introduction for Parents and Carers*. Human Horizon Series. London: Souvenir Press.

Eisermann MM, DeLaRaillère A, Dellatolas G et al. (2003) Infantile spasms in Down syndrome—effects of delayed anticonvulsive treatment. *Epilepsy Res* 55: 21–27. doi: 10.1016/S0920-1211(03)00088-3.

Ferlazzo E, Adjien CK, Guerrini R et al. (2009) Lennox-Gastaut syndrome with late-onset and prominent reflex seizures in trisomy 21 patients. *Epilepsia* 50: 1587–1595. doi: 10.1111/j.1528-1167.2008.01944.x.

Galli M, Cimolin V, Patti P et al. (2010) Quantifying established clinical assessment measures using 3D-movement analysis in individuals with Down syndrome. *Disabil Rehabil* 32: 1768–1774.

Guéant J-L, Anello G, Bosco P et al. (2005) Homocysteine and related genetic polymorphisms in Down's syndrome IQ. *J Neurol Neurosurg Psychiatry* 76: 706–709. doi: 10.1136/jnnp.2004.039875.

Jarrold C, Baddeley A D and Phillips CE (2002) Verbal short-term memory in Down syndrome: A Problem of memory, audition, or speech? *Journal of Speech, Language, and Hearing Research* 45: 531–544.

Jea A, Smith ER, Robertson R, Scott RM (2005) Moyamoya syndrome associated with Down syndrome: Outcome after surgical revascularization. *Pediatrics* 116: e694–e701. doi: 10.1542/peds.2005-0568.

Jover M, Ayoun C, Beron C, Carlier M (2010) Specific grasp characteristics of children with trisomy 21. *Dev Psychobiol* 52: 782–793. doi: 10.1002/dev.20474.

Kent RD, Vorperian HK (2013) Speech impairment in Down syndrome: A review. *J Speech Lang Hear Res* 56: 178–210. doi: 10.1044/1092-4388(2012/12-0148).

Lott IT (2012) Neurological phenotypes for Down syndrome across the life span. *Prog Brain Res* 197: 101–121. doi: 10.1016/B978-0-444-54299-1.00006-6.

Lott IT, Dierssen M (2010) Cognitive deficits and associated neurological complications in individuals with Down's syndrome. *Lancet Neurol* 9: 623–633. doi: 10.1016/S1474-4422(10)70112-5.

Rigoldi C, Galli M, Albertini G (2001) Gait development during lifespan in subjects with Down syndrome. *Res Dev Disabil* 32: 158–163.

Scott RM, Smith ER (2009) Moyamoya disease and Moyamoya syndrome. *N Engl J Med* 360: 1226–1237.

18

Part 2: Developmental, Psychological and Psychiatric Function

Jeremy Turk

Introduction

This section will explore the range of developmental, temperamental, psychological, and psychiatric behaviours seen in young people with Down syndrome.

Intelligence

In infancy the discrepancy between intellectual functioning in individuals with Down syndrome and their typically developing peers may be minimal (Carr 1970). However, by the pre-school years, children with Down syndrome have been reported as displaying deficits in means-end thinking (Fidler et al. 2005). By commencement of school, around 5 years of age, developmental impairment is common with a mean IQ of about 60 and a range from approximately 25–70. In the UK increasing numbers of children with Down syndrome are educated in mainstream schools, with the benefit of an Educational Healthcare Plan (EHC) or another means of provision for resource. This can provide special educational input, adaptation of the curriculum, small group and individual tuition and attention to the specific profile of educational and adaptive behaviour needs. A minority will still require education in special schools, usually those with resources, facilities and professional expertise to meet the educational requirements of pupils and students with a moderate or severe learning disability. The presence of associated challenging behaviours makes specialist schooling more likely. Early stimulation programmes may enhance development, at least temporarily (Carr 1988), though evidence for longer-term developmental gains is sparse. Visuomotor skills and tactile discrimination may be areas of particularly special need throughout childhood.

Fidler (2005) has argued that some aspects of the Down syndrome behavioural phenotype are already evident in infants and toddlers. She cites emerging relative strengths in visual processing, receptive language and non-verbal social functioning. In contrast she identifies relative weaknesses in gross motor and expressive language skills. In addition, children with Down syndrome, on parental reports, have been found to have less attentional focusing, less inhibitory control and less sadness than children with typical development (Nygaard et al. 2002). Also, it has been suggested that a limited repertoire of strategies for coping with frustration may lead to greater dependence on adults for guidance, with correspondingly fewer goal-directed strategies including assistance-seeking and cognitive self-soothing (Jahromi et al. 2008).

During the school years visuospatial processing skills exceed verbal ones, with working memory and verbal short-term and long-term memory deficits (Vicari 2006). Towards adolescence maintenance of existing skills can prove problematic with persistence of counter productive strategies for novel problem solving (Wishart 1993). Quality of care, warmth of nurturing and consistent continuing parent/carer educational efforts to complement those of school are associated with greater developmental and cognitive gains. There is an association between the IQs of children with Down syndrome and the academic and professional attainments of their parents (see Chapters 2 and 19).

Levels of maladaptive behaviours during childhood are somewhat less than expected (Dykens et al. 2002). However, sibling behavioural problems are more common where the brother or sister with Down syndrome has disturbed behaviour (Gath and Gumley 1987). Most areas of cognitive functioning can be predicted on the basis of overall levels of intellectual functioning. However, relative weaknesses have been found consistently to be associated with expressive language, syntactic/morphosyntactic processing and verbal working memory (Silverman 2007).

Other research has highlighted significant delays in non-verbal cognitive development with specific deficits in speech, language production, auditory short-term memory and verbal working memory (Chapman and Hesketh 2000). In contrast, adaptive behaviours appear to be relatively preserved. Weaknesses in hippocampal functions have been proposed as explaining the above profiles of strengths and needs (Pennington et al. 2003).

Social, language and communication development

Receptive language skills reportedly exceed expressive ones (Roberts et al. 2007). Syntax appears to be particularly problematic. High rates of pro-social behaviours such as sharing, staying on task, patience, group activity participation and accepting redirection have been observed (Walz and Benson 2002). This can extend to the use of social strategies to engage the conversational/interactional partner and distract them from the task in hand (Pitcairn and Wishart 1994).

Personality and temperament

There have been longstanding suggestions that children and young people with Down syndrome have a characteristic profile of temperament and personality. Increased good-naturedness, contentedness, and warmth of personality have been described. In addition many have been said to show endearing yet challenging degrees of stubbornness, oppositionality and defiance frequently (Visootsak and Sherman 2007) in association with good degrees of awareness and understanding of other people's mental, including emotional, states. This has been supported by research exploring systematic comparisons with siblings and with other similarly aged children with similar degrees of intellectual impairment (Gibbs and Thorpe 1983). Research has been hampered by concerns relating to the applicability of standard temperament scales to children with Down syndrome (Gibbs et al. 1987). However, these findings are consistent with the original descriptions by Langdon Down of people with Down syndrome displaying 'considerable powers of imitation even bordering on being mimics'. To these he added the traits of humour, a lively sense of the ridiculous, obstinacy and amiability. Nonetheless some children with Down syndrome can be aggressive and difficult.

Young people with Down syndrome have higher rates of problem behaviours than children matched on age, sex and socio-economic status, who do not have intellectual disability (Coe et al. 1999). In particular attention deficit, non-compliance, thought disorder and social withdrawal were observed. A study of age-related trends in psychopathology identified that while rates of externalizing behaviours were low, rates of internalizing behaviours were significantly higher in older adolescents, consistent with the increasing frequency of depression in this age group (Dykens et al. 2002). However, when compared with children with other genetic conditions (in this instance Prader-Willi syndrome and Angelman syndrome), the children with Down syndrome showed good social skills and low ratings of problem behaviours, including hyperactivity (Chertkoff Walz and Benson 2002).

Neurodevelopmental disorders
Both autism spectrum conditions (Rasmussen et al. 2001) and attention-deficit–hyperactivity disorder (ADHD) (Green et al. 1989) are more common in individuals with Down syndrome than in the general population, even though they may occur less often than expected for the average IQ level. This is in line with the trend for intellectual disability to be associated with increased rates and severities of most psychiatric and neurodevelopmental disabilities. These conditions often go undiagnosed and untreated, because of the associated challenging behaviours being attributed to intellectual disability. It may also be that the personality stereotype masks the presence of an autism spectrum condition, emphasizing the need to be alert clinically to the possibility of important neurodevelopmentally determined social and communication disorders in this client group.

ATTENTION-DEFICIT–HYPERACTIVITY DISORDER
Approximately 1 in 20 children with Down syndrome in the USA is diagnosed with ADHD (Coe et al. 1999). Ekstein et al. (2011) have rated the presence of ADHD in individuals with Down syndrome to be as high as 44%. Rates have also been reported as increased in the UK, compared with other children with similar levels of intellectual disability of unknown aetiology (Turk 1998). Brown et al. (2003) found shorter and less frequent periods of sustained attention in toddlers with Down syndrome compared with those with Williams syndrome and others matched on chronological and mental ages. Rates of hyperactivity have been reported to diminish as individuals enter adolescence (Stores et al. 1998). Children and young people with Down syndrome who have severe ADHD can often respond well to regular psychostimulant medication such as methylphenidate and dexamphetamine (see also Chapter 19). However, particularly careful medical monitoring is required because of the raised rate of cardiovascular disease in Down syndrome, and the pressor effects of psychostimulants. Regular monitoring of height, weight, pulse and blood pressure is required along with regular systematic enquiries about sleep, appetite, chest pain, palpitations and breathlessness, headaches, fainting, dizziness, abdominal pain, nervous tics and twitches and emotional lability. Children with autistic tendencies may have their social

impairments accentuated by stimulant medication, and occasionally paradoxical excitation can occur.

> *Alex is a 10-year-old boy with Down syndrome and mild cognitive impairment. He was making progress academically, socially and linguistically. He attends his local mainstream primary school, known to be interested and skilled in meeting the needs of children with developmental disabilities. His motor activity levels and inattentiveness were continuing to be a cause of substantial concern. He found it difficult to settle to any tasks and required one-to-one attention and support, pushed boundaries of allowable behaviours and could at times be stubborn, oppositional and defiant. His parents reported that he had always had a diminished attention span, flitting from task to task within minutes, easily becoming distracted suddenly and impulsively by some other activity or happening. His concentration span could be up to ten minutes on school work with one-to-one assistance. Alex had also begun to be able to spend more than half an hour on board games with assistance from adults. However, even at these times he could not sit still, constantly fidgeted and remained persistently restless, impulsive and distractible, no matter where he was or who he was with. His sleep pattern and mealtime behaviour were good. His parents had applied a variety of appropriate measures and programmes over a substantial period of time, including star charts, other incentive-based programmes, and breaking down activities into manageable chunks. All these efforts had met with limited success. His local CAMHS service reviewed him and judged his presentation to be consistent with attention-deficit–hyperactivity disorder.*
>
> *After checking for medical contra-indications Alex was commenced on a low dose of modified-release methylphenidate (a psychostimulant), in the form of Equasym XL 10mg each morning. Parents reported immediate gratifying and persisting behavioural benefits. These comprised enhanced attentiveness, mental focusing, compliance, concentration and freedom from restlessness, fidgetiness, impulsiveness and distractibility. Alex still needed high degrees of structure, predictability of routine with clear expectations, and boundaries for allowable behaviour. Appetite and sleep remained good. He experienced no headaches, chest pains, palpitations, breathlessness, abdominal pain, tics or twitching. Parents reported that he was possibly slightly more emotionally labile with a slightly increased propensity to cry when upset; but this was not a substantial problem. Weight, height, pulse and blood pressure remained satisfactory. Alex's school communication book confirmed his substantial classroom and lunchtime behavioural improvements with lots of stickers obtained for hard work and good behaviour. He remained very happy in himself, albeit still somewhat impulsive in pressing lift buttons and racing down corridors!*

Autism spectrum conditions

As many as 10% of children with Down syndrome have a diagnosable autism spectrum condition (Turk and Graham 1997). Risk factors for autism in children with Down syndrome include seizures—particularly West syndrome, early hypothyroidism, post-cardiac surgery complications, lower IQ and first- or second-degree relatives with the autism phenotype (Dykens 2007). The dual diagnoses of Down syndrome and autism may predispose to a distinctive set of aberrant behaviours marked by characteristic, odd and bizarre stereotypic behaviours, anxiety and social withdrawal (Carter et al. 2007). Children with Down syndrome who have an autism spectrum disorder receive a diagnosis at an older age than their peers, and parents and carers may experience considerable difficulty in obtaining the diagnosis (Howlin et al. 1995).

Mood disorders

Throughout childhood, psychopathology is less frequent and less severe than for other children with similar developmental abilities (Dykens et al. 2002). However, in adolescence people with Down syndrome are more prone to clinical depression than those in the general population (Collacott et al. 1998, McCarthy and Boyd 2001). This association is maintained even when the effects of adverse life events and daily hassles have been accounted for. Biological and behavioural features are said to be more common than cognitive and emotional content. Social withdrawal, mutism, psychomotor retardation, low mood, passivity, decreased appetite and insomnia have all been documented as frequently occurring.

Jamie has Down syndrome with a mild-to-moderate intellectual disability. He presented at the age of 16½ to child and adolescent mental health developmental disability services having been in and out of school for 3 years, prior to commencing residential specialist provision. Efforts at day schooling had floundered. Jamie had benefited academically and socially from mainstream education but had become emotionally distressed with absconding, physical violence and risk-taking behaviours. Fluoxetine had been prescribed for clinical depression. This triggered psychotic experiences. He was admitted to hospital and looked after by psychiatry services. The fluoxetine was discontinued. In the 4 months which followed he settled and thrived. He was identified as having fine motor difficulties, noise intolerance, information processing problems and poorly developed language comprehension skills. An unsuccessful residential school placement followed. Here he became highly anxious, obsessive, stubborn, oppositional and defiant with frequent physically dangerous, chaotic and disorganized tantrums. Jamie would plead to be restrained and would be contrite and remorseful thereafter. All agreed that Jamie was an emotionally warm, loving, caring, considerate, sensitive and thoughtful individual who was always well-meaning.

Placement in a highly specialist boarding school produced marked improvements. He developed anger management and self-calming skills, and benefited from structured and predictable routines, sensory integration therapy, visual prompts, reminders and memory check-lists. He was commenced on risperidone 0.5mg each morning with extra doses as needed. Increased appetite and weight gain necessitated discontinuation. Jamie managed with continuing psychological, educational, occupational and speech and language therapy inputs.

Five months later he was progressing well. He was well-behaved, cooperative and compliant with only occasional tantrums. Weight had diminished, but he experienced repeated, frequent, distressing memories and imagery relating to earlier familial strife. Detailed questioning revealed that these episodes had been underlying many of the earlier challenging behaviours. Post-traumatic stress disorder was diagnosed, and cognitive-behavioural therapy recommended. However, Jamie's mental state deteriorated and he struggled with temper and self-control. There were daily behavioural outbursts, social withdrawal, and frequent, persistent, distressing mental flashbacks and obsessional ruminations. Escalating anxiety states with associated challenging behaviours, plus now clearly identifiable mood swings, were identified as being consistent with a cyclical (bipolar) mood disorder. Carbamazepine was commenced, initially 50mg twice daily, and increased slowly to 200mg twice daily. This produced substantially improved mood stability. Persisting anxiety, agitation, mood swings and tantrums were managed by psychological approaches and medication fine-tuning. Later evaluation confirmed that Jamie fulfilled criteria for an autism spectrum condition. This allowed for recommendations regarding autism-friendly education programmes, and school and living circumstances. Aged 18 Jamie was transferred to local services for adults with intellectual disability and mental health challenges. His psychiatric status is now stable.

Sleep

Sleep disorders are common in children and young people, and even more so in those with developmental disabilities (Turk 2010). In Down syndrome, although sleep problems are rarer than in other children with intellectual disability, they are still far more common than in the general population and contribute to parental stress, poor parent–child relationships and family cohesion problems (Sloper et al. 1991). Carter et al. (2009) found that, compared with children from the general population, children with Down syndrome were reported to have significantly greater bedtime resistance, sleep anxiety, night waking, parasomnias, sleep disordered breathing and day-time sleepiness. Amongst children 4 years and older who had Down syndrome, 66% rarely fell asleep in their own beds, 55% were always restless during sleep and 40% usually woke at least once during the night. Seventy-eight percent seemed tired during the day at least 2 days per week, suggesting inadequate sleep. The authors concluded that parents of children with Down syndrome report universal sleep problems (see also Chapter 4).

Children with Down syndrome may suffer with periodic airways obstruction and associated apnoea because of upper airway structural anomalies (Stebbens et al. 1991). Upper airway obstruction, aggravated by enlarged tonsils and obesity, may explain raised rates of restless sleep, repeated night-time waking and early morning waking (Stores et al. 1996) as well as raised rates of day-time problem behaviours, in particular irritability, hyperactivity and stereotypies (see Chapter 9 for detail). Initial managements, once medical contributors have been identified and treated, should be sleep hygiene and behavioural processes, including applied behavioural analysis (Feeley and Jones 2006). Melatonin is being used increasingly for sleep induction problems (Turk 2003) and has been reported as beneficial for individuals with autism spectrum conditions who have sleep induction problems (Garstang and Wallis 2006, Malow et al. 2012). However, a recent report suggests that improvements in sleep onset latency may be minimal with sleep duration remaining relatively unchanged and child behaviour and family functioning not improving significantly (Gringras et al. 2012). Where repeated night-time waking is problematic, the alpha 2 agonist clonidine may be useful as an evening prescription, particularly in those with features of ADHD (Ingrassia and Turk 2005).

Prognosis

Problem behaviours in childhood predict such behaviours in adults with Down syndrome (McCarthy and Boyd 2001). The prevalence and predictors of mental health needs and service use in adolescents with intellectual disabilities have been explored (Hassiotis and Turk 2012). For adolescents with intellectual disability generally, prevalence rates for mental illness rose from 51% as reported by parents to 67% as judged by clinical interviews. Caseness was associated with low adaptive functioning, diagnosis of autism and family history of mental illness. High scores on parent reports of participant mental ill-health showed negative correlations with adaptive functioning scores. However, only approximately half of the participants had sought help for their mental health needs. Five out of the total study population of 75 had Down syndrome. Vineland Adaptive Behaviour Scale composite score, the presence of autism and family history of mental illness significantly predicted caseness. The most common diagnoses were conduct disorder, ASD, ADHD and emotional disorder.

Interventions and supports

Addressing the educational, social and emotional needs of children and young people with Down syndrome is of paramount importance. Many will respond to these inputs, thereby not requiring specialist mental health intervention. Where challenging behaviours do occur, these should in the first instance be addressed by functional behavioural assessments, positive behavioural supports and applied behaviour analysis (Feeley and Jones 2006). Speech and language therapy, and occupational therapy, particularly sensory integration work, can be crucial. Occasionally, medication may be warranted (Bernard and Turk 2009), for example psychostimulants or clonidine for ADHD, selective serotonin reuptake inhibitors or serotonin and noradrenaline reuptake inhibitors for major depressive disorder, traditional antiepileptic drugs as mood and behaviour stabilizers, and rarely atypical antipsychotics such as risperidone, quetiapine and aripiprazole for severe tics, Tourette syndrome and early onset psychoses. However, there is nothing to suggest that cognitive-behavioural psychotherapeutic techniques cannot be useful in this client group (Turk 2004).

Most recently, interest has developed in the possibility of targeted medications that may act on central neurotransmitter pathways that are critical to the developmental, emotional and behavioural challenges experienced by children and young people with Down syndrome. Research has focused on agents that antagonize the central nervous system inhibitory effects of gamma amino butyric acid (GABA) (Braudeau et al. 2011). However, preliminary promising studies with mouse models require considerable further exploration.

In addition, the risk of precipitating epilepsy and heightened anxiety states needs to be balanced against possible learning and information processing enhancements (Silva and Ehninger 2009).

Key points

- In Down syndrome the relative cognitive strengths are visual processing, receptive language and non-verbal social functioning; relative weaknesses are gross motor and expressive language skills.
- Personality and temperament traits include increased good-naturedness, contentedness and warmth of personality linked at times with challenging degrees of stubbornness, oppositionality and defiance.
- Problem behaviours are more common than in children with typical development.
- Sleep disorders are common and require full assessment.
- The principle features of ADHD are persistent, enduring and all-pervasive inattentiveness, restlessness, fidgetiness, impulsiveness and distractibility in association with marked overactivity.
- Risk factors for autism include seizures, early hypothyroidism, post-cardiac surgery complications, lower IQ and first- or second-degree relatives with the autism phenotype.
- In adolescence people with Down syndrome are more prone to clinical depression than those in the general population.
- Challenging behaviours require functional behavioural assessments, positive behavioural supports, applied behaviour analysis along with a full assessment of educational strengths and weaknesses.

REFERENCES

Bernard S, Turk J (2009) *Developing Mental Health Services for Children & Adolescents with Learning Disabilities; a Toolkit for Clinicians*. London: Royal College of Psychiatrists. Chapter 8, *Medical* 42–48.

Braudeau J, Delatour B, Duchon A et al. (2011) Specific targeting of the GABA-A receptor α5 subtype by a selective inverse agonist restores cognitive deficits in Down syndrome mice. *J Psychopharmacol* 25: 1030–1042.

Brown JH, Johnson MH, Paterson SJ, Gilmore R, Longhi E, Karmiloff-Smith A (2003) Spatial representation and attention in toddlers with Williams syndrome and Down syndrome. *Neuropsychologia* 41: 1037–1046.

Carr J (1970) Mental and motor development in young Mongol children. *J Ment Defic Res* 14: 205–220.

Carr J (1988) Six weeks to twenty-one years old: A longitudinal study of children with Down's syndrome and their families. *J Child Psychol Psychiatry* 29: 407–432.

Carter JC, Capone GT, Gray RM, Cox CS, Kauffman WE (2007) Autistic-spectrum disorders in Down syndrome: Further delineation and distinction from other behavioral abnormalities. *Am J Med Genet B Neuropsychiatr Genet* 144B: 87–94.

Carter M, McCaughey E, Annaz D, Hill CM (2009) Sleep problems in a Down syndrome population. *Arch Dis Child* 94: 308–310.

Chapman R, Hesketh L (2000) Behavioural phenotype of individuals with Down syndrome. *Ment Retard Dev Disabil Res Rev* 6: 84–95.

Chertkoff Walz N, Benson BA (2002) Behavioral phenotypes in children with Down syndrome, Prader-Willi syndrome, or Angelman syndrome. *J Dev Phys Disabil* 14: 307–321.

Coe DA, Matson JL, Russell DW et al. (1999) Behavior problems of children with Down syndrome and life events. *J Autism Dev Disord* 29: 149–156.

Collacott RA, Cooper S-A, Branford D, McGrother C (1998) Behaviour phenotype for Down's syndrome. *Br J Psychiatry* 172: 85–89.

Dykens EM (2007) Psychiatric and behavioral disorders in persons with Down syndrome. *Ment Retard Dev Disabil Res Rev* 13: 272–278.

Dykens EM, Shah B, Sagun J, Beck T, King BH (2002) Maladaptive behaviour in children & adolescents with Down's syndrome. *J Intellect Disabil Res* 46: 484–492.

Ekstein S, Glick B, Weill M, Kay B, Berger I (2011) Down syndrome and attention deficit/hyperactivity disorder (ADHD). *J Child Neurol* 26: 1290–1295.

Feeley K, Jones E (2006) Addressing challenging behaviour in children with Down syndrome: The use of applied behaviour analysis for assessment and intervention. *Down Syndr Res Pract* 11: 64–77.

Fidler D (2005) The emerging Down syndrome behavioral phenotype in early childhood: Implications for practice. *Infants Young Child* 18: 86–103.

Fidler DJ, Philofsky A, Hepburn S, Rogers S (2005) Nonverbal requesting and problem solving in toddlers with Down syndrome. *Am J Ment Retard* 110: 312–322.

Garstang J, Wallis M (2006) Randomized control trial of melatonin for children with autistic spectrum disorders and sleep problems. *Child Care Health Dev* 32: 585–589.

Gath A, Gumley D (1987) Down's syndrome and the family: Follow-up of children first seen in infancy. *Dev Med Child Neurol* 26: 500–508.

Gibbs MV, Reeves D, Cunningham CC (1987) The application of temperament questionnaires to a British sample: Issues of reliability and validity. *J Child Psychol Psychiatry* 28: 61–77.

Gibbs MV, Thorpe JG (1983) Personality stereotype of non-institutionalised Down syndrome children. *Am J Ment Defic* 87: 601–605.

Green JM, Dennis J, Bennets LA (1989) Attention disorder in a group of young Down's syndrome children. *J Ment Defic Res* 33: 105–122.

Gringras P, Gamble C, Jones AP et al. (2012) Melatonin for sleep problems in children with neurodevelopmental disorders: Randomised double-masked placebo controlled trial. *Br Med J* 345: e6664.

Hassiotis A, Turk J (2012) Mental health needs in adolescents with intellectual disabilities: Cross-sectional survey of a service sample. *J Appl Res Intellect Disabil* 25: 252–261.

Howlin P, Wing L, Gould J (1995) The recognition of autism in children with Down syndrome – implications for intervention and some speculations about pathology. *Dev Med Child Neurol* 37: 406–414.

Ingrassia A, Turk J (2005) The use of clonidine for severe and intractable sleep problems in children with neurodevelopmental disorders: A case series. *Eur Child Adolesc Psychiatry* 14: 34–40.

Jahromi LB, Gulsrud A, Kasari C (2008) Emotional competence in children with Down syndrome. *Am J Ment Retard* 113: 32–43.

Malow B, Adkins KW, McGrew SG et al. (2012) Melatonin for sleep in children with autism: A controlled trial examining dose, tolerability and outcomes. *J Autism Dev Disord* 42: 1729–1737.

McCarthy J, Boyd J (2001) Psychopathology and young people with Down's syndrome: Childhood predictors and adult outcome of disorder. *J Intellect Disabil Res* 45: 99–105.

Nygaard E, Smith L, Torgersen AM (2002) Temperament in children with Down syndrome and prematurely born children. *Scand J Psychol* 43: 61–71.

Pennington BF, Moon J, Edgin J, Stedron J, Nadel L (2003) The neuropsychology of Down syndrome: Evidence for hippocampal dysfunction. *Child Dev* 74: 75–93.

Pitcairn TK, Wishart JG (1994) Reactions of young children with Down's syndrome to an impossible task. *Br J Dev Psychol* 12: 485–489.

Rasmussen P, Börjesson O, Wentz E, Gillberg C (2001) Autistic disorders in Down syndrome: Background factors and clinical correlates. *Dev Med Child Neurol* 43: 750–754.

Roberts JE, Price J, Malkin C (2007) Language and communication development in Down syndrome. *Ment Retard Dev Disabil Res Rev* 13: 26–35.

Silva AJ, Ehninger D (2009) Adult reversal of cognitive phenotypes in neurodevelopmental disorders. *J Neurodev Disord* 1: 150–157.

Silverman W (2007) Down syndrome: Cognitive phenotype. *Ment Retard Dev Disabil Res Rev* 13: 228–236.

Sloper S, Knussen C, Turner S, Cunningham C (1991) Factors related to stress and satisfaction with life in families of children with Down's syndrome. *J Child Psychol Psychiatry* 32: 655–676.

Stebbens VA, Dennis J, Samuels MP, Croft CB, Southall DP (1991) Sleep related upper airway obstruction in a cohort with Down's syndrome. *Arch Dis Child* 66: 1333–1338.

Stores R, Stores G, Buckley S (1996) The pattern of sleep problems in children with Down's syndrome and other intellectual disabilities. *J Appl Res Intellect Disabil* 9: 145–159.

Stores R, Stores G, Fellows B, Buckley S (1998) Daytime behavioural problems and maternal distress in children with Down's syndrome, their siblings and non-intellectually disabled and other intellectually disabled peers. *J Intellect Disabil Res* 42: 228–237.

Turk J (1998) Fragile X syndrome and attentional deficits. *J Appl Res Intellect Disabil* 11: 175–191.

Turk J (2003) Melatonin supplementation for severe and intractable sleep disturbance in young people with developmental disabilities: Short review and commentary *J Med Genet* 40: 793–796.

Turk J (2004) Children with developmental disabilities & their parents. In: Graham P, editor. *Cognitive Behaviour Therapy for Children & Families*, 2nd ed, 244–262. Cambridge: Cambridge University Press.

Turk J (2010) Sleep disorders in children and adolescents with learning disabilities and their management. *Adv Ment Health Learn Disabil* 4: 50–59.

Turk J, Graham P (1997) Fragile X syndrome, autism and autistic features. *Autism* 1: 175–197.

Vicari S (2006) Motor development & neuropsychological patterns in persons with Down syndrome. *Behav Genet* 36: 355–364.

Visootsak J, Sherman S (2007) Neuropsychiatric and behavioral aspects of trisomy 21. *Curr Psychiatry Rep* 9: 135–140.

Walz NC, Benson BA (2002) Behavioural phenotype in children with Down syndrome, Prader-Willi syndrome, or Angelman syndrome. *J Dev Phys Disabil* 14: 307–321.

Wishart J (1993) The development of learning difficulties in children with Down's syndrome. *J Intellect Disabil Res* 37: 389–403.

18

Part 3: Mental Health and Dementia in Adults with Down Syndrome

Tiina Annus, Liam Reese Wilson and Anthony Holland

Introduction

Individuals with Down syndrome are more prone than the average person to age-related cognitive decline and are at high risk of developing dementia that replicates the clinical features of Alzheimer disease (Beacher et al. 2010). Such health risks are of increasing importance as the life expectancy of people with Down syndrome has significantly improved over the last 100 years (Roizen and Patterson 2003). In the early 1900s, few survived beyond the age of 10 years (Holland and Oliver 1995), whereas now it exceeds 50 years, with at least 20% of adults with Down syndrome now aged more than 55 years (Zigman and Lott 2007, Handen et al. 2012). The emphasis is now directed towards preventative health checks through screening. General practitioners now offer annual health screening to adults with Down syndrome as they age. Since the development of dementia is very likely to be in this ageing population, any suggestion of functional decline should lead to a check for depression, thyroid disorders, sensory impairments and dementia (see Royal College of Psychiatrist and British Psychological Society Best Practice Guidance 2009). Further decline in adult life particularly when due to the onset of dementia leads to greater dependence on carers, greater morbidity and a poorer quality of life (McCarron et al. 2005) (see Chapter 4).

The mental health of adults with Down syndrome

The association of Alzheimer disease with Down syndrome is so well recognized now that there is a danger that other mental health explanations for behavioural and possibly functional changes (listed above) are missed. Within the broad community of people with learning disabilities, prevalence rates of behaviour problems (often referred to as challenging behaviour) and mental ill-health have been found to be high. The co-occurrence of autistic spectrum disorder, the severity of the intellectual disability and the presence of sensory and other impairments contribute to the nature and severity of the risk (Cooper et al. 2007). Different conceptual models including those of applied behavioural analysis, the occurrence of comorbid disorders and a consequence of developmental arrest may account for problem behaviours and/or mental ill-health issues. Syndrome-specific behavioural phenotype studies also shed light on comorbidities or problem behaviours (Arron et al. 2011). In Down syndrome mental health problems are probably not increased and are even claimed to be decreased (see below). Clinical assessment requires gleaning information from parents and careers, as well as detailed and continuing observations of a person's behaviour and mental state. The task is always to integrate what is known about the person, with established and theoretically sound models of understanding, to ensure appropriate intervention.

The definitive study of Mantry et al. (2008) investigated the incidence and prevalence of mental ill-health in 186 adults (aged 16 years and older). Using a longitudinal design over 2 years they found a point prevalence of mental ill-health (excluding specific phobias) of 19.9% using the modified diagnostic criteria, DC-LD. The 2-year incidence of mental ill-health of any type was 9%. Lower rates were recorded using the more stringent DSM-IV-TR criteria. Depressive episodes were most common. Prevalence and incidence rates in Down syndrome were lower than in other causes of intellectual disability with standardized prevalence rates of 0.6 or 0.4 and standardized incidence ratio for mental ill-health of 0.9, when organic disorders are excluded. No cases of ADHD, psychotic or bipolar disorders were observed. There may be a biologically determined protective factor(s) specific to Down syndrome. However, problem behaviours, affective and anxiety disorders were still significant problems, along with organic disorders such as dementia. There is evidence for behaviour and personality changes, and possibly affective disorder, serving as very early signs of the developing dementia but further study is required (Ball et al. 2006, 2010).

Prevalence of dementia in adults with Down syndrome

The diagnosis of Alzheimer disease is challenging in the presence of intellectual disability and comorbid sensory impairment, particularly when a person's previous level of functioning is unknown (Strydom et al. 2010). The first symptoms may not necessarily be deficits in memory but changes in behaviour and personality (Holland and Oliver 1995, 1998, Holland et al. 2000, Ball et al. 2006). For these and other methodological reasons, clinical studies investigating age-related prevalence of Alzheimer disease dementia in adults with Down syndrome have reported inconsistent results (see Fig. 18c.1). A population-based study by Holland et al. (1998) found that the prevalence of Alzheimer disease in Down syndrome was 3.4% for those aged 30–39, 10.3% for those aged 40–49 and 40% in those over 50 years of age, with other studies reporting similar, if slightly lower, rates of prevalence (Tyrrell et al. 2001, Coppus et al. 2006). The percentage of individuals reported to have both Down syndrome and Alzheimer disease in their 60s varies considerably more (Strydom et al. 2010). The prevalence of Alzheimer disease for this age group may be as low as 25% (Coppus et al. 2006) or as high as 77% (Visser et al. 1997), a discrepancy which is mainly attributable to small participant numbers (Fig. 18c.1).

Schupf et al. (1998) took the analysis even further and investigated the sex differences in age at onset and risk of Alzheimer disease. Men with Down syndrome were three times more likely than women to develop Alzheimer disease with earlier onset, perhaps an hormonal effect. Although neuropathology is present in nearly 100% of those with Down syndrome over the age of 50 years, the prevalence does not appear to reach 100% as might be expected if Alzheimer disease was a fully penetrant genetic disorder.

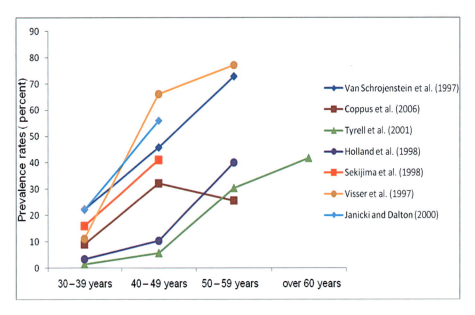

Fig. 18:3.1 Data from studies investigating age-specific prevalence rates of dementia in adults with Down syndrome.

Clinical presentation of Alzheimer disease in Down syndrome

Holland and colleagues (Holland et al. 2000, Ball et al. 2010) suggest that the early course of the clinical symptoms of Alzheimer disease in Down syndrome differs from that in the general population and manifests as changes in personality and behaviour as opposed to memory impairment. The authors used a selection of tests including a modified version of the Cambridge Examination for Mental Disorders of the Elderly (since published under the name CAMDEX-DS, Cambridge University Press). They found that the early changes of dementia were those pertaining to personality and behaviour (such as increased apathy, decreased empathy or concern for other people, or perseveration). This could be due to developmentally smaller frontal lobes, which with frontal lobe pathology compromises reserve capacity predisposing to a 'frontal-like' dementia (fronto-temporal dementia [FTD]). A follow-up study 18 months later demonstrated that adults with FTD were likely to progress to a full diagnosis of Alzheimer disease (Holland et al. 2000). The highest incidence of FTD was in younger groups, whereas for Alzheimer disease it was in the older groups, supporting the hypothesis that a frontal-like syndrome precedes dementia in this population.

Aylward et al. (1997) proposed that baseline functioning in intellectual disability is so low that it obscures the initial changes of Alzheimer disease, such as memory loss. However, findings by Ball et al. (2006) support an alternative mechanism. The authors administered a battery of neuropsychological tests probing executive function and memory, and a comprehensive caregiver interview, to correlate changes in personality and behaviour with a neuropsychological measure (such as executive function). Participants exhibiting personality and behaviour changes sufficient for a diagnosis of FTD also showed significant impairment in executive function but not in memory. These findings offer further support for the FTD-like symptoms being more than just an artefact of intellectual disability comorbidity. Furthermore, Adams and Oliver (2010) demonstrated that deficits in executive function alone were present in people with Down syndrome who had cognitive decline over 16 months. As expected, executive function impairment was associated with behavioural changes but not memory decline, again indicating that changes in behaviour and executive function precede the memory deficit in Alzheimer disease in Down syndrome.

The observed acquired deficit in frontal lobe functioning (Lott and Head 2001) may be due to early amyloid deposition and/or the underdevelopment of the frontal lobes in Down syndrome brains (Contestabile et al. 2010). Evidence from volumetric magnetic resonance imaging (MRI) studies suggests that the brain weight is much lower for age in comparison with typically developing individuals. The reduction in grey and white-matter density (including the frontal lobes) continues throughout life (Teipel et al. 2004, Suzuki 2007, Beacher et al. 2010, Menghini et al. 2011). It is attributed to accelerated brain ageing (de la Monte 1989, de la Monte and Hedley-Whyte 1990, Mann 1991). This predisposes individuals with Down syndrome to age-related cognitive decline, when compared with age-matched comparison individuals (Capone 2001, Beacher et al. 2010).

Azizeh et al. (2000) demonstrated that the earliest accumulation of β-amyloid (Aβ) neuropathology occurs in the superficial layers of the frontal and entorhinal cortices of people with Down syndrome, in keeping with FTD-like symptoms early on in the disease process. However, evidence for this hypothesis is limited and opposed by numerous other studies that have reported the distribution of Aβ in Down syndrome to be comparable to that in the general population (Mann et al. 1984, Braak and Braak 1991, and Mann 1998). Ball et al. (2010), drawing on ideas first put forward by Alexander et al. (1986) and Tekin and Cummings (2002), proffered a theoretical explanation that goes beyond the reserve capacity hypothesis and suggests the frontal-like symptoms arise due to disruption of the functional architecture of basal ganglia thalamocortical networks. Thus, it is clear the frontal lobes in Down syndrome are premorbidly abnormal and therefore probably at greater risk of damage from neuropathology relative to other areas but it is not certain. The exact cause and mechanism for this frontal profile of Alzheimer disease in Down syndrome has yet to be elucidated.

Alzheimer disease neuropathology in Down syndrome

Post-mortem studies in those over 40 suggest that people with Down syndrome almost uniformly develop neuropathological features that resemble Alzheimer disease in the general population. An early accumulation of amyloid plaques containing the pathogenic peptide Aβ and the presence of hyperphosphorylated tau proteins are typical findings (Mann et al. 1984, Wisniewski et al. 1985). Soluble Aβ42 (42 amino acid long Aβ peptide) has been shown to be present in the brains of fetuses with Down syndrome from as early as 21 weeks' gestation (Teller et al. 1996). Trisomy for chromosome 21 genes implicated in Alzheimer disease is clearly linked to this enhanced risk: the extra copy of the amyloid precursor protein (APP) gene contributes to the overproduction of the pathological Aβ peptide in brain and plasma. This causes Aβ to aggregate, form plaques and contribute to the downstream pathological cascade culminating in full blown Alzheimer disease (Wisniewski et al. 1985, Mann 1988, Mann 2006). Mutations in the APP gene have been linked to early onset familial Alzheimer disease in the general population (see Alzheimer disease gene mutation database on http://www.molgen.ua.ac.be/admutations/). Trisomy for myo-inositol (mI) transporter protein in Down syndrome causes an increase in brain mI, a compound that modulates neuronal development and survival, signal transduction, protein C activation and amyloid deposition. This is associated with reduced overall cognitive ability and brain reserve capacity (McLaurin et al. 1998, Beacher et al. 2005, Foy et al. 2011). Therefore, in Down syndrome amyloid plaques and neurofibrillary tangles (NFTs) may appear in the brain as early as in adolescence, and universally by the age of 40 years (Mann et al. 1984, Wisniewski et al. 1985).

Amyloid cascade hypothesis

The pathogenesis of Alzheimer disease remains uncertain but Aβ is considered to play a central role. The amyloid cascade hypothesis proposed by Hardy and Higgins (1992) proposes that the pathological process is triggered by abnormal APP metabolism. This in turn leads to progressive accumulation of fibrillar aggregates of APP peptide products. These Aβ deposits and pathological species of tau protein, called NFT, are toxic to the neurons and trigger cellular processes that lead to synaptic dysfunction and cell death (Selkoe 1991, Hardy and Higgins 1992). APP proteolysis can follow one of two pathways, the first of which produces Aβ and is believed to initiate the pathological cascade. The alternative, non-amyloidogenic pathway cleaves APP to produce the innocuous p3 peptide and amyloid intracellular domain (AICD) (Cole and Vassar 2007, Haass and Selkoe 2007, Querfurth and LaFerla 2010) (Fig. 18c.2). However, the aforementioned pathological cascade begins with the cleavage of APP by beta-site APP-cleaving enzyme-1 (BACE-1), followed by subsequent enzymatic cleavage by β-secretase, producing the aggregation-prone Aβ peptide and intracellular AICD (Querfurth and LaFerla 2010).

β-amyloid and tau protein

Aβ peptides can be between 38 and 43 amino acids long and spontaneously self-aggregate into multiple different forms (Querfurth and LaFerla 2010). One form consists of oligomers (2–6 peptides) that can exist in either soluble form (monomers and dimers) or coalesce into intermediate assemblies (3–6 peptides) (McLean et al. 1999, Haass and Selkoe 2007, Jin et al. 2011). Some evidence indicates that the oligomeric forms of Aβ are even more neurotoxic than fibrillar plaques as they cause disruption of synapses and eventually neuronal death (Haass and Selkoe 2007). Aβ can also present in insoluble fibrillar form and, by self-arranging into β-sheet structure, form the core of the amyloid deposits (De Strooper 2010). Consistent with the amyloid cascade hypothesis, large amounts of Aβ peptides (especially Aβ40/42) are toxic to neurons and are responsible for the initiation of the pathological cascade leading to clinical Alzheimer disease (see above). At the cellular level, Aβ may exert its neurotoxic effects in a variety of ways, including disruption of synaptic

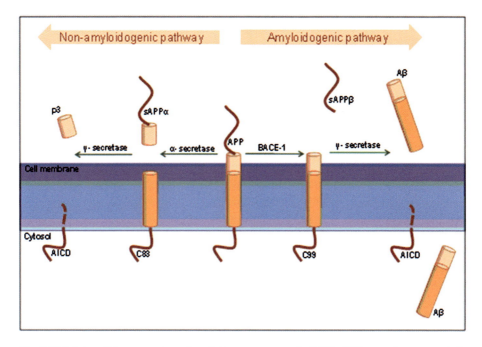

Fig. 18:3.2 Intracellular processing of amyloid precursor protein (APP). APP can undergo proteolytic processing via two pathways. Cleavage by β-secretase occurs within the Aβ domain and generates a large soluble APP (sAPPβ) ectodomain and an 83-residue C-terminal fragment C83. Further cleavage of C83 by β-secretase generates the non-amyloidogenic extracellular peptide p3 and the amyloid intracellular domain (AICD). Alternatively, cleavage of APP by beta-site APP-cleaving enzyme-1 (BACE-1) occurs at the beginning of the Aβ domain, liberating a shorter soluble APP (sAPPβ) and longer C-terminal fragment C99. Further proteolytic digestion of C99 by β-secretase generates the amyloidogenic soluble Aβ peptide and AICD. Proteolytic cleavage of sAPPβ by β-secretases yields either 40 amino acid (Aβ40) or 42 amino acid (Aβ42) long Aβ peptides (Querfurth and LaFerla 2010). The figure is adapted with permission from Wilson et al. (2014).

transmission, mitochondrial function and calcium homeostasis, hyperphosphorylation of tau protein and their assembly into NFTs, production of reactive oxygen species and expression of apoptotic genes, culminating in neuronal dysfunction and cell death (Hardy and Higgins 1992, Bamberger and Landreth 2001, Caricasole et al. 2003, Lustbader et al. 2004). However, the majority of evidence indicates that degree of atrophy seen in the Alzheimer disease brain cannot be explained by the toxicity of Aβ alone (Hardy 2009). Tau is a soluble microtubule associated protein that supports axonal transport of vesicles and organelles. In Alzheimer disease, tau becomes hyperphosphorylated, which attenuates its affinity for microtubules and promotes the formation of neurotoxic NFTs (Mehta 2006, Wolfe 2009, Jin et al. 2011). How tau becomes hyperphosphorylated is unclear. Recent evidence has demonstrated tau to be the primary cause of the neuronal damage; its level in the form of NFTs correlates better with clinical dementia than Aβ load (Braak and Braak 1991, Wolfe 2009).

Imaging β-amyloid in the Down syndrome brain

Landt et al. (2011) conducted a pilot study to determine the safety, feasibility and tolerability of positron emission tomography (PET) in people with Down syndrome. It was found to be safe and acceptable and furthermore, an enjoyable experience for the participants. The ethical and methodological challenges involved, in addition to the positive feedback from study participants, are considered by D'Abrera et al. (2011). In line with the neuropathological data, Landt and colleagues (2011) also found that amyloid binding was substantially higher in older individuals with Down syndrome. All participants over the age of 45 (*n* = 5) were found to have amyloid binding in at least five of the six defined brain regions. Four of these participants already had a diagnosis of Alzheimer disease. Three younger individuals between 25 and 36 years of age were negative for amyloid binding. A similar study was conducted by Handen et al. (2012), but only adults with Down syndrome without dementia participated. Nevertheless, two participants, aged 38 and 44 years, were found to have increased amyloid binding in comparison to cognitively normal individuals who did not have Down syndrome. In agreement with the Landt et al. (2011) findings, no amyloid binding was seen in the younger individuals (aged between 20 and 35 years).

Interventions and treatments

Any changes in behaviour recognized by the person themselves, family member or support worker as being new and atypical require detailed assessment. This should lead to a formulation and diagnosis of any comorbid mental or physical disorder which will guide appropriate intervention.

INTERVENTIONS FOR MENTAL ILL-HEALTH

Approaches to the treatment of mental ill-health are broadly similar to those used in the general population: within a bio-psycho-social framework the potential precipitants of ill-health and the relational and environmental factors that may be contributing and maintaining the abnormal mental state (e.g. low mood) are addressed. For people with intellectual disabilities, there is rather limited evidence about the effectiveness of some of the mainstream psychological treatments (Taylor et al. 2005, Willner 2006). Cognitive behavioural approaches are reported to be helpful in anxiety disorders, particularly following trauma (Stenfert Kroese and Thomas 2006), and for the treatment of aggression in people with mild intellectual disabilities (Taylor et al. 2005). Such approaches may well need the modification of the material and of the language used. Psychiatric medications may also be effective, where there is a clear comorbid psychiatric illness. People with neurodevelopmental disorders may have atypical wanted and unwanted effects. The guidance is to start at a lower dose and build up carefully according to clinical response.

INTERVENTIONS FOR DEMENTIA

In the absence of a pharmacological intervention that has any demonstrable effect in alleviating the symptoms of Alzheimer disease in Down syndrome, approaches that focus on care-giving and adaptation of environment are most likely to help. The Royal College of

Psychiatrists and the British Psychological Society (2009) have indicated that efficacy will depend largely on early and accurate diagnosis, as well an understanding of how associated behavioural problems can be managed without compromising the dignity of the affected person (Dodd et al. 2009). Approaches used include modifying the way staff and family interact, changes to the physical environment and ensuring that the person's physical health is maintained (see Chapter 4 for more detail). For staff working in services for people with intellectual disability, one difficulty is to switch focus from helping those they support to acquire new skills to acknowledging that Alzheimer disease is a progressive disorder of the brain that will inevitably lead to loss of skills. Cognitive and functional assessments may helpfully be repeated at intervals so as to inform the communication and support strategies that are being used.

Several drugs licensed for the treatment of Alzheimer disease have been studied in Down syndrome. Donepezil, an acetylcholinesterase inhibitor, has been shown to slow the rate of decline in people with Down syndrome and Alzheimer disease. However, the results should be viewed with caution, as many studies suffer from small sample sizes (see Chapter 19).

In the general population benefit is established for donepezil in people with Alzheimer disease. In their study of 431 people randomized either to donepezil or placebo for 54 weeks, the treated group maintained a higher level of function for 72% longer (Mohs et al. 2001). Roizen (2005) in her review of complementary and alternative therapies for Down syndrome identified five studies of the drug but four of these were grossly under powered with between 4 and 19 participants. To illustrate, Kishnani et al. (1999) conducted a study in which only four adults with Down syndrome took part: two diagnosed with Alzheimer disease and two young adults without Alzheimer disease. The authors reported all four participants to have improved on the Vineland Alzheimer Adaptive Behaviour Scale. However, the lack of a placebo-only control group limits the extent to which these findings can be reliably interpreted. Lott et al. (2002) had similar low numbers (nine treated with six controls). The improvements seen in dementia scores for the donepezil group may not be entirely reliable!

A thorough 24-week long double-blind placebo-controlled trial of donepezil in adults with Down syndrome and Alzheimer disease was conducted by Prasher et al. (2002). The sample size was small with only 27 participants. The donepezil group had a non-significant reduction in deterioration in the Dementia Scale for Mentally Retarded Persons (DMR) (50% vs 69% respectively), the Severe Impairment Battery and the Adapted Behavioural Scale but the Neuro-Psychiatry Inventory scores showed less improvement when compared with the placebo group. A number of unwanted side effects were reported including diarrhoea, insomnia, fatigue and nausea. However, in a subsequent open label study the same participant groups showed significant differences in their performance on DMR after 2 years with benefit seen in the treatment group (50% in the treatment group showed DMR improvement; 31% in controls).

A randomized double-blind placebo-controlled trial of memantine (an NMDA-glutamate receptor antagonist) conducted by Hanney et al. (2012) was sizeable and well controlled, with 72 participants in the experimental group and 74 controls. The authors concluded memantine to be ineffective as a treatment for Alzheimer disease in Down syndrome. This raised concerns over the possibility that other drugs effective against Alzheimer disease in the general population may not be beneficial in Down syndrome. Lockrow and colleagues (2011) have studied the drug in Ts65Dn mice. Whereas benefit for memory facilitation was demonstrated that the pathology of Alzheimer disease in the mice was in no way arrested, indicating the treated group maintained function for longer until the inevitable deterioration followed.

Conclusions and key points

The assessment and treatment of mental ill-health in adults with Down syndrome, requires sound clinical skills with respect to history taking, mental state and physical assessments and the choice of appropriate and necessary investigations.

Dementia offers added complexities particularly with respect to eliciting a history and consent to treatment. A team approach encompassing psychology and psychiatry services is required; diagnostic and functional approaches are of value.

Despite large advances in our understanding, effective treatments are yet to be developed. It may be that once clinical symptoms meeting the diagnostic criteria for Alzheimer disease are present, the brain neuropathology is so advanced it can no longer be reversed.

Previous studies on ageing and pathology in Down syndrome have done much to inform our current understanding of Alzheimer disease. More basic research is needed to pinpoint the window for intervention that will allow us to prevent and/or arrest the development of dementia.

Down syndrome will continue to serve as a unique and most natural of models for Alzheimer disease within the wider population; and people with Down syndrome engage enthusiastically as participants in research studies.

REFERENCES

Adams D, Oliver C (2010) The relationship between acquired impairments of executive function and behaviour change in adults with Down syndrome. *J Intellect Disabil Res* 54: 393–405.

Alexander GE, Delong MR, Strick PL (1986) Parallel organization of functionally segregated circuits linking basal ganglia and cortex. *Ann Rev Neurosci* 9: 357–381.

Arron K, Oliver C, MOSS J et al. (2011) The prevalence and phenomenology of self-injurious and aggressive behaviour in genetic syndrome. *J Intellect Disabil Res* 55: 109–120.

Aylward EH, Burt DB, Thorpe LU, Lai F, Dalton A (1997) Diagnosis of dementia in individuals with intellectual disability. *J Intellect Disabil Res* 41: 152–164.

Azizeh BY, Head E, Ibrahim MA et al. (2000) Molecular dating of senile plaques in the brains of individuals with Down syndrome and in aged dogs. *Exp Neurol* 163: 111–122.

Ball SL, Holland AJ, Hon J, Huppert FA, Treppner P, Watson PC (2006) Personality and behaviour changes mark the early stages of Alzheimer disease in adults with Down's syndrome: Findings from a prospective population-based study. *Int J Geriatr Psychiatry* 21: 661–673.

Ball SL, Holland AJ, Watson PC, Huppert FA (2010) Theoretical exploration of the neural bases of behavioural disinhibition, apathy and executive dysfunction in preclinical Alzheimer disease in people with Down's syndrome: Potential involvement of multiple frontal-subcortical neuronal circuits. *J Intellect Disabil Res* 54: 320–336.

Bamberger ME, Landreth GE (2001) Microglial interaction with beta-amyloid: Implications for the pathogenesis of Alzheimer disease. *Microsc Res Tech* 54: 59–70.

Beacher F, Daly E, Simmons A et al. (2010) Brain anatomy and ageing in non-demented adults with Down's syndrome: An in vivo MRI study. *Psychol Med* 40: 611–619.

Beacher F, Simmons A, Daly E et al. (2005) Hippocampal myo-inositol and cognitive ability in adults with Down syndrome: An in vivo proton magnetic resonance spectroscopy study. *Arch Gen Psychiatry* 62: 1360–1365.

Braak H, Braak E (1991) Neuropathological stageing of Alzheimer-related changes. *Acta Neuropathol* 82: 239–259.

Capone GT (2001) Down syndrome: Alzheimer diseasevances in molecular biology and the neurosciences. *J Dev Behav Pediatr* 22: 40–59.

Caricasole A, Copani A, Caruso A et al. (2003) The Wnt pathway, cell-cycle activation and beta-amyloid: Novel therapeutic strategies in Alzheimer disease? *Trends Pharmacol Sci* 24: 233–238.

Cole SL, Vassar R (2007) The Alzheimer disease beta-secretase enzyme, BACE-1. *Mol Neurodegener* 2: 22.

Contestabile A, Benfenati F, Gasparini L (2010) Communication breaks-Down: From neurodevelopment defects to cognitive disabilities in Down syndrome. *Prog Neurobiol* 91: 1–22.

Cooper SA, Smiley E, Morrison J et al. (2007) Mental ill-health in adults with intellectual disabilities: prevalence and associated factors. *Br J Psychiatry* 190: 27–35.

Coppus A, Evenhuis H, Verberne GJ et al. (2006) Dementia and mortality in persons with Down's syndrome. *J Intellect Disabil Res* 50: 768–777.

D'abrera JC, Holland AJ, Landt J, Stocks-Gee G, Zaman SH (2011) A neuroimaging proof of principle study of Down's syndrome and dementia: Ethical and methodological challenges in intrusive research. *J Intellect Disabil Res* 57: 105–118. doi: 10.1111/j.1365-2788.2011.01495.x.

De La Monte SM (1989) Quantitation of cerebral atrophy in preclinical and end-stage Alzheimer disease. *Ann Neurol* 25: 450–459.

De La Monte SM, Hedley-Whyte ET (1990) Small cerebral hemispheres in adults with Down's syndrome: Contributions of developmental arrest and lesions of Alzheimer disease. *J Neuropathol Exp Neurol* 49: 509–520.

De Strooper B (2010) Proteases and proteolysis in Alzheimer disease: A multifactorial view on the disease process. *Physiol Rev* 90: 465–494.

Dodd K, Bhaumik S, Benbow SM et al. (2009) *Dementia and People with Learning Disabilities: Guidance on the Assessment, Diagnosis, Treatment and Support of People with Learning Disabilities Who Develop Dementia*. Leicester: The British Psychological Society and the Royal College of Psychiatrists.

Foy CM, Daly EM, Glover A et al. (2011) Hippocampal proton MR spectroscopy in early Alzheimer disease and mild cognitive impairment. *Brain Topogr* 24: 316–322.

Haass C, Selkoe DJ (2007) Soluble protein oligomers in neurodegeneration: Lessons from the Alzheimer's amyloid beta-peptide. *Nat Rev Mol Cell Biol* 8: 101–112.

Handen BL, Cohen AD, Channamalappa U et al. (2012) Imaging brain amyloid in non-demented young adults with Down syndrome using pittsburgh compound B. *Alzheimer's Dement* 8: 496–501.

Hanney M, Prasher V, Williams N et al. (2012) Memantine for dementia in adults older than 40 years with Down's syndrome (MEADS): A randomized, double-blind, placebo-controlled trial. *Lancet* 379: 528–536.

Hardy J (2009) The amyloid hypothesis for Alzheimer disease: A critical reappraisal. *J Neurochem* 110: 1129–1134.

Hardy J, Higgins G (1992) Alzheimer disease: The amyloid cascade hypothesis. *Science* 256: 184–185.

Holland AJ, Oliver C (1995) Down's syndrome and the links with Alzheimer disease. *J Neurol Neurosurg Psychiatry* 59: 111–114.

Holland AJ, Hon J, Huppert FA, Stevens F (2000) Incidence and course of dementia in people with Down's syndrome: Findings from a population-based study. *J Intellect Disabil Res* 44: 138–146.

Holland AJ, Hon J, Huppert FA, Stevens F, Watson P (1998) Population-based study of the prevalence and presentation of dementia in adults with Down's syndrome. *Br J Psychiatry* 172: 493–498.

Jin M, Shepardon N, Yang T, Chen G, Walsh D, Selkoe DJ (2011) Soluble amyloid beta-protein dimers isolated from Alzheimer cortex directly induce tau hyperphosphorylation and neuritic degeneration. *Proc Natl Acad Sci USA* 108: 5819–5824.

Kishnani PS. Sullivan JA, Walter BK et al. (1999). Cholinergic therapy for Down's syndrome. *Lancet* 353: 1064–1065.

Landt J, D'abrera JC, Holland AJ et al. (2011) Using positron emission tomography and carbon 11-labeled Pittsburgh compound B to image brain fibrillar beta-amyloid in adults with Down syndrome: Safety, acceptability, and feasibility. *Arch Neurol* 68: 890–896.

Lockrow J, Bogera H, Bimonte-Nelson H, Granholm AC (2011) Effects of long-term memantine on memory and neuropathology in Ts65Dn mice, a model for Down syndrome. *Behav Brain Res* 221: 610–622. doi: 10.1016/j.bbr.2010.03.036.

Lott IT, Head E (2001) Down syndrome and Alzheimer disease: A link between development and aging. *Ment Retard Dev Disabil Res Rev* 7: 172–178.

Lott IT, Osann K, Doran E, Nelson L (2002) Down syndrome and Alzheimer disease: Response to donepezil. *Arch Neurol* 59: 1133–1136.

Lustbader JW, Cirilli M, Lin C et al. (2004) ABAD directly links Abeta to mitochondrial toxicity in Alzheimer disease. *Science* 304: 448–452.

Mann DM (1988) The pathological association between Down syndrome and Alzheimer disease. *Mech Ageing Dev* 43: 99–136.

Mann DM (1991) The topographic distribution of brain atrophy in Alzheimer disease. *Acta Neuropathol* 83: 81–86.

Mann DM (2006) Neuropathology of Alzheimer disease in Down's syndrome. In: Prasher VP, editor. *Down's Syndrome and Alzheimer Disease. Biological Correlates.* Oxford, Seattle: Radcliffe Publishing.

Mann DMA (1998) Dementia of frontal type and dementias with subcortical gliosis. *Brain Pathol* 8: 325–338.

Mann DMA, Yates PO, Marcyniuk B (1984) Alzheimer's presenile dementia, senile dementia of Alzheimer's type and Down's syndrome in middle age form an age related continuum of pathological changes. *Neuropathol Appl Neurobiol* 10: 185–207.

Mantry D, Cooper S-A, Smiley E et al. (2008) The prevalence and incidence of mental ill-health in adults with Down syndrome. *J Intellect Disabil Res* 52: 141–155.

Mccarron M, Gill M, Mccallion P, Begley C (2005) Health co-morbidities in ageing persons with Down syndrome and Alzheimer's dementia. *J Intellect Disabil Res* 49: 560–566.

Mclaurin J, Franklin T, Chakrabartty A, Fraser PE (1998) Phosphatidylinositol and inositol involvement in Alzheimer amyloid-beta fibril growth and arrest. *J Mol Biol* 278: 183–194.

Mclean CA, Cherny RA, Fraser FW et al. (1999) Soluble pool of Abeta amyloid as a determinant of severity of neurodegeneration in Alzheimer disease. *Ann Neurol* 46: 860–866.

Mehta PD (2006) Amyloid beta and tau proteins in Alzheimer disease and Down syndrome. In: Prasher VP, editor. *Down Syndrome and Alzheimer disease. Biological Correlates.* Oxford, Seattle: Radcliffe Publishing.

Menghini D, Costanzo F, Vicari S (2011) Relationship between brain and cognitive processes in Down syndrome. *Behav Genet* 41: 381–393.

Mohs RC, Doody RS, Morris JC et al. (2001) A 1-year, placebo-controlled preservation of function survival study of donepezil in AD patients. *Neurology* 57: 481–488.

Prasher VP, Huxley A, Haque MS (2002) A 24-week, double-blind, placebo-controlled trial of donepezil in patients with Down syndrome and Alzheimer disease—pilot study. *Int J Geriatr Psychiatry* 17: 270–278.

Querfurth HW, Laferla FM (2010) Alzheimer disease. *N Engl J Med* 362: 329 344.

Roizen NJ (2005) Complementary and alternative therapies for Down syndrome. *Ment Retard Dev Disabil Res Rev* 11: 149–155.

Roizen NJ, Patterson D (2003) Down's syndrome. *Lancet* 361: 1281–1289.

Royal College of Psychiatrist and British Psychological Society (2009) *Dementia and People with Learning Disabilities.* Leicester: The British Psychological Society. ISBN: 978-1-85433-493-0.

Schupf N, Kapell D, Nightingale B, Rodriguez A, Tycko B, Mayeux R (1998) Earlier onset of Alzheimer disease in men with Down syndrome. *Neurology* 50: 991–995.

Selkoe DJ (1991) The molecular pathology of Alzheimer disease. *Neuron* 6: 487–498.

Stenfert Kroese B and Thomas G (2006). Treating chronic nightmares of sexual assault survivors with an intellectual disability – Two descriptive case studies. *J Appl Res Intellect Disabil.* 19: 75–80.

Strydom A, Shooshtari S, Lee L et al. (2010) Dementia in older adults with intellectual disabilities— epidemiology, presentation, and diagnosis. *J Policy Pract Intellect Disabil* 7: 96–110.

Suzuki K (2007) Neuropathology of developmental abnormalities. *Brain Dev* 29: 129–141.

Taylor JL, Novaco RW, Gillmer BT et al. (2005) Individual cognitive-behavioural anger treatment for people with mild-borderline intellectual disabilities and histories of aggression: a controlled trial. *Br J Clin Psychol* 44:367–82.

Teipel SJ, Alexander GE, Schapiro MB, Moller HJ, Rapoport SI, Hampel H (2004) Age-related cortical grey matter reductions in non-demented Down's syndrome adults determined by MRI with voxel-based morphometry. *Brain* 127: 811–824.

Tekin S, Cummings JL (2002) Frontal–subcortical neuronal circuits and clinical neuropsychiatry: An update. *J Psychosom Res* 53: 647–654.

Teller JK, Russo C, Debusk LM et al. (1996) Presence of soluble amyloid beta-peptide precedes amyloid plaque formation in Down's syndrome. *Nat Med* 2: 93–95.

Tyrrell J, Cosgrave M, Mccarron M et al. (2001) Dementia in people with Down's syndrome. *Int J Geriatr Psychiatry* 16: 1168–1174.

Visser FE, Aldenkamp AP, Van Huffelen AC, Kuilman M, Overweg J, Van Wijk J (1997) Prospective study of the prevalence of Alzheimer-type dementia in institutionalized individuals with Down syndrome. *Am J Ment Retard* 101: 400–412.

Willner P (2006) The effectiveness of psychotherapeutic interventions for people with learning disabilities: a critical overview. *J Intellect Disabil Res* 49: 73–85.

Wilson LR, Annus T, Zaman S, Holland AJ (2014) Understanding the process: Links between Down's syndrome and dementia. In: Watchman K, editor. *Intellectual Disability and Dementia*. London: Jessica Kingsley Publishers.

Wisniewski KE, Wisniewski HM, Wen GY (1985) Occurrence of neuropathological changes and dementia of Alzheimer disease in Down's syndrome. *Ann Neurol* 17: 278–282.

Wolfe MS (2009) Tau mutations in neurodegenerative diseases. *J Biol Chem* 284: 6021–6025.

Zigman WB, Lott IT (2007) Alzheimer disease in Down syndrome: Neurobiology and risk. *Ment Retard Dev Disabil Res Rev* 13: 237–246.

19

INTERVENTION AND ALTERNATIVE THERAPIES: MEDICINE, MYTH AND MAGICAL BELIEF

Richard Newton

What do parents want for their children?

There are a few exceptions, but the vast majority of parents hope for a child with typical development who will reach a potential appropriate for the family's expectation and enjoy a fulfilling life. To achieve this what is needed throughout life is

Love—to add a sense of security and bolster self-esteem with home a safe haven to return to when the going gets tough;

Encouragement—so that children (and adults) can be urged or coaxed into situations they find challenging and learn from the experience; and

Opportunity—so that love and encouragement can be put to work.

Most parents will do all they can to ensure their child reaches this potential. This emotion is felt particularly keenly by parents of a child with a developmental impairment. Part of this is the natural feeling; part of it is based on a yearning 'to put the problem right'. In some cases, sustained pathological grief related to the birth of a child with disability may be a continuing negative influence on the individual parent and family life. This may need intervention in its own right but this chapter will deal with interventions for the children themselves, the biologically plausible and implausible and how we might measure success. Meanwhile, it is as well to remember that for any child on earth to succeed whether they have developmental impairment or not they need that love, opportunity and encouragement.

What is the rationale and scope for intervention? How might we help?

Mainstream medicine and alternative therapies have used two approaches. The first is to alter the environment in which the child learns (opportunity and encouragement). Interventions have been devised to alter either the quality or quantity of contact the teacher (including parents) has with the child.

The other approach has been to administer medication or a potion of some sort so as to alter the child's metabolism in a beneficial way. The evidence for both approaches will be examined but first the rationale for biochemical intervention will be explored.

We learnt in Chapter 2 how advances in knowledge have led us to modify our perception of the biochemical world. At one time, it was thought that one gene produced one protein which in turn helped an individual cell to function efficiently. In 2014, we now know that many genes interact (rather than one gene) to synthesize protein, and that these epigenetic mechanisms are an integral part of healthy cell function. The additional copy leads to an overexpression of 30–50% of chromosome 21 genes. This upregulation of genetic activity can trigger a deregulation in the expression of non-chromosome 21 genes. There may actually be downregulation of some target genes. It is easy to see how this system disruption quickly becomes ever more complex and multidimensional. A host of transcriptional and posttranscriptional alterations produce abnormal phenotypes in almost all tissue.

To date, this has been studied mainly in the mouse. Functional analysis of chromosome 21 encoded proteins indicates their involvement in up to 87 biological processes with 81 different functions and a localization pattern in 26 cellular compartments (Fillat and Altafaj 2012). Five microRNAs have also been identified on 21q but their function is currently unknown. As different tissues will be disrupted in different ways, there can be no one single approach to putting it right. Furthermore, the timing of the intervention (prenatal, postnatal or adult) is likely to be critical.

For the moment, different target genes and their association with specific functions (e.g. cognition) are being identified for possible modulation. Meanwhile, a number of gene therapy vectors are being tested to ensure safety and lack of toxicity. Promising progress is being made in some areas and clinical trials are now being undertaken in Down syndrome-associated phenotypes such as Alzheimer disease in non-Down syndrome individuals. For the moment, though, this research is very much at a preliminary stage and the murine model is the centre of focus.

Gene expression studies (the Down syndrome transcriptome) have led to useful insight into how the transcriptome of cells may vary not only between different anatomical locations within the brain but also at different ages. This science along with advances in proteomics has allowed scientists a much better understanding (which is still growing) of morphological and cellular changes within brain structures, for example, neuronal proliferation in neural cell precursors of Ts64Dn (the commonly used murine model) has been shown to be impaired as a result of inhibition of the Sonic hedgehog (Shh) pathway. This may occur through overexpression of a fragment of amyloid precursor protein (also important in Alzheimer disease). This proliferation defect may be associated with the lack of solid brain tumours seen in Down syndrome (especially medulloblastoma and neuroblastoma). This constrained nerve cell proliferation, which is likely to contribute to cognitive impairment in Down syndrome, may also protect against these tumours (Créau 2012).

This is but one example of many disruptions in function identified by this sort of science. Others include excitation–inhibition imbalance, shown to play a central role in brain malfunction involving neurotransmitter inhibition and a reduction of cortical interneurones. The fact that different parts of the brain may be disrupted by different mechanisms at the same time and then through different mechanisms with the passing of time serves only to emphasize how complex a quest for effective intervention is likely to be. This growth of knowledge has led to the number of therapeutic approaches in Down syndrome mouse models to increase rapidly along with accompanying outcome measures for behavioural rescue. However, but little is known about the molecular and cellular consequences of these treatments and only through greater knowledge of this will they ever be able to be used in affected humans.

What is the best way to structure a scientific study to demonstrate benefit?
The strongest design would be a randomized controlled trial in which participants with Down syndrome are allocated either to have the intervention, or a placebo (where medication is concerned), or some sort of interaction which is far less active than the teaching method under study (and therefore much less likely to be effective). The period of intervention should extend over many months so that the opportunity for accelerated improvement, or deterioration (compared with the control group), is sufficient. The outcome measure (say a formal standardized test of cognitive ability) should be clear and the person doing the testing should be blinded from whether the participant received the intervention or was in the control group. The numbers in the intervention and control group should be sufficient to be able to show a difference in the outcome measure so that the probability of that particular result having happened by chance is less than 5% (1 in 20). The number required to meet this standard can be defined through a power calculation. For example, to detect a 6-point (0.5 standard deviation) IQ difference on a two-sided test, a p value of 0.05 and a desired power of 0.8, the sample size would have to be 126 (63 with Down syndrome in one arm and 63 controls). No study to date has met these criteria (see below).

What interventions have been studied to date?
DRUGS
Drugs for Dementia
Alzheimer disease is characterized neurochemically by deficits in neurotransmitters including acetylcholine, noradrenalin and serotonin. The goal of drug treatment is to enhance selective cholinergic transmission by stimulating cholinergic receptors or by reducing acetylcholine metabolism by inhibiting cholinesterase action. The drugs studied to date are donepezil and memantine. The results of these underpowered studies are given in Chapter 18, Part 3.

Antioxidants
Both development and ageing in Down syndrome are associated with oxidative stress. Several chromosome 21 genes are associated with oxidative stress through their overexpression, leading to the propagation of reactive oxygen species. Mitochondrial dysfunction seems to be central in this adverse biological process (Lott 2012).

Lott et al. (2011) carried out a randomized double-blind placebo-controlled trial to assess whether daily antioxidant supplementation (900IU of alpha-tocopherol, 200mg of ascorbic acid and 600mg of alpha-lipoic acid) was effective, safe and tolerable for 53 participants with Down syndrome and Alzheimer disease. They were assessed at six monthly intervals with a battery of neuropsychological tests throughout the 2-year study. No benefit was demonstrated.

Ellis and colleagues (2008) assessed whether supplementation with antioxidants or folinic acid (or both) improved the psychomotor and language development of children with Down syndrome under 7 months. They compared daily oral supplementation with antioxidants (selenium 10μg, zinc 5mg, vitamin A 0.9mg, vitamin E 100mg and vitamin C 50mg), folinic acid (0.1mg), antioxidants and folinic acid combined, or placebo and found no significant difference in developmental outcome at 18 months.

Tianoa et al. (2012) studied prolonged coenzyme Q10 treatment in participants with Down syndrome and its effect on DNA oxidation. Their outcome measures were not related to neural function but rather biochemical surrogates for oxidative stress. Some benefit was demonstrated at 10 months (but not at 6 months) but there is no evidence here that benefit conferred on the studied lymphocytes might be translated into benefit for neural function. The same can be said of the study by Miles and colleagues (2007) who demonstrated that the pro-oxidant state in plasma of children with trisomy 21 as assessed by ubiquinol-10: Total coenzyme Q10 ratio may be normalized with ubiquinol-10 supplementation.

We conclude, despite there being strong evidence for oxidative stress and a central role in the impairment of function and ultimate deterioration in Down syndrome, there is no evidence to date that we can ameliorate this through antioxidant treatment. Newer generation antioxidants may be round the corner and worthy of further study.

Drugs for Cognition

Piracetam: Piracetam is a cyclic derivative of gamma-amino butyric acid. In a number of animal models, piracetam has been shown to improve cognitive performance but this effect was not demonstrated in humans. Lobaugh and colleagues (2001) studied 25 participants, aged 6–13 years, with Down syndrome in a double-blind crossover study. Piracetam did not significantly improve cognitive performance over placebo use. Seven of the 25 had unwanted effects.

Donepezil: Kishnani et al. (2010) published a 10-week randomized double-blind placebo-controlled multicentre study of donepezil in Down syndrome. The intervention was 2.5–10mg a day in children aged 10–17 years. A number of neuropsychometric measures were used but this placebo-controlled trial failed to show any benefit for the intervention.

Fluoxetine: Fluoxetine is used in clinical practice as an antidepressant and it inhibits serotonin (5HT) reuptake. Bianchi and colleagues (2010) demonstrated that early pharmacotherapy could correct neurogenesis and behavioural impairment in Ts65Dn mice. This was in concordance with the work of Clark and colleagues (2006) who in the same mouse model demonstrated increased neurogenesis in the hippocampus following use of the drug. However, Heinen and colleagues (2012) using the drug in adult mice found no benefit. These studies perhaps demonstrate critical windows of opportunity for therapeutic intervention in a biological model that is changing with time. To date, no human study is available.

Risperidone: The successful use of risperidone to target behaviour such as aggression, disruptiveness, self-injury, stereotypy and social withdrawal has been dealt with in Chapter 18b.

Other drugs: Roizen (2005) in her review draws attention to the fact that vasopressin and pituitary extract were assessed in two studies involving but nine children with Down syndrome: six in one and three in the other. The small numbers make it difficult to make a judgement on any effect on cognitive outcome. Growth hormone has been demonstrated to produce an increase in growth velocity (the idea was to improve self-esteem) but none of the publications define final height and it appears treated children will reach their ultimate height sooner than otherwise but final height is not enhanced.

Combination nutritional therapies: 'U' series, Haps, Caps, MSB+; NuTriVene-D; antioxidants; vitamins A, B6, thiamine, niacin, C, E; minerals: selenium, zinc. It is 11 years since Salman (2002) undertook a systematic review of trials relating dietary supplements to cognitive outcome in Down syndrome. He identified over 28 000 studies from which he selected 428 as possibly relevant. He included studies if all the participants had Down syndrome; the intervention included the use of drugs and/or dietary supplements; cognitive function was used as an outcome measure; the trials were controlled with a placebo group running concurrently or in a crossover design; and/or there was randomization or pseudo-randomization of the participants. Eleven studies met these criteria and involved 373 randomized participants. Follow-up ranged from 1.3 to 36 months. None of these studies demonstrated a beneficial effect. No significant studies have been published subsequently other than those already mentioned above.

The new treatment made available from the 'Changing Minds Foundation', including regular doses of fluoxetine, dexmethylphenidate, ginkgo biloba, phosphatidylcholine, body bio-balanced oil and folinic acid, is another example of expectations being raised. No evidence for efficacy is forwarded; indeed, scientific studies have not been carried out on this combination of drugs. There remains the potential for harm and significant unwanted effects.

Interventions involving manipulation or an invasive procedure

CELL THERAPY

This involves the injection of freeze-dried or lyophilized cells derived from fetal tissues of sheep and rabbits. It is widespread in continental Europe. It is illegal in the USA and carries the theoretical risk of prion or viral transmission, allergic or hypersensitivity reactions. The proponents usually delivering this at high cost suggest that it improves cognitive, social and language ability along with improvement in dysmorphic features. A Canadian double-blind prospective study of 59 participants and an English study of 10 participants in the intervention group and 10 in the control group failed to show a benefit (Roizen 2005). The rationale is ostensibly that injected fetal cells migrate to target organs and restore defective genes, biochemical substrates and enzymes. Given the difficulties slowly being overcome with stem cell therapy in mainstream science, this can clearly carry no biological rationale. Furthermore, the proposed mechanism is rather implausible in a condition that is already centred on overexpression rather than underexpression of genes.

PLASTIC SURGERY

This was widely advocated in Europe 20 or so years ago. The idea was to 'improve' facial appearance so that the person subjected to the operation would be less likely to be recognized as having Down syndrome. This, in turn, ostensibly would help their social integration. Thankfully, most human beings are not quite as shallow as that and respond to a person rather than a facial appearance. The operation was often accompanied by reducing the size of what is often a large tongue so as to improve speech. As indicated in Chapter 18a, however, the speech and language difficulties in Down syndrome are multidimensional and the rationale of this approach is flawed as shown by objective postoperative studies (Roizen 2005). Plastic surgery, therefore, cannot be recommended in any generic sense, which is not to say in specific instances it may be for a clear medical indication.

CRANIAL OSTEOPATHY

Mainline osteopathy is a respected discipline and a profession allied to medicine. Cranial osteopathy is not. The central rationale for cranio-osteopathy in intellectual disability in general and Down syndrome in particular relies on a few oft-repeated central tenets: brain development may be delayed or impaired by restriction within the skull (this is, of course, true when there is preterm suture fusion but untrue when there is not); reiteration of a hypothesis raised by an osteopath known as Nicholas J R Handoll as a fact (as if the hypothesis were proven) that 'postnatal hypoxia causes much of the disability of Down syndrome and that osteopathic treatment may be used effectively to reduce it'; manipulation of the skull may realign the nasal passages and upper airway to secure better drainage and minimize the risk of obstructive apnoea thereby abating hypoxia; manipulation around the temporal bone with relief of congestion improves blood flow to the brain. In 2002, Hartman (an anatomist) and Norton (a physiologist), both academics at the College of Osteopathic Medicine, University of New England, reviewed evidence for interexaminer reliability in cranio-osteopathy. The paper explains how diagnosis and intervention by osteopaths is explained by a biological model known as the 'Primary Respiratory Mechanism'. Ostensibly, the Primary Respiratory Mechanism refers to intrinsic rhythmic movements of the brain (which are independent of respiratory and cardiovascular rhythms) which cause rhythmic fluctuations of cerebrospinal fluid and specific relational changes among dural membranes, cranial bones and the sacrum. Furthermore, purportedly osteopaths with special skills can palpate this rhythm throughout the body. The authors point out that neurons lack the microstructure to be able to produce such movement. They then review six published assessments of interobserver reliability by which cranial osteopaths identify parameters relevant to diagnosis. Five of the reports focused on the cranial rhythm frequency showing interexaminer reliability of approximately zero and the sixth report in their opinion was badly flawed.

Cranial osteopaths also claim articular mobility between skull bones. In the words of the authors, 'These claims are so completely lacking in scientific support they border on ridiculous'. Most craniofacial and maxillary facial surgeons would agree with this.

That is not to say the immature skull cannot be remodelled. We know this from the observation that children with hypotonia (no matter what the cause) spend a long time lying on their backs and resting the weight of their skull on their occiputs. The occiput becomes flat. Once they tone up and start to sit, the gravitational forces through the skull alter and nature remodels the skull to its usual shape. This is achieved, however, through weeks of constant gravitational force, not through five or six intermittent treatments. The intervention is explained on one typical website:

Using light touch, practitioners assess the quality of the patient's Cranial Rhythm and compare it to what they consider to be a normal rhythm. They can then judge the state of the patient's body and how well it is functioning. During a session, the practitioner will delicately manipulate the cranial and spinal bones in order to restore the cranial rhythm, boost blood circulation and drain lymph and sinus fluids in the head . . .

Neither this site nor any other explains the method of manipulation, the target for the manipulation or the likely resulting physiological mechanism that might restore normality. So the intervention is not defined, interrelater performance shown to be unreliable and the underlying physiological and anatomical facts implausible. One has to conclude this intervention cannot be recommended.

OTHER THERAPIES

Many other experiences are offered to disabled children with the suffix 'therapy'. These include massage therapy, hydrotherapy, music therapy, aromatherapy, neurologically based movement programmes (including a recent vogue for bouncy castles) and animal therapy (therapeutic horseback riding). In a child with typical development, these would be named massage, horse riding, swimming and music; the suffix 'therapy' would disappear. All these things should be encouraged for people with Down syndrome because they offer opportunity and encouragement, an experience of life that enhances learning opportunity. Parents should resist the temptation to pay over the odds for these 'interventions'. If any of them are clinically indicated (and sometimes they are, e.g. music therapy for a particular psychological issue), then access can usually be achieved through the National Health Service.

Early intervention

Having seen the complexity of the biochemical genetics and how difficult it will be to manipulate them in an effective way, we come back to how professionals might help parents create their own encouragement and opportunity (they probably do not need help to provide the love!). The subject of early intervention has been reviewed by Christine Bonnier (2008). It is a term that broadly speaking denotes early educational strategies and encompasses all interventions that promote normal development including organizational, therapeutic and environment-modifying measures such as early stimulation programmes (I dislike the word 'stimulation'. What they really mean by stimulation is fun, opportunity and encouragement). Evidence for a beneficial effect has been patchy. Most often, studies have shown early benefit that is not sustained long-term. One Swedish study (Nidcap) did show longer-term benefit (Kleberg et al. 2006) but this was determined at least in part by maternal education. Overall the data suggest that early intervention programmes have positive effects, although scientific proof of efficacy is not available for all the strategies. Most benefit comes from programmes encouraging play between parents and children.

The study offering the best methodological rigor, probably unequalled, came from the Manchester Down syndrome cohort study (Cunningham 1987). This study involved 181 families with a recently born child with Down syndrome. The intervention involved the provision of accurate information on Down syndrome; emotional support for the parents; the provision of information on local services; information on how to get the best out of these services; and, lastly, advocacy for parents on how they should approach services. Intervention for the child was related to health and the psychological and educational needs of infants with Down syndrome. Within the cohort there were a number of subcohort groups, the design providing four training variables to analyse according to group, age of starting, intensity of intervention and visiting rate. Bailey Scales of Infant Development provided the outcome measure up to the age of 2–2.5 years and subsequently the Stanford Binet Intelligence Scale was used. Multivariate analysis looked at the relative influence on developmental scores of significant variables.

No association between motor development and intervention strategy was found. Impaired motor development was more often related to attendant medical problems. This makes clinical sense; we often have to wait for any child with an intellectual disability to 'tone up' (often into the second year of life) before they can make steady progress. In relation to cognition, the most striking association was the effect of parental education/school-leaving age. The effect appeared by 2 years and had increasing impact through to school entry. The females were more advanced than the males and first children more advanced than subsequent children (both as within the general population). In contrast, specialist elements of intensity and highly structured programmes brought only short-term gain and no lasting effect. That is, intense coaching will bring a short-term gain but will not overcome the compounding effect of the underlying cognitive impairment. The brain will consolidate learning (during a period of performance unreliability) and then only be ready to learn a new task when the underlying biological substrate allows. This period seems to be unaltered by the intervention. The results emphasize the importance of multivariate analysis in these sorts of studies.

Interestingly, families who had the most intense in-study training were more likely to have their children in mainstream preschool or primary school placement. This was independent of the mental age of the child and clearly reflected better parental advocacy skills in that group.

The same point of short-term gain from coaching but no consolidated long-term benefit can be taken from the work of Burgoyne and colleagues (2012). This was a randomized controlled trial studying the efficacy of a reading and language intervention delivered by teaching assistants who gave 40-minute sessions each over 40 weeks to children with Down syndrome. After 20 weeks of intervention, the intervention group showed significantly greater progress than the waiting control group for measures of single-word reading, letter-sound knowledge, phoneme blending and taught expressive vocabulary. Having said that, the gain in single-word reading was but 2.5 words. Although statistically significant, clearly this measureable effect was not important. Furthermore, after the passing of a further 20 weeks (the waiting group now having received their own intervention) there was no significant difference between the groups. That is, the early intervention group had to consolidate their learning before being able to pass on to the further acquisition of skills. The initial gains did not transfer to other skills (non-word reading, spelling, standardized expressive and receptive vocabulary, expressive intervention and grammar).

Key points

- The complexities of the molecular genetic abnormalities in Down syndrome indicate that we are not going to find a 'magic bullet' soon.
- Educational intervention studies demonstrate some short-term gains which are not consolidated.
- The factors that determine good cognitive performance in a population with Down syndrome are the same as those for the general population.
- What all children (and adults) need to reach their potential, including those with Down syndrome, is love, opportunity and encouragement.

REFERENCES

Bianchi P, Ciani E, Guidi S et al. (2010) Early pharmacotherapy restores neurogenesis and cognitive performance in the Ts65Dn mouse model for Down syndrome. *J Neurosci* 30: 8769–8779. doi: 10.1523/JNEUROSCI.0534-10.2010.

Bonnier C (2008) Evaluation of early stimulation programs for enhancing brain development. *Acta Paediatr* 97: 853–858. doi:10.1111/j.1651-2227.2008.00834.x.

Burgoyne K, Duff FJ, Clarke PJ, Buckley S, Snowling MJ, Hulme C (2012) Efficacy of a reading and language intervention for children with Down syndrome: A randomized controlled trial. *J Child Psychol Psychiatry* 53: 1044–1053. doi: 10.1111/j.1469-7610.2012.02557.x.

Clark S, Schwalbe J, Stasko MR, Yarowsky PJ, Costa ACS (2006) Fluoxetine rescues deficient neurogenesis in hippocampus of the Ts65Dn mouse model for Down syndrome. *Exp Neurol* 200: 256–261.

Créau N (2012) Molecular and cellular alterations in Down syndrome: Toward the identification of targets for therapeutics. *Neur Plast* Article ID 171639, 14 pages. doi: 10.1155/2012/171639.

Cunningham C (1987) Early intervention in Down's syndrome. In: Hosking G, Murphy G, editors. *Prevention of Mental Handicap: A World View*, vol. 112, 165–182. London: Royal Society of Medicine Series, International Congress and Symposium Series.

Ellis JM, Tan KH, Gilbert RE et al. (2008) Supplementation with antioxidants and folinic acid for children with Down's syndrome: Randomised controlled trial *BMJ* 336: 594–597. doi: 10.1136/bmj.39465.544028.AE.

Fillat C, Altafaj X (2012) Gene therapy for Down syndrome. *Prog Brain Res* 197: 237–247.

Hartman SE, Norton JM (2002) Inter-examiner reliability and cranial osteopathy. *Sci Rev Alt Med* 6: 23–34.

Heinen M, Hettich MM, Ryan DP, Schnell S, Paesler K, Ehninger D (2012) Adult-onset fluoxetine treatment does not improve behavioral impairments and may have adverse effects on the Ts65Dn mouse model of Down syndrome. *Neur Plast* 2012, Article ID 467251, 10 pages. doi: 10.1155/2012/467251.

Kishnani PS, Heller JH, Spiridigliozzi GA, et al. (2010) Donepezil for treatment of cognitive dysfunction in children with Down syndrome aged 10–17. *Am J Med Genet A* 152A: 3028–3035. doi: 10.1002/ajmg.a.33730.

Kleberg A, Hellstrom-Westras L, Widstrom AM (2006) Mother's perception of Newborn Individualized Developmental Care and Assessment Program (NIDCAP) as compared to conventional care. *Early Hum Dev* 15: PMID: 17112689.

Lobaugh NJ, Karaskov V, Rombough V et al. (2001) Piracetam therapy does not enhance cognitive functioning in children with Down syndrome. *Arch Pediatr Adolesc Med* 155: 442–448.

Lott IT (2012) Antioxidants in Down syndrome. *Biochim Biophys Acta* 1822: 657–663.

Lott IT, Doran E, Nguyen VQ, Tournay A, Head E, Gillen DL (2011) Down syndrome and dementia: A randomized, controlled trial of antioxidant supplementation. *Am J Med Genet A* 155A: 1939–1948.

Miles MV, Patterson BJ, Chalfonte-Evans ML et al. (2007) Coenzyme Q10 (ubiquinol-10) supplementation improves oxidative imbalance in children with trisomy 21. *Pediatr Neurol* 37: 398–403.

Roizen NJ (2005) Complementary and alternative therapies for Down syndrome. *Ment Retard Dev Disabil Res Rev* 11: 149–155.

Salman S (2002) Systematic review of the effect of therapeutic dietary supplements and drugs on cognitive function in subjects with Down syndrome. *Eur J Paediatr Neurol* 6: 213–219. doi: 10.1053/ejpn.2002.0596.

Tianoa L, Padellab L, Santorob L et al. (2012) Prolonged coenzyme Q10 treatment in Down syndrome patients, effect on DNA oxidation. *Neurobiol Aging* 33: 626.e1–626.e8.

20
PERSPECTIVES

Richard Newton

Through these pages, we have learnt that the biology of Down syndrome is complex, multidimensional and probably changes constantly throughout life from conception to old age. The notion that one gene gives one gene product no longer holds true. Epigenetic mechanisms maintain cell function and in Down syndrome the trisomy disrupts the usual intracellular gene orientation, which may itself distort transcriptome function. It seems unlikely that any biological or pharmacological intervention is going fundamentally to alter the disordered cell function in Down syndrome any time soon. The genetic research must continue: Why are solid tumours and coronary artery disease so rare in Down syndrome and why is the ageing process and Alzheimer disease accelerated? Study of these conditions along with autoimmune disorders, thyroid disease and many others will be of benefit not only to people with Down syndrome but the population at large.

Doctors and professionals allied to medicine must avoid the trap of 'diagnostic over-shadowing'. We must strive for early interventions to prevent secondary disadvantage—for example, the recognition and treatment of arthropathy, thyroid replacement therapy or restoring function through cardiac surgery in children with congenital heart disease. The future of this work must be to continue to develop and refine guidelines and standards so that health surveillance might lead to early diagnosis and intervention for the benefit of a vulnerable group of people.

Meanwhile, we have learnt that knowledge, be it motor, cognition, speech and language, social, cannot be forced into brains which are not in a biological state of readiness to receive it. When a human brain is ready to learn, it will learn given the opportunity. So intensive anything—vitamins, therapies, teaching courses—for young people with Down syndrome is not the order of the day. What the research tells us is that determinants of outcome in Down syndrome are the same as in the general population, birth order, maternal education and so on. This is good as it takes the pressure off parents. They should not feel they are missing a trick, that they should be doing more. What is good for any child is good for children with Down syndrome—love, opportunity and encouragement.

This applies to adults too, but here we have an even bigger challenge in creating opportunity. The principles of the World Health Organization's International Classification of Functioning, Disability and Health, for Children and Youth (ICF-CY; WHO 2007) should apply throughout life. As health professionals, we feel comfortable with part 1 of this classification which deals with functioning and disability. That is our home ground. We should also endeavour to bring sustained improvements in relation to part 2 which deals with contextual issues. Participation restrictions and environmental factors may limit both opportunity and encouragement. We can help individuals to feel more comfortable in life situations outside the home. It is within our power to remove unnecessary restrictions ('the doctor said he should never do this'). We also need to be advocates for people with a disability by promoting a good physical, social and attitudinal environment in which people can live and conduct their lives. Incentives and policies are often termed 'Inclusion' as if the default position is exclusion. Whenever an opportunity comes along to promote more positive attitudes and action, we should take it. We can do this through teaching, writing and our dealings with educational and social services, local and national politicians so as to instigate concerted change. Through these means, the context as well as body function will change for the benefit of all people with a disability.

APPENDIX 1
MEDICAL SURVEILLANCE
AND GUIDELINES

Liz Marder

Throughout this book we have described how health and development may differ in those with Down syndrome compared with the general population. We have shown how some medical conditions are more common in people with Down syndrome than in the general population, and how some may present differently.

When babies are born with Down syndrome (or the diagnosis is being considered antenatally), parents need prompt information about the syndrome and services that their child may need. Medical assessment is required to identify congenital anomalies that need immediate or subsequent medical intervention. Children with Down syndrome should have a programme of regular medical review to enable early identification and management of medical problems. Referral onto specialist services such as cardiology, ophthalmology and ENT surgery will be required for many. The multidisciplinary health team, particularly speech and language therapists, will need to be involved to encouragement development and early educational intervention should be offered. Families will need advice and sign-posting with regard to social care, benefits and to support organizations.

The need for medical surveillance tailored specifically to the medical conditions prevalent in Down syndrome should continue throughout life. It is important that those with Down syndrome are also included in the screening programmes that are offered to the general population. Particular note should be taken of conditions where presentation or management may differ from the general population or, alternatively, where presentation is as for others, but where diagnosis is missed as symptoms are assumed to be part of the syndrome or other coexisting medical conditions—so-called 'diagnostic overshadowing'. The situation may be complicated by the associated intellectual disability as individuals with Down syndrome may be less able to recognize or bring to the attention of others, symptoms that may indicate comorbid conditions.

A number of guidelines have been developed to describe the surveillance that should be provided for people with Down syndrome. There is a high degree of agreement and overlap between the recommendations in these guidelines, though each has a slightly different focus and is geared to a different audience. Generally, these guidelines are based on a consensus of opinion based upon available literature and experience, as the evidence base for some recommendations is limited given the paucity of research in the field.

All those with Down syndrome should be offered a programme of health care which takes into account the factors described above. However, the model of service provision will differ for different age groups, from country to country, between different health care systems and may also vary according to individual preference and need.

Medical surveillance for children

There are a number of different models of service provision for children. In the UK, care may be offered within hospital or community paediatric services and in child development centres. A paediatrician should be involved to provide a holistic overview, involving other specialists as needed. In some areas, there are dedicated Down syndrome clinics or services. The programme of surveillance may be informed by the following guidelines:

Down Syndrome Medical Interest Group UK and Ireland

(http://www.dsmig.org.uk/publications/guidelines.html)

Guidelines for basic essential medical surveillance which set out a minimum standard of basic medical surveillance—which we consider essential and realistically achievable within the framework of health care services in the UK and Ireland—include guidelines on hearing, vision, heart disease, thyroid disorder, cervical spine instability and growth. The health checks advised at various ages are summarized in a chart in the special insert for babies born with Down syndrome for the UK Personal Child Health Record available at: (http://www.healthforallchildren.com/wp-content/uploads/2013/04/A5-Downs-Instrucs-charts-full-copy.pdf)

Work is continuing in England under the auspices of the Royal College of Paediatrics and Child Health to produce a national service specification for Down syndrome, as guidance to those who commission services.

A draft version is currently available at: (http://www.bacdis.org.uk/policy/documents/DownSyndrome.pdf)

American Academy of Pediatrics Health Supervision for Children with Down Syndrome

(http://pediatrics.aappublications.org/content/early/2011/07/21/peds.2011-1605)

Designed to help paediatricians care for children with Down syndrome and their families, organized by issues likely to be important at different ages 0–21 years. They emphasize the importance of monitoring, screening and diagnosing those medical conditions known to result in significant morbidity or mortality in this population.

European Down Syndrome Association Health Care Guidelines for People with Down Syndrome

(http://www.edsa.eu/files/essentials/edsa_essentials_2_healthcare.pdf)

These guidelines include current recommendations at different ages, with justification as to why they are recommended.

Local Guidelines

In many areas local guidelines have also been developed, for example, Nottingham Guidelines for the Management of Children with Down Syndrome: (https://www.nuh.nhs.uk/handlers/downloads.ashx?id=48953). This guideline suggests the appropriate management, referrals, tests and so forth at each stage, from prenatal diagnosis, neonatal care and throughout childhood and adolescence. The aim is to ensure that all children with Down syndrome in Nottingham receive a comprehensive service which can be provided in the most appropriate place according to the needs and wishes of the child and family.

Medical surveillance for adults

General medical care for adults with Down syndrome is commonly provided from primary care, with referral onto specialist services for specific conditions only. There are few Down syndrome-specific adult services in the UK where general practitioners are most likely to provide health surveillance, sometimes with involvement of adult intellectual disability teams particularly for those with mental health needs.

Specific guidelines for adults with Down syndrome are less well established than those for children, although the American Academy of Pediatrics and the European Down Syndrome Association guidelines both include recommendations for adults.

In the UK, annual health checks for people with intellectual disability are recommended and general practitioners are incentivized to carry these out. The Royal College of General Practitioners publish guidance on these checks which includes recommendations specific to Down syndrome: (http://www.rcgp.org.uk/clinical-and-research/clinical-resources/learning-disabilities.aspx)

The UK Down's Syndrome Association has developed a health book for adults with Down syndrome to help guide practitioners through the necessary health checks and signpost them to further information on Down syndrome-related health conditions: (http://www.downs-syndrome.org.uk/campaigns/annual-health-checks)

In addition to the surveillance programmes recommended specifically for those with Down syndrome, the usual screening programmes offered to the general population should be followed. This may sometimes prove to be a challenge because of difficulties with understanding, communication or behaviour. A pragmatic approach should be taken, considering the individuals' needs and the likely risk and impact of the conditions being screened for. For example, the cancer risk profile is different in Down syndrome, with many solid tumours (except testicular cancer—see Chapter 14) being less common. Routine screening usually offered for breast, cervical or prostate cancer may therefore be less important for this group (unless there is a family history or other risk factors).

APPENDIX 2
SOME ADDITIONAL RESOURCES
FOR FAMILIES

In clinic, it is often helpful to let families know what information is available on particular topics. We have collated a list of potentially useful guidance. It is centred on practice and resources available in the UK but we know many support groups for Down syndrome around the world offer a similar portfolio.

The Down's Syndrome Association (England, Wales and Northern Ireland)
(www.downs-syndrome.org.uk)

The DSA provides access to a range of resources covering health, welfare benefits, education and social care from http://www.downs-syndrome.org.uk. The website has a useful search facility but is easy to navigate by clicking on the appropriate tab, with links at times to resources on other sites.

The following resources are available for new parents

Booklet for new parents
New baby FAQ's
Down syndrome leaflet for friends and family
Information booklet—an Early Support manual
Local Down syndrome support group—for local support
Benefits 0–3—for guidance on government allowances

There is advice on siblings and there reactions, with links to two useful books:

- *the Sibling Slam Book: What it' Really Like to Have a brother or Sister with Special Needs* by Don Meyer and David Gallaher (Woodbine House, 2005).
- *Fasten Your Seatbelt* - written exclusively for teens with a brother or sister with Down syndrome by Brian Skoto and Susan Levine (Woodbine House, 2009)

DSA health series

This is a range of information leaflets about health and medical conditions written for parents and carers. Topics include:

- Ageing and its consequences
- Alzheimer disease
- Bereavement
- Gastrointestinal problems in children
- Managing sleep problems in children
- Diabetes
- Eye problems in children
- Oral health care
- Continuing pregnancy with a diagnosis of Down syndrome
- Depression
- Thyroid disorder
- Neck instability
- Epileptic spasms in children
- Sexual health

On speech, language and communication:
(http://www.downs-syndrome.org.uk/for-new-parents/faqs/speech-and-language/)

This information is suitable for families, school staff and speech and language therapists:

Dysfluency, stammering, getting stuck: Practical activities and strategies to help with dysfluency and stammering as well as new Makaton symbols.

Supporting people who have Down's syndrome to overcome communication difficulties: Information for schools and colleges, community groups and services, employers, care staff, professionals and families about what we can all do to tackle the challenges that people who have Down syndrome face when communicating.

Factsheet for Speech and Language Practical Activities
To access these please put Bold title into your search engine and select dsa option.

Other DSA Resources

Education
To match the Health series, there is a series to help families and schools.

Child development
For information on the development of children with Down's syndrome and ideas for how you can help at home, see the website page 'Growing Up'.

Stages of education
Pages on the different stages of education provide a brief guide to education from early years to further education. There are links to useful resources and further information on.

- Early Years
- Primary

- Secondary
- Further Education

Behaviour
Practical tips are provided to help parents support their child to behave well

Teenagers and Young Adults
This series of pages addresses issues such as sex and relationships, wanting independence, good personal hygiene, needing personal space and building good self-esteem. Topics addressed include:

- Planning for Adulthood
- Self-Esteem
- Self-Talk
- Puberty
- Making Choices
- Staying Safe Online
- Thinking About Work
- Things To Do
- Talking About Leaving Home

Dementia/Alzheimer's Disease
There is a series of web-pages with useful information on the following:
- What is Alzheimer's disease?
- Is Alzheimer's disease inevitable for people with Down's syndrome?
- Can other conditions look like Alzheimer's disease?
- What are the symptoms that may indicate dementia?
- Is it difficult to diagnosis dementia in someone with Down's syndrome?
- What is a baseline assessment?
- Down's syndrome, specific issues
- I suspect my relative may have dementia, who do I turn to for help?
- Are there any specific dementia services for people with Down's syndrome?
- Where should people with Down's syndrome and dementia live?
- Where to get support after your relative has received a diagnosis of dementia

Social Care Series
The following factsheets are available for planning child and adult support and services:
  1: Preparing for a Community Care Assessment
  2: Asking for a Community Care Assessment
  3: Asking for a Carer's Assessment
  4: Getting the Care Plan Right
  5: Preparing for a Social Care/Children's Act Assessment of your child

Supported Living Series
FAQs - Thinking About Supported Living
Preparing for Supported Living
FAQs – Handling Problems
www.housingandsupport.org.uk.

WorkFit (http://www.housingandsupport.org.uk/home)
An employment project connecting employers to employees with Down's syndrome.

Housing and Support Alliance (http://www.housingandsupport.org.uk/home)
Housing opportunities for people with learning disabilities.

Foundation for People with Learning Disabilities
Thinking Ahead – a planning guide for families is available at
www.fpld.org.uk/our-work/family-friends-community/thinking-ahead/

Down's Heart Group (http://www.dhg.org.uk/information/)
This website provides non-medical people with good quality information about the heart conditions and associated topics. Written from a parent's perspective all items of a medical nature have been checked for accuracy by professionals in the appropriate medical field. The web-site covers different forms of congenital heart disease, investigation, the different operations used and possible complications. There are useful sections on many other topics including dental care, health checks, travel advice and the difficult topic of grief.

INDEX

Page references in *italics* refer to material in tables or boxes.

Other titles from Mac Keith Press www.mackeith.co.uk

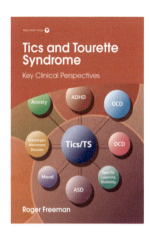

Tics and Tourette Syndrome: Key Clinical Perspectives
Roger Freeman

2015 ▪ 304pp ▪ softback ▪ 978-1-909962-41-5

£55.95/ €72.95 / $90.00

Written by a world-renowned expert in developmental neurology, this book will be of practical use to clinicians who may encounter tic disorders and Tourette syndrome that complicate the management of their patients. It contains wide-ranging discussion of tics that occur alone or in other conditions such as ADHD, DCD, and ASD. It includes extensive information on stereotypic movement disorder and other repetitive movements which are often confused with tics.

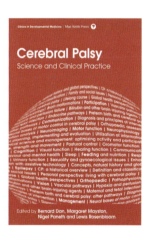

Cerebral Palsy: Science and Clinical Practice
Bernard Dan, Margaret Mayston, Nigel Paneth
and Lewis Rosenbloom (Editors)

Clinics in Developmental Medicine
2014 ▪ 712pp ▪ hardback ▪ 978-1-909962-38-5
£190.00 / €235.80 / $299.95

The only complete, scientifically rigorous, fully integrated reference giving a wide ranging and in-depth perspective on cerebral palsy and related neurodevelopment disabilities. It considers all aspects of cerebral palsy from the causes to clinical problems and their implications for individuals. Leading scientists present the evidence on the role of pre-term birth, inflammation, hypoxia, endocrinological and other pathways. They explore opportunities for neuroprotection leading to clinical applications.

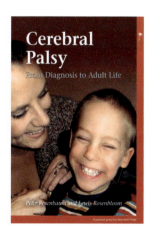

Cerebral Palsy: From Diagnosis to Adult Life
Peter L. Rosenbaum and Lewis Rosenbloom

A practical guide from Mac Keith Press
2012 ▪ 224pp ▪ softback ▪ 978-1-908316-50-9
£29.95 / €36.00 / $50.00

This book has been designed to provide readers with an understanding of cerebral palsy as a developmental as well as a neurological condition. It details the nature of cerebral palsy, its causes and its clinical manifestations. Using clear, accessible language (supported by an extensive glossary) the authors have blended current science with metaphor to explain the biomedical underpinnings of cerebral palsy.
.

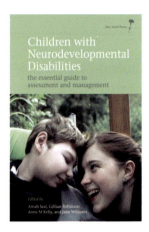

Children with Neurodevelopmental Disabilities: the essential guide to assessment and management
Arnab Seal, Gillian Robinson, Anne M. Kelly
and Jane Williams (Editors)

2013 ▪ 744pp ▪ softback ▪ 978-1-908316-62-2
£65.00 / €78.00 / $99.95

A comprehensive textbook on the practice of paediatric neurodisability, written by practitioners and experts in the field. Using a problem-oriented approach, the authors give best-practice guidance, and centre on the needs of the child and family, working in partnership with multi-disciplinary, multi-agency teams. It provides a ready reference for managing problems encountered in the paediatric clinic.

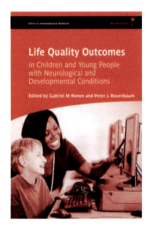

Life Quality Outcomes in Children and Young People with Neurological and Developmental Conditions
Gabriel M. Ronen and Peter L. Rosenbaum (Editors)

Clinics in Developmental Medicine
2013 ▪ 394pp ▪ hardback ▪ 978-1-908316-58-5
£95.00 / €120.70 / $149.95

Healthcare professionals need to understand their patients' views of their condition and its effects on their health and well-being. This book builds on the World Health Organization's concepts of 'health', 'functioning' and 'quality of life' for young people with neurodisabilities: it emphasises the importance of engaging with patients in the identification of both treatment goals and their evaluation. Uniquely, it enables healthcare professionals to find critically reviewed outcomes-related information.

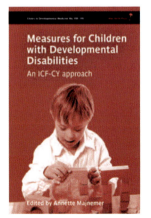

Measures for Children with Developmental Disabilities
An ICF-CY approach
Annette Majnemer (Editor)

Clinics in Developmental Medicine No 194-195
2012 ▪ 552pp ▪ hardback ▪ 978-1-908316-45-5
£154.00 / €184.80 / $235.00

This title presents and reviews outcome measures across a wide range of attributes that are applicable to children and adolescents with developmental disabilities. It uses the children and youth version of the International Classification of Functioning, Disability and Health (ICF-CY) as a framework for organizing the various measures into sections and chapters. Each chapter coincides with domains within the WHO framework of Body Functions, Activities and Participation, and

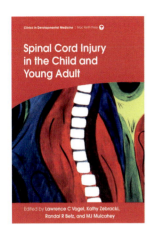

Spinal Cord Injury in the Child and Young Adult
Lawrence C Vogel, Kathy Zebracki, Randall R Betz and MJ Mulcahey (Editors)

Clinics in Developmental Medicine
2014 ▪ 460pp ▪ hardback ▪ 978-1-909962-34-7
£125.00 / €155.10 / $206.50

Compared to adult-onset spinal cord injury (SCI), individuals with childhood-onset SCI are unique in several ways. First, as a result of their younger age at injury and longer lifespan, individuals with pediatric-onset SCI are particularly susceptible to long-term complications related to a sedentary lifestyle. This book is intended for clinicians of all disciplines who may only occasionally care for young people with SCI to those who specialize in SCI as well as clinical and basic researchers in the SCI field.

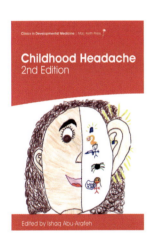

Childhood Headache, 2nd Edition
Ishaq Abu-Arafeh (Editor)

Clinics in Developmental Medicine
2013 ▪ 352pp ▪ hardback ▪ 978-1-908316-75-2
£95.00 / €115.20 / $154.95

Headache is a common problem which has a significant impact on children's quality of life. *Childhood Headache* is a comprehensive source of knowledge and guidance to practising clinicians looking after children with headache that includes many clinical examples to illustrate the difficulties in diagnosis or options for treatment. It is also a resource for researchers who are looking for a full analysis of the published studies.

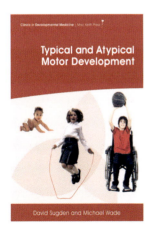

Typical and Atypical Motor Development
David Sugden and Michael Wade

Clinics in Developmental Medicine
2013 ▪ 400pp ▪ hardback ▪ 978-1-908316-55-4
£145.00 / €180.00 / $234.95

Sugden and Wade, leading authors in this area, comprehensively cover motor development and motor impairment, drawing on sources in medicine and health-related studies, motor learning and developmental psychology. A theme that runs through the book is that movement outcomes are a complex transaction of child resources, the context in which movement takes place, and the manner in which tasks are presented.

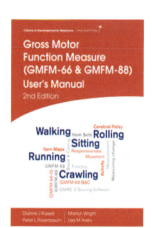

Gross Motor Function Measure (GMFM-66 and GMFM-88) User's Manual, 2nd Edition

Dianne J. Russell, Peter L. Rosenbaum, Marilyn Wright, Lisa M. Avery

Clinics in Developmental Medicine
2013 ▪ 304pp ▪ spiral-bound softback ▪ 978-1-908316-88-2
£70.00 / €84.00 / $115.00

The Gross Motor Function Measure (GMFM) has become the best evaluative measure of motor function designed for quantifying change in the gross motor abilities of children with cerebral palsy. The new version of the scoring programme has now been released, and includes two abbreviated methods of estimating GMFM-66 scores using the GMFM-66-Item sets and the GMFM-66-Basal & Ceiling. This new edition builds on the wide success of the first edition.

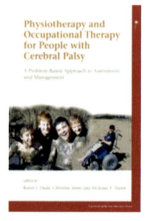

Physiotherapy and Occupational Therapy for People with Cerebral Palsy

Karen J. Dodd, Christine Imms, Nicholas F. Taylor (Editors)

A practical guide from Mac Keith Press
2010 ▪ 320pp ▪ softback ▪ 978-1-898683-68-1
£29.95/ €36.00 / $41.99

This book is a practical resource for physiotherapists and occupational therapists who support people with cerebral palsy, helping them to solve the problems with movement and other impairments that so often accompany cerebral palsy, so that they can be more active and better able to participate in roles such as study, work, recreation and relationships

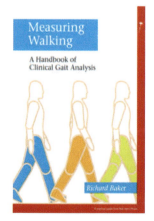

Measuring Walking: A Handbook of Clinical Gait Analysis

Richard Baker

A practical guide from Mac Keith Press
2013 ▪ 248pp ▪ softback ▪ 978-1-908316-66-0
£49.95 / €60.60 / $84.95

This book is a practical guide to instrumented clinical gait analysis covering all aspects of routine service provision. It reinforces what is coming to be regarded as the conventional approach to clinical gait analysis. Data capture, processing and biomechanical interpretation are all described with an emphasis on ensuring high quality results. There are also chapters on how to set up and maintain clinical gait analysis services and laboratories.